Applying Medication
Math Skills

DEDICATION

. . . dedicated to our respective families for their patience and support . . .

Mom, Dad, Tom, Kelli, Morgan, Ian, West Mountain Kibo, Securro, and Peggy

&

Mom, Dad, Becky, Jonathan, Krystle, Michael, Rosie, Katarina, Alexandra, and Katherine

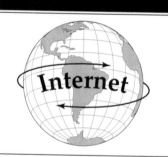

Applying Medication Math Skills

A Dimensional Analysis Approach

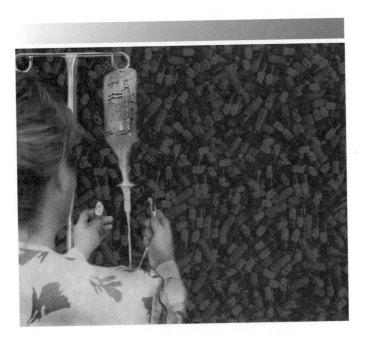

KAREN CLEMENT-O'BRIEN MS, RN

Education Specialist
Department of Education and Development
Albany Medical Center
Albany, NY

GARY M. LAWLER, MA, BS, AS

Professor of Mathematics
Adirondack Community College
Queensbury, NY

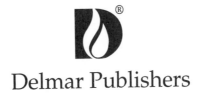

Delmar Publishers

an International Thomson Publishing company I(T)P®

Albany • Bonn • Boston • Cincinnati • Detroit • London • Madrid
Melbourne • Mexico City • New York • Pacific Grove • Paris • San Francisco
Singapore • Tokyo • Toronto • Washington

Cover Design: Timothy J. Conners

Delmar Staff
Publisher: William Brottmiller
Acquisitions Editor: Marion Waldman
Project Editor: Patricia Gillivan
Production Coordinator: Sandy Woods
Art and Design Coordinator: Timothy J. Conners
Editorial Assistant: Diane Speece

COPYRIGHT © 1999

an International Thomson Publishing company I(T)P®

By Delmar Publishers
an International Thomson Publishing Company, Inc.

The ITP logo is a trademark under license.

Printed in the United States of America

For more information, contact:

Delmar Publishers
3 Columbia Circle, Box 15015
Albany, New York 12212-5015

International Thomson Publishing Europe
Berkshire House
168-173 High Holborn
London, WC1V7AA
United Kingdom

Nelson ITP, Australia
102 Dodds Street
South Melbourne,
Victoria, 3205 Australia

Nelson Canada
1120 Birchmont Road
Scarborough, Ontario
M1K 5G4, Canada

International Thomson Publishing France
Tour Maine-Montparnasse
33 Avenue du Maine
75755 Paris Cedex 15, France

International Thomson Editores
Seneca 53
Colonia Polanco
11560 Mexico D. F. Mexico

International Thomson Publishing GmbH
Königswinterer Straße 418
53227 Bonn
Germany

International Thomson Publishing Asia
60 Albert Street
#15-01 Albert Complex
Singapore 189969

International Thomson Publishing Japan
Hirakawa-cho Kyowa Building, 3F
2-2-1 Hirakawa-cho, Chiyoda-ku,
Tokyo 102, Japan

ITE Spain/ Paraninfo
Calle Magallanes, 25
28015-Madrid, Espana

1 2 3 4 5 6 7 8 9 10 XXX 03 02 01 00 99 98

Library of Congress Cataloging-in-Publication Data

Clement-O'Brien, Karen.
    Applying medication math skills : a dimensional analysis
approach / Karen Clement-O'Brien, Gary M. Lawler.
        p. cm.
    Includes index.
    ISBN 0-7668-0050-4
    1. Pharmaceutical arithmetic.   I. Lawler, Gary M.   II. Title.
RS75.C54 1999
615'.14'01513--dc21   98-8415
                                                        CIP
                                                        rev.

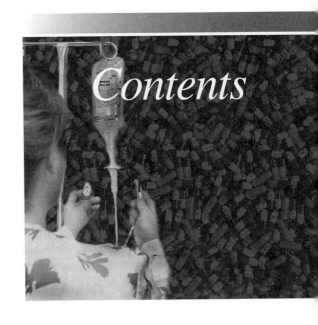

Contents

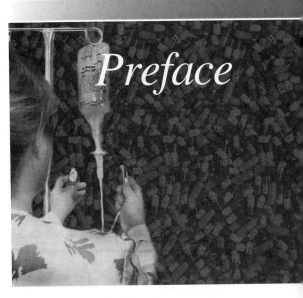

Preface

As a result of a growing need to provide nursing and health sciences students with a strong arithmetic background, we embarked on the journey of preparing this book. To ensure that students would enter required science courses for nursing with comprehensive problem-solving and computation skills, the mathematics and nursing divisions of Adirondack Community College teamed up to develop a team-taught course. The course was taught without a textbook because the content of the course was not covered thoroughly in any of the available books. We believed we could streamline learning for the student of the health sciences by promoting a single-method approach to problem solving and calculating.

This publication is unique. It is designed for the prechemistry, prebiology student, and the nursing student, as well as the graduate nurse. It introduces mathematic concepts and shows how they are applied in the health sciences. Learning activities are included in every chapter to assist with difficult concepts. These sections suggest as many hands-on activities and manipulatives as necessary to make the arithmetic come alive.

As you proceed through the book, note that the first chapters are the groundwork. They help you to relearn or review concepts that you may not have used in a while. Many of our students are returning adult learners and may not have used this previously learned knowledge in quite some time.

Our "Dimensional Analysis" chapter is the magic chapter! Once this concept is incorporated, you will see the subsequent consistency applied in calculation throughout the book. We believe very strongly in this method of solving clinical problems. All medication, intravenous/infusion, and client-related calculations can be solved in the same way. We believe the *factor-label* method of calculation takes much of the guesswork out of clinical calculations. Most books have a different "formula" for each application, however we promote a single method for all. It takes the doubtfulness, which you may have experienced, out of ratios and proportions.

Our method is extremely dependent on the *units* of the quantity. We believe that throughout computations, you should be very aware of what you are trying to solve. This is accomplished by labeling all quantities and recognizing what you are trying to solve for from the beginning. The dimensional analysis method provides a means to solve all computations for the correct *units* by preparing the equation with units of the quantities. We believe strongly in written work, calculator nondependent learning. In the health care area, one cannot always have the luxury of a calculator or the time to rely on one. After arriving at the answer, evaluate the answer: Ask yourself, *Does my answer make sense? Is the answer appropriate?* We believe that this evaluation step is important. The learner needs to take responsibility for verifying the answer.

Thus, the calculation of all problems requires:

1. What are the units of my answer?
2. Start the factor-label equation with the given.
3. Set up the equation according to the units desired.
4. Label your answer.
5. Ask yourself, *Does my answer make sense?*

Throughout the text we make use of common abbreviations used in nursing/health care. We vary the notations that are commonly accepted to familiarize the learner with different forms.

Organization

The organization of the chapters is based on the progression of concepts. Part I, Review of Mathematics, assists the learner to develop problem-solving skills and review any previously learned arithmetic concepts in detail. Part II, Dosage Calculation, takes the nursing and health care worker through nursing applications that promote problem solving and development of judgment in adapting to the needs of the individual patient. Part III, Advanced Mathematics, contains concepts used in the science and nursing disciplines. This section assists in preparing the learner with the arithmetic needed to develop these concepts. The Appendixes are resources that are intended to be used from the very beginning to develop the learners' knowledge base.

Chapter Elements

The chapter elements focus on the learner's need for practice and active learning.

Objectives   The objectives help the learner to focus on the intent of each chapter and clarify the purpose.

Introduction   The introduction briefly explains why each chapter is important. It gives meaning to the text to follow.

Examples   The examples provided, after discussion of new concepts, take the learner, step-by-step, through the problem-solving process, depicting the steps required in planning to solve a calculation.

Practice Exercises   The practice exercises give the learner the opportunity to solve questions similar to the content and examples that have just been presented.

Key Points   Key points depict the very most important, crucial aspects of the content that is being presented. If the learner needs to review quickly, this feature gets to the point!

Remember Boxes   The remember boxes are similar to *key points*, but may not be depicting the crucial concepts. This feature provides a summary or quick reference to presented content and concepts.

Learning Activities   Learning activities are the *laboratory experience*. The science and nursing disciplines foster experimental, *hands-on* learning that keep arithmetic real. The designed activities bring real-world situations to the learning process. We have provided as many health science applications as we could think of to assist the learner to transfer arithmetic and problem-solving skills. From the very first chapter, applications, although very minor, are used for the student to transfer the arithmetic to an applied situation. As the book grows, so does the nature and quantity of laboratory exercises. Built into the applications is our philosophy of promoting problem solving, interpreting word problems, and evaluating the results of the computations.

Chapter Review Exercises   Chapter review exercises are just what they say they are. These exercises provide the learner with examples that review all the concepts presented in the chapter.

Critical Thinking   Critical thinking exercises stretch the content and concepts to clinical situations even farther. These exercises call upon the student to problem solve an application question in a clinical situation. The nursing professional, besides proficiency in calculating, needs to be able to make clinical judgments about actions to take when the preparation or administration of medications and solutions is not completely clear.

CD-ROM

The CD ROM is an interactive multimedia presentation that is designed for individual, self-paced learning at home or in the computer lab.

Features include:

- Tutorial to help you get started
- 300-word glossary
- Audio pronunciation of drug names
- Testing assessment tool with scoring capabilities
- Review questions with answers and rationales
- Practice problems with answers and rationales
- Critical thinking skills
- Color photographs
- 160 Drug labels
- Audio pronunciation of common sound-alike drug names
- Intuitive and attractive interface
- Help feature
- Toll-free technical support
- Plus Flash!™, an electronic flash card proßgram

So, now you should have everything you need to go forward. We wish you the best of luck in your goals and endeavors.

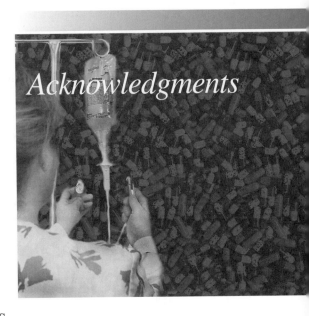

Acknowledgments

Reviewers

Elizabeth A. Chandler, BA, BS, MS
Nursing Faculty
Quincy College
Quincy, MA

Deborah R. Garrison, RN, PhD
Assistant Clinical Professor
Texas Woman's University College of Nursing
Denton, TX

Connie Hauser, RNC, MSN
Director of Education
Tuomey Healthcare System
Sumter, SC

Dianne L. Josephson, RN, MSN
Nursing and Continuing Education Faculty
El Paso Community College
El Paso, TX

Williams Lederman, RN, BSN, MA
Professor of Nursing
Glen Oaks Community College
Centerville, MI

Elaine Ridgeway, RN, MSN
Assistant Professor and Head
Department of Associate Degree Nursing
Clayton College and State University
Morrow, GA

Pamela J. Singer, RN, MSN
Professor, Nursing Education
Miami–Dade Community College
Miami, FL

Manufacturers

The following companies provided technical data, reporting forms, photographs, drug labels, package inserts, package labels, or packaging to illustrate examples and problems:

Abbott Laboratories, Abbott Park, IL

Adria Laboratories, Columbus, OH

Albany Medical Center Hospital, Albany, NY

Astra USA, Inc., Westborough, MA

Bristol-Myers Institutional Products, Evansville, IN

Bristol-Myers Squibb Company, Princeton, NJ

Burroughs Wellcome Company, Research Triangle Park, NC

Forest Pharmaceuticals, Inc., St. Louis, MO

Lederle Laboratories, A Division of American Cyanamid Company, Wayne, NJ

Muro Pharmaceuticals, Tewksbury, MA

Sandoz Pharmaceuticals Corporation, East Hanover, NJ

Smith Kline & French Laboratories, A Division of Smithkline Beckman Corporation, Philadelphia, PA

Warner-Lambert Company, Morris Plains, NJ

Review of Mathematics

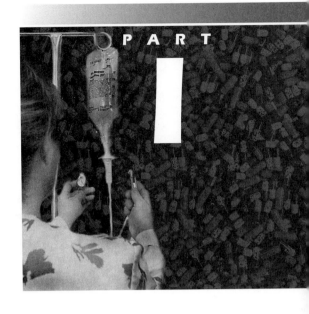

Arithmetic Pretest

1. Perform the following operation on signed numbers:

a. $7 + (-2) =$ _____

b. $(-2) + (-3) =$ _____

c. $3 + (-8) =$ _____

d. $(-5) - 2 =$ _____

e. $(-3) - (-5) =$ _____

f. $(-5) \times 2 =$ _____

g. $(-3) \times (-5) =$ _____

h. $0 - (-3) =$ _____

i. $12 \div (-2) =$ _____

j. $(-4) \div (-2) =$ _____

k. $0 \div (-6) =$ _____

l. $0 \times 7 =$ _____

2. Perform the following operations on fractions:

a. $\frac{2}{3} + \frac{1}{4} + \frac{1}{6} =$ ____

b. $2\frac{1}{3} - \frac{5}{6} =$ ____

c. $\left(3\frac{2}{5}\right) \times \left(\frac{1}{5}\right) =$ ____

d. $\left(3\frac{2}{5}\right) \div \left(\frac{1}{5}\right) =$ ____

3. Perform the following operations on decimals:

a. $1.3566 + 7.9887 + 5.2 =$ _____

b. $5 - 0.387 =$ _____

c. $(1.0011) \times (2.2) =$ _____

d. $(1.1) \div (0.05) =$ _____

4. Convert the following percentages to decimals:

a. $2.1\% =$ _·021_   move Decimal Ⓛ 2 places

b. $0.45\% =$ _____

5. Convert the following decimals to percentages:

a. $0.009 =$ _·9%_   move Decimal Ⓡ 2 places

b. $0.375 =$ _____

Operations on Signed Numbers

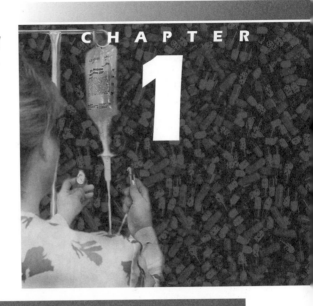

CHAPTER 1

OBJECTIVES

Upon completion of this chapter, you will be able to:

- Conceptualize signed numbers with the assistance of the number line.
- Perform operations on signed numbers.
- Apply signed numbers to temperature and fluid balance situations.

Introduction

Why do we need numbers? Simply, to count. Every civilization since ancient times has had its own method of counting. The symbols that were used and the language surrounding numbers have evolved. Numbers such as zero and the negative numbers date back to the ancient Babylonian civilizations. However, they were not formalized until the sixteenth century.

Once numbers (for counting) were being used, operations on numbers evolved. The ancient Egyptians used numbers and measurement to calculate the area of the land they owned. Each year the Nile would overflow its banks and wash away part of their land. The landowners wanted to recalculate the amount of land they owned so as not to be paying taxes on land they no longer had.

What is the connection to health care? Medicine and nursing have been practiced in many forms for thousands of years. Early Hebrews and Egyptians recorded the practice of hygiene, sanitation, surgery, and nursing procedures such as dressing care, care of patients with tetanus, and assisting women in child bearing. What about counting and numbers in health care? The earliest formal counting system in health care is the Apothecary system. Its origins date back to prehistoric times when a grain of wheat was used for counting. This system of measurement was refined by the Egyptians, Babylonians, Greeks, and Romans. The modern version of the Apothecary system was formalized during the fourteenth century in France and is still in limited use today while being replaced by the metric system.

Signed Numbers

There are three sets of numbers necessary in applied areas. Those numbers are:

- Counting numbers: 1, 2, 3, 4, 5, 6, 7, 8, 9, 10, . . .
- Zero: 0
- Negative (counting) numbers: –1, –2, –3, –4, –5, –6, –7, . . .

We can order the preceding numbers by considering the number line—a visual look at these numbers. The number line has 0 at the center with the counting numbers to the right and the negative counting numbers to the left. The number line shown below may not look familiar, but we have several examples of it in everyday life. The ruler or meter stick is an example of a number line with only some of the positive numbers used. A thermometer can also be considered a number line with 0° positioned as 0 is on the line.

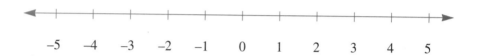

Notice that position on the number line can help us determine which of two numbers is larger in value. As you move to the right on the number line the numbers get larger. Therefore, –1 is larger than –5 because –1 is to the right of –5 on the number line. We have a way of writing this using the "greater than" or "less than" symbol.

KEY POINT

Symbol	Meaning	Example
>	greater than	5 > 2 (5 is greater than 2)
		–1 > –5 (–1 is greater than –5)
<	less than	1 < 5 (1 is less than 5)
		–2 < 3 (–2 is less than 3)
		–4 < –3 (–4 is less than –3)

Note: Recognize that the symbol (whether > or <) always points to the smaller number.

PRACTICE EXERCISE 1.A

Insert the symbol < or > as appropriate between the following pairs of numbers:

1. 2 ___ 5

2. –3 ___ 0

3. 7 ___ –4

4. –3 ___ –2

5. –5 ___ 5

6. –2 ___ –4

Addition and Subtraction

We are now ready to begin operations on these numbers. The first operation to consider is addition, which is denoted by +.

KEY POINT

To ADD two numbers: Find the first number on the number line. If the second number is:

positive—move that many spaces to the *right* on the line.

negative—move that many spaces to the *left* on the line.

EXAMPLE: $(-3) + 5$

Locate -3 on the line.

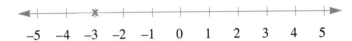

Now move 5 spaces to the right (for 5).

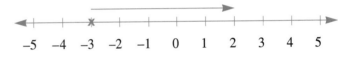

So, $(-3) + 5 = 2$

EXAMPLE: $(-1) + (-3)$

Locate -1 on the line.

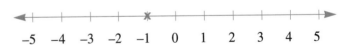

Now move 3 spaces to the left (for -3).

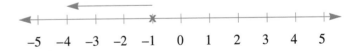

So, $(-1) + (-3) = -4$

Note that the use of parentheses around any number does not change its value—the parentheses are there only for clarity.

The second operation is subtraction, denoted by $-$. Subtraction is defined in terms of addition. Therefore, we can use the number line to subtract only when we have changed the subtraction back to addition.

> **KEY POINT**
>
> To subtract two numbers a, b we define:
>
> $$a - b = a + (-b)$$

This is read *a subtract b is equal to a added to the opposite of b*. If b is 2, its opposite is –2. If b is –5, its opposite is 5. Therefore, if we have 5 – 2, it may be written as 5 + (–2), and the number line may be used to determine that the answer is 3. Although this definition may not be needed with the subtraction of two positive numbers as in this example, it is the most useful when working with subtraction involving negative numbers.

EXAMPLE: $-2 - (3) = -2 + (-3)$

So, we can use the number line to locate –2:

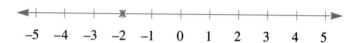

and now move 3 spaces to the LEFT (for –3).

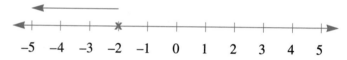

So, $-2 - (3) = -5$

Consider $5 - 7 = 5 + (-7) = -2$ using the number line. Also, we may use practical situations to help with these problems. Consider the original problem 5 – 7. Think of money and a checking account. If we have only $5 in the bank and write a check for $7, we are behind $2. So, 5 – 7 = –2 (behind $2). You may also think of temperature. If it is 5° out and the temperature drops 7°, it is now 2° below zero (–2°)—or –2.

EXAMPLE: $2 - (-4) = 2 + (4) = 6$

Recall that we must take the opposite of the number following the subtraction sign as we change to addition—the opposite of –4 is 4. We have the least intuition about subtracting negative numbers, so it is best not to guess—just change the subtraction to addition and use the number line as need be.

EXAMPLE: $-3 - (-7) = -3 + (7) = 4$

Again, we may think about the –3 + (7) as if we are $3 behind at the bank and we make a deposit (add) of $7. We are now $4 to the good—the 4.

PRACTICE EXERCISE 1.B

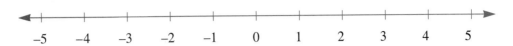

$$-5 \quad -4 \quad -3 \quad -2 \quad -1 \quad 0 \quad 1 \quad 2 \quad 3 \quad 4 \quad 5$$

Use the number line to add the following numbers:

1. $1 + 3 =$ **2.** $-2 + 7 =$ **3.** $-3 + (-2) =$ **4.** $0 + (-4) =$ **5.** $5 + (-3) =$

Subtract the following numbers:

6. $-3 - (2) =$ **7.** $5 - 9 =$ **8.** $2 - (-4) =$ **9.** $0 - 5 =$ **10.** $-1 - (-6) =$

Multiplication and Division

We are now ready to consider the operations of multiplication, which is denoted by $\times$, and division, which is denoted by $\div$. There is no need to consider these separately as the operations follow very similar patterns.

Consider the possibility of writing six bad checks each for $5. This would mean that we were $30 behind: –30. So, $6 \times (-5) = -30$. Notice that the two numbers involved had different signs—one was positive and the other was negative. What if you multiply two negative numbers? The result is positive. Consider the following example to illustrate this idea.

Consider multiplying $(-6) \times (-5)$. Recall that –6 is the opposite of +6—that is $-6 = -(6)$. We can write $(-6) \times (-5)$ as $-[6 \times (-5)]$—that is, as the *opposite* of "6 times –5." We know from our previous example that $6 \times (-5) = -30$. Therefore, its opposite is 30. So, $(-6) \times (-5) = 30$. Notice that multiplying two negative numbers (both have the same sign) results in a positive number. Recognize that this is also true when multiplying two positive numbers (same signs).

The same rules apply to division. Therefore, we have the following results:

> **KEY POINT**
>
> To multiply or divide two numbers:
>
> • If the two numbers have the same sign, the result is positive.
>
> • If the two numbers have different signs, the result is negative.

EXAMPLES: $2 \times 5 = 10$ (both numbers have the same sign)

$-2 \times 5 = -10$ (the numbers have different signs)

$-2 \times (-5) = 10$ (both numbers have the same sign)

$-10 \div (-5) = 2$ (both numbers have the same sign)

$10 \div (-5) = -2$ (the numbers have different signs)

When multiplying a number by 0, the result is always 0. If you divide 0 by any (nonzero) number, the result is 0 as well.

EXAMPLES: $0 \times (-5) = 0$

$0 \div 7 = 0$

PRACTICE EXERCISE 1.C

Multiply the following numbers:

1. $2 \times (-5) =$ **2.** $(-3) \times (-4) =$ **3.** $(3) \times (4) =$ **4.** $0 \times (-4) =$

Divide the following numbers:

5. $-6 \div 2 =$ **6.** $-10 \div (-2) =$ **7.** $4 \div 1 =$ **8.** $0 \div (-5) =$

To review the operations discussed, we must recognize that addition/subtraction and multiplication/division are very different operations with their own governing rules. When adding or subtracting we may rely on the number line to help us. Recall that all subtractions may be converted to additions. In multiplication and division the sign of the answer is dependent on the signs of the original numbers—whether they are the same or different signs.

R E V I E W

To ADD

1. Locate the first number on the number line.

2. If the second number is:

> POSITIVE—move to the RIGHT.
>
> NEGATIVE—move to the LEFT.

To SUBTRACT

Change the problem to addition by adding the opposite of the second number to the first: $a - b = a + (-b)$.

To MULTIPLY

Consider the signs of the two numbers.

> If the signs are the:
>
> > SAME—the answer is POSITIVE
> >
> > DIFFERENT—the answer is NEGATIVE.

To DIVIDE

Consider the signs of the two numbers.

> If the signs are the:
>
> > SAME—the answer is POSITIVE.
> >
> > DIFFERENT—the answer is NEGATIVE.

Uses of Signed Numbers

The concept of signed numbers is utilized in various ways in the allied health sciences.

Thermometers

Outdoor Winter Temperature: Have you ever read an outdoor thermometer that measured a negative number? Whether you are reading Fahrenheit or Celsius, the reading could be negative during the colder months of the year in a northern climate (see Figure 1-1). The thermometer indicates the temperature is below zero.

Chemical Reactions

During your chemistry courses, as you study the properties and composition of matter, various experiments will require the study of energy and heat changes. These studies will yield various signed numbers. Many chemical reactions are accompanied by energy changes. An exothermic reaction releases or evolves heat. Heat flows from the reaction mixture into the surroundings. The effect is an increase in the temperature of the immediate area about the reactants. When natural gas, which is mostly methane, burns, the heat provides the means to cook on a gas range or boil water on a Bunsen burner. Heat is expended. The number that will best express this heat loss will have a negative sign.

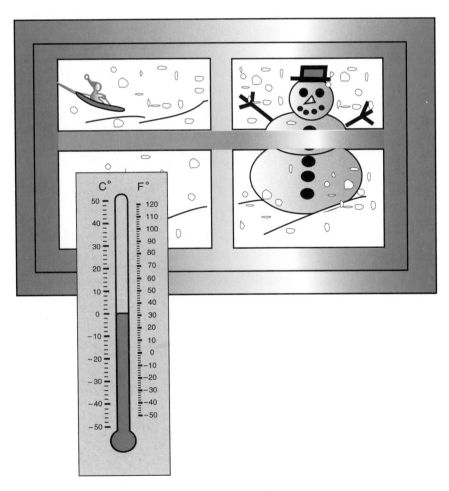

FIGURE 1-1
Fahrenheit/Celsius Thermometer Displays Positive and Negative Numbers.

A reaction that is endothermic absorbs heat, such as ice melting. Heat flows into the reaction mixture from the surroundings. Heat energy is absorbed by the ice. This number would be expressed as a positive number.

Consider the difference in energy between the products and the reactants of a reaction. Generally we can represent reactions of this nature by considering enthalpy, *heat content,* which is given the symbol H. For reactions at constant pressure, that of the atmosphere, the heat flow is equal to the difference between the enthalpy of the products and that of the reactants. Using Q_p to represent the heat flow and ΔH for the enthalpy difference:

$$Q_p = H \text{ products} - H \text{ reactants} = \Delta H$$

As you utilize this *Law of Conservation of Energy* in your science courses, this equation will illustrate that energy is neither created nor destroyed. During exothermic reactions there is always a decrease in enthalpy, so $\Delta H < 0$. This number is expressed with a negative sign.

Body Temperature

Body temperature is assessed utilizing either the Fahrenheit temperature scale or the Celsius temperature scale. Although we do not measure negative body temperatures, we do refer to subnormal temperatures. A temperature that is less than normal body temperature, which is 98.6°F (37°C), is described as subnormal (see Chapter 21).

Newborns frequently have a less-than-normal body temperature during the first few hours of life. Because of heat loss and an immature temperature-regulating system, they may have difficulty maintaining a normal body temperature. Temperature-controlled isolette chambers assist in maintaining a normal body temperature in the infant who is at risk for greater temperature variations.

Intravenous Therapy

The concept of signed numbers is also utilized when assessing an intravenous infusion. A client may be receiving intravenous fluids for various reasons. The fluid is infused through a tubing and small catheter that is placed in a peripheral vein. The infusion of fluid requires monitoring by the nurse (see Figure 1-2).

KEY POINT

At this point we need to introduce the unit of measure that is used in allied health to monitor fluids. Intravenous fluids, as well as any other fluids in health care, are monitored and assessed in cubic centimeters (cc or cm³). You will see these notations used continuously throughout this book and your allied health career. We interpret the volume of 1 cubic centimeter of H_2O to be equal to 1 millimeter (ml) of H_2O. A milliliter is 1/1,000 of a liter (L). These relationships will be discussed in much greater detail in subsequent chapters. A liter of intravenous (IV) fluid has 1,000 cc or ml of fluid. A liter is said to be approximately equal to 1 quart. A quart has 32 ounces (denoted by ℥). There are 30 cc or ml in 1 ounce. A liquid medicine cup used to administer medications to clients is 1 ounce or 30 cc.

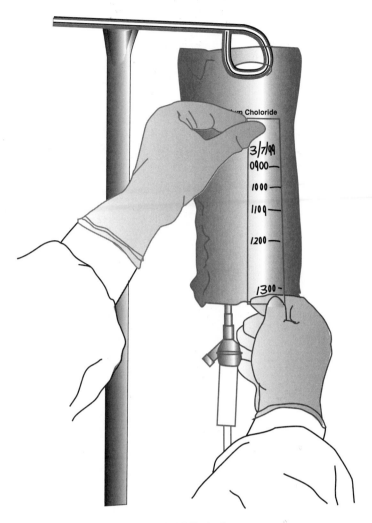

FIGURE 1-2
Monitoring Intravenous Infusion

The nurse needs to assess the quantities of IV fluids that have been utilized in the treatment of the client as well as the amount that remains to be administered. The nurse needs to ask two questions:

1. How much intravenous fluid did the patient receive?

2. How much fluid remains in the bag?

When reading the intravenous fluid bag or bottle, you must pay close attention to the calibrations along the side of the container (see Figure 1-3). The container may have calibrations that correspond to the amount that has infused. This type of container, Figure 1-3(A), starts with 0 at the top of the bottle. Another type of container, Figure 1-3(B), is labeled with the total volume to be infused at the top, with 0 at the bottom. There is also a third type, Figure 1-3(C), which has both types of scales on either side of the container. When reading the container, pay close attention to the scale you are reading. Let us assess the following IV infusion for amount of fluid infused and amount remaining:

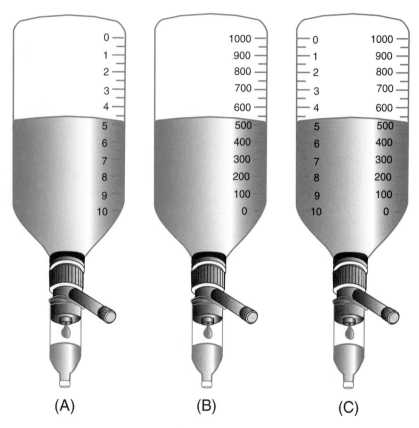

FIGURE 1-3

Reading Intravenous Containers for Volume Infused: (A) Numbering on container reflects amount infused. (B) Numbering requires subtraction from the total volume number at the top of the bag. (C) Numbering allows you to cross-check one scale with the other—A and B scale on the same container.

EXAMPLE: At 0700, the client's intravenous infusion was initiated at a rate of 100 cc per hour (cc/hr). A 1 liter (1,000 cc) container was used. At the end of the nurse's shift of work, 1500, he needed to report to the oncoming nurse the status of the infusion (see Figure 1-4):

1. How much intravenous fluid was infused at 1500? Your answer should be 800 cc!

2. How much intravenous fluid remains in the container?

In question 1 it was expected that you would refer to the figure and look at the bottle for your answer, but for question 2 it is expected that you would use your knowledge of signed numbers and show an equation. The amount infused, 800 cc, is gone from the bag or minus from the volume you started with. This number has a negative sign. Although this is simple mental arithmetic, the illustration of this calculation is the first step in showing the importance of understanding where your answer comes

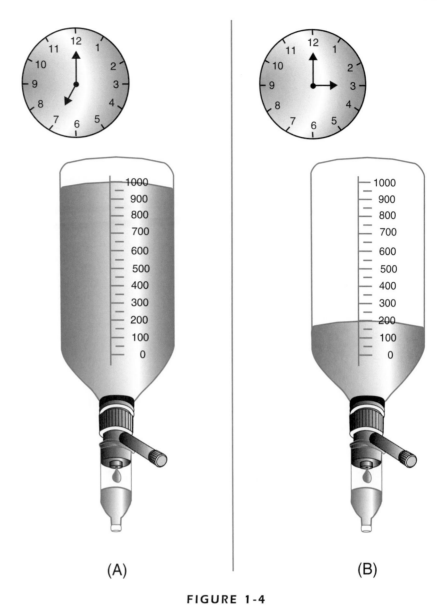

FIGURE 1-4

Determining Amount Infused: (A) 1,000 cc at 0700; (B) 200 cc at 1500.

from. Therefore, the amount remaining in the container can be assessed using the equation:

$$1,000 \text{ cc} - 800 \text{ cc} =$$

$$1,000 \text{ cc} + (-800 \text{ cc}) = 200 \text{ cc}$$

(total volume) + (amount infused) = (amount remaining)

Intake and Output/Net Fluid Balance

Another example in health care of the concept of signed numbers is utilized during the calculation of net fluid balance. In order to assess the fluid status of clients who are ill or receiving intensive treatments, close recording, monitoring, and evaluation of all fluids entering the body and leaving the body must be made (see Figure 1-5).

Albany Medical Center

Date: _____

INTAKE AND OUTPUT

PATIENT IDENTIFICATION PLATE

LEFT IN BAG

	0700		1500		2300	
#	SOLUTION/RATE	AMT.	# SOLUTION/RATE	AMT.	# SOLUTION/RATE	AMT.

TIME	INTAKE								COMMENTS	OUTPUT					INITIALS
	FEEDINGS	SOL. #	INF.	SOL. #	INF.	SOL. #	INF.								
TOTAL															

SIGNATURE _____

INITIALS/STATUS _____

95335 1090

FIGURE 1-5

Intake and Output Record

Intake (I) includes any fluids consumed by the body. This includes by mouth (per oral or po), peripheral and central infusion, feeding tubes, and irrigants, usually tallied after a 24-hour period. Output (O) includes any fluids removed from the body. This includes urine, liquid stool, emesis, or any drained body fluids.

When assessing net fluid balance, 24-hour totals of I&O for approximately a 3-day period are evaluated. Recall that these fluids are measured in cc or ml. Let's look at the following:

EXAMPLE: On 9/3 the patient took in a total of 1,100 cc of fluids and put out 600 cc. The net fluid balance is determined by using your knowledge of signed numbers. The intake has a positive sign and has been added to the body of the patient. The output has a negative sign and represents what has been lost from the body. Considering these two numbers, the equation thus formed yields the net fluid balance.

Date	24-Hour Total Intake	24-Hour Output
9/3	1,100	–600
9/4	1,000	–700
9/5	1,230	–650

For 9/3, the net fluid balance is 500 ml:

$$1,100 + (-600) = 500.$$

For 9/4, the net fluid balance is 300 ml:

$$1,000 + (-700) = 300.$$

For 9/5, the net fluid balance is 580 ml:

$$1,230 + (-650) = 580.$$

Looking at the net fluid balance for 1 day does not tell us much about the individual's fluid status. The information is much more valuable when we look at a period of 3 days.

Date	Net Fluid Balance
9/3	500
9/4	300
9/5	580
	1,380 ml

By calculating the total for 3 days, we know overall whether the patient is losing or retaining fluids. If the net fluid balance is a negative number, then the patient is losing more fluids than he is taking in. If the net balance is a positive number, then the patient is retaining more than he is putting out. In this example, the patient is in chronic renal failure and will require invasive measures to relieve the body tissues of the retained fluids.

> **KEY POINT**
>
> Ideally, the net fluid balance should be approximately zero. The intake and output numbers should balance out each other, such as the following recordings of a healthy individual:
>
> | Date | Intake | Output | Net Balance |
> |------|--------|--------|-------------|
> | 9/3 | 1,750 | −1,690 | = 60 |
> | 9/4 | 1,830 | −1,920 | = −90 |
> | 9/5 | 1,900 | −1,780 | = 120 |
> | | | | 90 ml |

LEARNING ACTIVITIES

This first lab is designed for you to begin to apply your objectives. Begin the problem-solving process. Remember, how you arrive at your answer is as important as the answer itself. Show all arithmetic computations where you have been prompted to do so.

1. Indicate the temperature reading on the line for each thermometer. Remember to consider the sign of each number.

a. _____ b. _____ c. _____

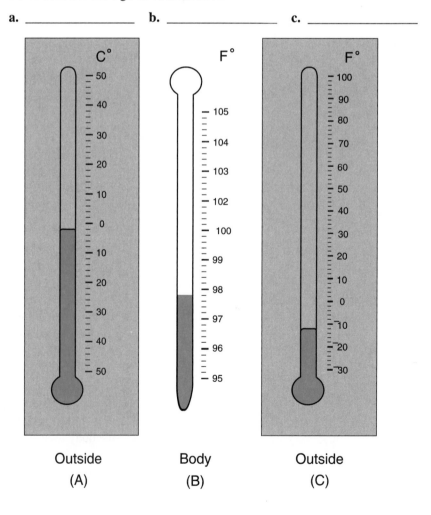

Outside (A)   Body (B)   Outside (C)

2. Read the bottle and answer the questions.

    a. How much solution has infused?

    b. How much solution remains in the IV bottle? (Show your calculation.)

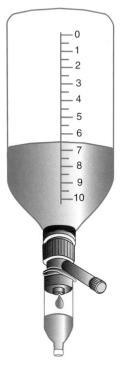

3. Read the bottle and answer the questions.

    a. How much solution has infused?

    b. How much solution remains in the IV bottle? (Show your calculation.)

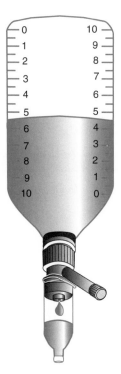

CHAPTER REVIEW EXERCISES

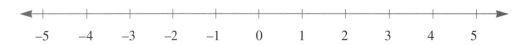

Add, subtract, multiply, or divide as indicated.

1. $(-2) \times (-5) =$ _____

2. $(-2) + (-5) =$ _____

3. $-8 \div (-2) =$ _____

4. $2 - 6 =$ _____

5. $(-3) + (-5) =$ _____

6. $6 - 8 =$ _____

7. $(-3) \times 5 =$ _____

8. $-2 + (-3) =$ _____

9. $(-8) \div (-8) =$ _____

10. $8 - (-3) =$ _____

11. $-2 + 3 =$ _____

12. $-3 - (-4) =$ _____

13. $-12 \div (-3) =$ _____

14. $(-2) \times (-7) =$ _____

15. $-6 - (-12) =$ _____

16. $3 - 9 =$ _____

17. $0 \div (-3) =$ _____

18. $6 - (-4) =$ _____

19. $9 + (-5) =$ _____

20. $-2 \times 8 =$ _____

21. $-4 \div (-1) =$ _____

22. $(-6) - 5 =$ _____

23. $7 \times (-3) =$ _____

24. $-3 + 7 =$ _____

25. $10 \div (-2) =$ _____

26. $0 - (-7) =$ _____

27. $(-5) \times 0 =$ _____

28. $8 + (-3) =$ _____

29. $0 \div (-15) =$ _____

30. $(-3) \times 6 =$ _____

31. $(-3) \times (-4) =$ _____

32. $-4 + (-9) =$ _____

33. $-3 - 5 =$ _____

34. $(-1) + 7 =$ _____

35. $(-6) \times 4 =$ _____

36. $-6 \div 2 =$ _____

37. $-3 \times (-7) =$ _____

38. $-5 + 10 =$ _____

39. $-6 \div (-6) =$ _____

40. $12 \div (-4) =$ _____

Use either the > or < sign between the following pairs of numbers:

41. -3 ___ 3

42. 2 ___ 0

43. -2 ___ 0

44. -5 ___ -6

45. 4 ___ 10

46. -100 ___ -101

CRITICAL THINKING

For questions 1 through 6, interpret the following abbreviations using Appendix 1:

1. gr

2. F

3. gtt

4. BP

5. ℳ

6. ℥

7. If an order reads to give medicine for a systolic BP > 180 and a diastolic BP > 90, interpret the meaning of the order.

8. Express the following using the > or < sign: Give acetaminophen for temperature above 101°.

9. Show equations for each answer:

   a. Compute Mr. Snow's net fluid balance for yesterday. His intake was 800 cc and his output totaled 600 cc.

   b. Today Mr. Snow drank 1,000 cc of liquid. After lunch, he felt nauseous and vomited approximately 400 cc. He excreted 900 cc of urine today. What is Mr. Snow's net fluid balance for today?

   c. What is Mr. Snow's net fluid balance for yesterday and today?

   d. Mr. Snow continues to vomit more fluids. Intravenous therapy is initiated to replace his losses. By the end of the following day, he has had 1,500 cc of IV fluids and 100 cc by mouth; he has vomited 400 cc and urinated 1,000 cc. What is his fluid balance for this day? What is his net fluid balance for the 3 days?

10. Consider making an equation of the following situation: Your friend goes on vacation to Howe Caverns, New York, an underground cavern with eerie rock formations, 200 feet below the earth's surface. You, on the other hand, tour the Whiteface Mountain Olympic Ski Area and take the chairlift ride to the top of the mountain with an elevation of 4,867 feet. How much higher is Whiteface Mountain than Howe Caverns? (*Careful:* What are the signs of these numbers? Show your work. Make an equation.)

11. You owe $137 to the college bookstore. Your savings account has $289. What will be your net worth when you pay your bill?

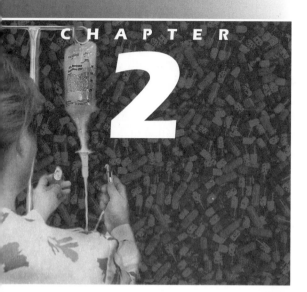

Fractions

OBJECTIVES

Upon completion of this chapter, you will be able to:

- Utilize the terms denoting fractional forms of numbers.
- Perform operations on fractions.
- Interpret fractional equations.
- Utilize fractional number forms when reading patient care orders.

Introduction

The fractional notation that we are all somewhat familiar with today was developed primarily during the Middle Ages by Arab civilizations, although the idea concerning fractional parts was evident in most ancient civilizations. Whether we paid ¼ of our earnings in taxes, or ½ of our crop was destroyed by a flood, the use of fractional parts has always been important.

Fractions

Fractions are simply a ratio of one whole number to another whole number with or without a sign (i.e., either positive or negative). Consider probably the most familiar fraction: one half. It is written in its fractional form as:

$\frac{1}{2}$ where 1 is called the numerator and 2 is called the denominator.

One half is also written as 1/2. The notation here is horizontal rather than the traditional vertical notation written above. One half, and all fractions in which the value of the numerator is smaller than the denominator, is called a proper fraction.

$\frac{2}{3}$, $\frac{11}{12}$, $\frac{5}{6}$, (or 2/3, 11/12, or 5/6) are all examples of proper fractions.

Fractions in which the value of the numerator is larger than the value of the denominator are called improper fractions.

$\frac{3}{2}$, $\frac{7}{3}$, $\frac{6}{5}$, (or 3/2, 7/3, or 6/5) are all examples of improper fractions.

Improper fractions, for our purposes are not generally used as final answers. In an application, since it does not make sense to speak about "3/2 tablets," we will convert these improper fractions to mixed numbers. Mixed numbers, by their very name, imply there is a mix of two numbers, in this case separated by an implied addition.

For example, to reduce 3/2 to a mixed number we simply divide 3 by 2 and what results is 1 with a remainder of 1—or a quotient of $1\frac{1}{2}$. Recall that the remainder must be placed over the divisor (the number you are dividing by). This process can be done by division as follows:

$$3/2 \text{ or } \frac{3}{2} \rightarrow 2\overline{)3}$$

$$2\overline{)3} \begin{array}{c} 1 \\ \underline{2} \\ 1 \end{array} = 1\ 1/2 \ (1 \text{ and } 1/2)$$

So, rather than saying we would give a patient 3/2 tablets, we would give the patient one and one-half tablets ($1\frac{1}{2}$). Therefore, all answers we work with will either be in proper or mixed form.

EXAMPLE: Reduce 8/3 to a mixed number.

$$3\overline{)8} \rightarrow 3\overline{)8} \begin{array}{c} 2 \\ \underline{6} \\ 2 \end{array} = 2\frac{2}{3} \text{ or } 2\ 2/3$$

PRACTICE EXERCISE 2.A

1. Identify the following fractions as either *proper, improper, or mixed:*

   a. $\frac{13}{12}$ **b.** 3/4   **c.** $\frac{8}{9}$ **d.** 3 2/3   **e.** 7/6   **f.** $4\frac{1}{2}$

2. Convert the following *improper* fractions to *mixed* numbers:

   a. $\frac{13}{12}$ **b.** 7/2   **c.** 7/6   **d.** $\frac{31}{3}$

When working with fractions, we always wish to represent the answer in its simplest form. That form, beyond the conversion to mixed numbers already discussed, assures that there are no numbers in common to the numerator and denominator. This process is referred to as reducing the fraction to lowest terms.

In order to consider some examples of reducing to lowest terms, we first must make a few observations:

> **KEY POINT**
>
> • Any number multiplied or divided by 1 has a value that remains the same.
>
> • Any number (other than zero) divided by itself has a value of 1.

EXAMPLE: Reduce $\frac{12}{26}$ to lowest terms.

Notice that there is a factor of 2 in both the numerator and the denominator—that is, both the top and bottom of the fraction are evenly divisible by 2. Therefore

$$\frac{12}{26} = \frac{6 \times 2}{13 \times 2} = \frac{6}{13} \times \frac{2}{2} = \frac{6}{13} \times 1 = \frac{6}{13}$$

We can also consider the portion of the equation:

$$\frac{6}{13} \times \frac{2}{2}$$

and *cancel* the $\frac{2}{2}$ which is another way of removing the factor of 1 that we multiplied by in the previous equation.

$$\frac{6}{13} \times \frac{\overset{1}{\cancel{2}}}{\underset{1}{\cancel{2}}} = \frac{6}{13}$$

The answer still remains $\frac{6}{13}$.

EXAMPLE: Reduce $\frac{24}{32}$ to the lowest terms.

$$\frac{24}{32} = \frac{3 \times 8}{4 \times 8} = \frac{3}{4} \times \frac{8}{8} = \frac{3}{4} \times 1 = \frac{3}{4}$$

So, the common factor in the numerator and the denominator was 8. Suppose that we did not notice the largest common factor (8)? Suppose we only noticed a 4. Consider below:

$$\frac{24}{32} = \frac{6 \times 4}{8 \times 4} = \frac{6}{8} \times \frac{4}{4} = \frac{6}{8} \times 1 = \frac{6}{8} = \frac{3 \times 2}{4 \times 2} = \frac{3}{4} \times \frac{2}{2} = \frac{3}{4}$$

So, if we do not see the largest common factor on the first try, we may continue the process until we have removed all common factors and have the fraction in simplest form.

EXAMPLE: Reduce $\frac{27}{6}$ to the lowest terms.

First we can convert the fraction from an improper fraction to a mixed number.

$$\frac{27}{6} = 6\overline{)27} = 4\frac{3}{6}$$
$$\phantom{\frac{27}{6} = 6)}\underline{24}$$
$$\phantom{\frac{27}{6} = 6)2}3$$

Now we can reduce the proper fraction 3/6 to its lowest form.

$$4\frac{3}{6} = 4\frac{1 \times 3}{2 \times 3} = 4\frac{1}{2} \times \frac{3}{3} = 4\frac{1}{2}$$

PRACTICE EXERCISE 2.B

Simplify the following fractions to the lowest terms:

1. $\dfrac{18}{27}$　　　**2.** $\dfrac{35}{25}$　　　**3.** $\dfrac{18}{12}$　　　**4.** $\dfrac{8}{6}$　　　**5.** $\dfrac{12}{18}$　　　**6.** $\dfrac{250}{75}$

The main purpose of this chapter is to review the concepts and processes involved in operations on fractions. Before we can begin that work there is one idea that we need to consider: converting from mixed numbers to improper fractions. Although, as stated our *answers* will always be in the form of either improper fractions or mixed numbers, it is often important for us to be able to convert to an improper fraction for ease of calculation.

Let us consider the mixed number 4½. As read, the mixed number is "four and one half." The *and* implies an addition. So, consider the following:

$$4\tfrac{1}{2} = 4\tfrac{1}{2} = 4 + \frac{1}{2} = \frac{4\times 2}{1\times 2} + \frac{1}{2} = \frac{8}{2} + \frac{1}{2} = \frac{9}{2}$$

The main idea is to change the whole number 4 into a fraction by placing a 1 in the denominator (does not change the value), and multiplying the numerator and denominator by the same value (the value in the denominator of the improper fraction). The result is that 4½ is the same as 9/2.

A faster way to obtain the same result using the same theory is to consider the following:

KEY POINT

To *convert* a *mixed* number to an *improper* fraction:

1. Multiply the whole number portion by the denominator of the proper fraction.

2. Add to that number the numerator of the proper fraction.

3. Place the result over the denominator of the original improper fraction.

EXAMPLE:　　Convert 5¾ to an improper fraction.

Multiply the 5 by 4 → $5 \times 4 = 20$

Add the 3 → $20 + 3 = 23$

Place 23 over 4 → $\dfrac{23}{4}$

Therefore, $5\tfrac{3}{4} = \dfrac{23}{4}$

Or, $5\tfrac{3}{4} = \dfrac{5\times 4 + 3}{4} = \dfrac{23}{4}$

EXAMPLE: Convert 6⅔ to an improper fraction.

$$6⅔ = \frac{6 \times 3 + 2}{3} = \frac{20}{3}$$

PRACTICE EXERCISE 2.C

Convert the following mixed numbers to improper fractions:

1. $2\frac{1}{2}$ **2.** $5\frac{6}{7}$ **3.** $3\frac{2}{3}$ **4.** $1\frac{3}{4}$

Multiplication and Division

Often when we consider operations, as in Chapter 1, we begin with addition (and subtraction). However, in working with fractions the easiest operation to consider is multiplication, so we shall begin there.

To multiply two fractions, we simply multiply numerator times numerator and denominator times denominator. The fractions must both be either improper or proper fractions (no mixed numbers).

KEY POINT

To multiply two fractions $\frac{a}{c} \times \frac{b}{d}$:

$$\frac{a}{c} \times \frac{b}{d} = \frac{a \times b}{c \times d}$$

EXAMPLE: $\frac{2}{3} \times \frac{5}{6} = \frac{2 \times 5}{3 \times 6} = \frac{10}{18} = \frac{5}{9} \times \frac{2}{2} = \frac{5}{9} \times 1 = \frac{5}{9}$

Recognize that we should not leave the answer 10/18 as it is not in the lowest terms. That is why we continue to reduce the fraction to the lowest terms, yielding the answer 5/9.

Also, we may recognize that there was a common factor within the problem that led to the reduction to the lowest terms already mentioned. Can we avoid that and still come to the answer? Yes. We need to remove the 2/2 located in the problem as we are multiplying (cancel the 2's). See the following:

$$\frac{\overset{1}{\cancel{2}}}{3} \times \frac{5}{\underset{3}{\cancel{6}}} = \frac{1 \times 5}{3 \times 3} = \frac{5}{9}$$

The canceling takes place as we divide one number in a numerator and one number in a denominator by 2.

Recall that a whole number can be written as a fraction by dividing the whole number by 1 (placing 1 in the denominator).

EXAMPLE: $\frac{3}{5} \times 2 = \frac{3}{5} \times \frac{2}{1} = \frac{3 \times 2}{5 \times 1} = \frac{6}{5} = 1\frac{1}{5}$

Notice there were no common factors in the numerator and denominator, so there was no opportunity to cancel. However, we did have to convert our answer as we ended up with an improper fraction.

Recall that if we have to multiply mixed numbers we first must convert them to improper fractions. This is because of the addition implied in "one *and* one half."

EXAMPLE: $1\frac{1}{2} \times 2\frac{2}{5} =$

$1\frac{1}{2} = \frac{1 \times 2 + 1}{2} = \frac{2 + 1}{2} = \frac{3}{2}$ and

$2\frac{2}{5} = \frac{2 \times 5 + 2}{5} = \frac{10 + 2}{5} = \frac{12}{5}$

So, $1\frac{1}{2} \times 2\frac{2}{5} = \frac{3}{\cancel{2}_1} \times \frac{\cancel{12}^6}{5} = \frac{3 \times 6}{1 \times 5} = \frac{18}{5} = 3\frac{3}{5}$

Notice that we canceled as there was a factor of 2 in both the numerator and denominator. Also, it was necessary to convert our answer since it was an improper fraction. What if we had not noticed the common factor? We would have had to reduce the improper fraction or the mixed number at the end of the problem. In general, it will tend to be easier if we can recognize the common factors early in the multiplication process rather than reducing at the end of the problem. Occasionally it is not apparent that there is a common factor as the numbers get larger.

PRACTICE EXERCISE 2.D

Multiply the following fractions. Be sure to reduce your answers to the lowest terms.

1. $\frac{3}{5} \times \frac{1}{2} =$ 2. $\frac{2}{3} \times \frac{5}{6} =$ 3. $\frac{3}{4} \times \frac{8}{11} =$ 4. $\frac{5}{2} \times 4 =$ 5. $1\frac{4}{5} \times 3\frac{1}{3} =$

We are now ready to consider division. Division of fractions is closely related to multiplication. Suppose we wish to divide:

$$\frac{4}{5} \div \frac{3}{2}$$

For the purposes of introduction we can write this fraction as the quotient of two fractions. When a fraction is written within a larger fraction we call it complex.

$$\frac{\frac{4}{5}}{\frac{3}{2}}$$

To simplify this complex fraction, we could make the denominator simple if we could multiply by some quantity that makes the denominator become 1. We can multiply by the reciprocal. The reciprocal of 3/2 is 2/3—that is, the numerator and denominator are reversed.

$$\frac{\frac{4}{5}\times\frac{2}{3}}{\frac{3}{2}\times\frac{2}{3}}=\frac{\frac{4}{5}\times\frac{2}{3}}{1}=\frac{4}{5}\times\frac{2}{3}=\frac{8}{15}$$

Because we can always use this idea of the reciprocal and the product of the reciprocals is always 1, the problem simply reduces to the following:

$$\frac{\frac{4}{5}}{\frac{3}{2}}=\frac{4}{5}\bigg/\frac{3}{2}=\frac{4}{5}\times\frac{2}{3}=\frac{8}{15}$$

Therefore, we can generalize:

KEY POINT

To divide two fractions a/c and b/d:

$$\frac{a}{c}\div\frac{b}{d}=\frac{a}{c}\times\frac{d}{b}=\frac{a\times d}{c\times b}$$

In other words, to divide two fractions, we multiply the first fraction by the reciprocal of the second fraction (the divisor).

EXAMPLE: $\frac{2}{3}\div\frac{3}{5}=\frac{2}{3}\times\frac{5}{3}=\frac{10}{9}=1\frac{1}{9}$

Note that we cannot cancel in division; however, we may cancel after we convert the division to multiplication.

EXAMPLE: Consider the following division problem:

$$\frac{1\frac{1}{2}}{\frac{2}{3}}$$

It will be easier to work with this problem if we change it into the form in the previous example. Also, as in multiplication, we will need to change the mixed number to an improper fraction.

$$1\frac{1}{2}\div\frac{2}{3}=\frac{3}{2}\times\frac{3}{2}=\frac{9}{4}=2\frac{1}{4}$$

EXAMPLE: Consider:

$$1\frac{5}{6} \div 5$$

In this problem, beyond changing the mixed number to an improper fraction, we will also need to write the whole number 5 in fractional form 5/1 so that we may be able to take its reciprocal. So,

$$1\frac{5}{6} \div 5 = \frac{11}{6} \div \frac{5}{1} = \frac{11}{6} \times \frac{1}{5} = \frac{11}{30}$$

The fraction 11/30 is certainly not an ordinary fraction. It is important that we begin to have an idea of value beyond getting an answer! Suppose you needed to measure 11/30 of an ounce?

You would need to recognize that this amount is approximately equivalent to 1/3 (10/30). With this idea we could measure the quantity fairly accurately.

PRACTICE EXERCISE 2.E

Divide the following fractions. Make sure that your answer is in lowest terms.

1. $\frac{1}{3} \div \frac{2}{5} =$ **2.** $\frac{3}{5} \div \frac{5}{2} =$ **3.** $1\frac{1}{2} \div 2\frac{1}{2} =$ **4.** $2\frac{2}{3} \div 1\frac{1}{9} =$ **5.** $2\frac{2}{5} \div 5 =$

6. What common fraction is the answer in question 5 approximately equal to?

Lowest Common Denominator—LCD

Before we move ahead to consider the operations of addition and subtraction, let us consider several ideas important to this work.

> ### KEY POINT
>
> If you multiply the numerator and denominator by the same number, the value of the fraction remains unchanged.

Why is this so? If we are multiplying *both* the numerator and denominator by the same number, we are multiplying the entire fraction by the number 1. Multiplication by 1 yields the same value with which we began.

Before we formally introduce the concept of adding fractions, let us explore a common problem that we can all probably answer:

EXAMPLE: $\frac{1}{3} + \frac{1}{3} = \frac{2}{3}$

Let us consider why this problem is so easy. Why can we answer it without any rules for addition? The reason is that this problem lies within our experience.

We may have considered a recipe that called for ⅓ cup of water. We started to make the mixture and then decided we wanted to make more. So, we had to add another third of a cup to the mixture. We used ⅔ of a cup of water. What makes this problem so easy (from an arithmetic standpoint)? You will notice that each fraction has the same denominator and essentially we add the numerators while keeping the same denominator. Note that we do *not* add the denominators. These are some key ideas in adding (or subtracting) fractions. However, what happens when we do not have the same denominators?

When we do not have the same denominators we need to convert the fractions while not changing their value to those that have the same denominators. The process is called *finding a common denominator,* or preferably *finding the lowest common denominator,* often notated as the LCD. The LCD is the smallest number evenly divisible by all denominators in the problem. It is important to recognize that this is only used in connection with the operations of addition and subtraction. We have already seen that multiplication and division required no such convention.

There are a host of methods for finding the LCD. We will consider several. The first method for finding the LCD is:

KEY POINT

Trial and error

As its name indicates, this method does not give us a specific strategy for finding the LCD, but instead allows us to find the value by using the concept of *finding the smallest number evenly divisible by all the denominators* and intuition.

EXAMPLE: Find the LCD of 1/2 and 1/4.

So, we need to find the smallest number evenly divisible by 2 and 4. That value is 4. We quickly note that the value for the LCD must be at least as large as the largest denominator. In this case, the largest is 4, and that divides the other denominator evenly.

EXAMPLE: Find the LCD of 1/3, 1/2, and 1/4.

We need to find the smallest number evenly divisible by 3, 2, and 4. The value is not 4. Four is the largest and it is evenly divisible by 2, but not 3. So, it must be something larger. The first whole number that divides evenly is 12. Therefore, the LCD is 12.

It is useful for us to have a more specific strategy to work with as well. Consider a second method for finding the LCD:

KEY POINT

Division strategy

   a. Write down all denominators horizontally.

   b. Find the smallest factor of at least one of the values. Divide the number into that one (or those ones) and write the quotient below. For those not evenly divisible, carry the value down.

   c. Continue the process in b until all quotients are 1. *Note:* Numbers may be used more than once. A hint of a list of numbers to try is 2, 3, 5, 7, 11, 13, etc. We may ask why is the number 4 not included on the list? If a number were divisible by 4, it would be divisible by 2 twice. Similarly, 6 is not on the list because a number divisible by 6 is also divisible by 2 and 3. (The numbers on the list are referred to as prime numbers.)

   d. The LCD is the *product* of all the divisors.

EXAMPLE: Find the LCD of 2/3, 1/2, and 3/4.

   a. Writing the denominators horizontally:

      3 2 4

   b. The smallest factor of at least one of the factors is 2.

$$2\overline{)\,3\,1\,2\,}^{\,3\,2\,4}$$

3 does not evenly divide by 2, so we carry it down. 2 divided by 2 is 1. 4 divided by 2 is 2.

   c. Since all quotients are not 1, we continue. Since there still is a factor of 2 in a number, we may use 2 again.

$$2\overline{)}^{\,3\,2\,4}$$

$$2\overline{)\,3\,1\,1\,}^{\,3\,1\,2}$$

3 again does not divide evenly by 2. We carry the 1 down, and 2 divided by 2 is 1.

     We still do not have 1s all the way across. The next number to try is 3.

$$2\overline{)}^{\,3\,2\,4}$$

$$2\overline{)}^{\,3\,1\,2}$$

$$3\overline{)\,1\,1\,1\,}^{\,3\,1\,1}$$

The quotients are all now 1.

d. The LCD is the product of the divisors: 2, 2, 3.

Therefore, the LCD is $2 \times 2 \times 3 = 12$.

EXAMPLE: Find the LCD of 1/2, 1/6, and 1/5.

Solution:

$$
\begin{array}{r}
2\overline{)\,2\ 6\ 5} \\[4pt]
3\overline{)\,1\ 3\ 5} \\[4pt]
5\overline{)\,1\ 1\ 1} \\
1\ 1\ 5
\end{array}
$$

So, the LCD is $2 \times 3 \times 5 = 30$.

PRACTICE EXERCISE 2.F

Find the lowest common denominator (LCD) for each of the following lists of fractions:

1. $\dfrac{1}{2}$, $\dfrac{5}{6}$ **2.** $\dfrac{1}{2}$, $\dfrac{2}{3}$, $\dfrac{3}{4}$ **3.** $\dfrac{3}{4}$, $\dfrac{5}{8}$, $\dfrac{2}{3}$ **4.** $\dfrac{1}{2}$, $\dfrac{1}{3}$, $\dfrac{2}{5}$ **5.** $\dfrac{3}{8}$, $\dfrac{2}{3}$, $\dfrac{4}{5}$

Once we have found the LCD for a group of fractions, before we can begin adding or subtracting, we have to convert each of those fractions to ones with the same common denominator. For this conversion we consider the denominator of each fraction separately. We need to find the value when multiplied by the given denominator that will yield the LCD. In other words, suppose the LCD is 12 and the fraction that we are working with is 2/3. We consider the 3 and say: "What do I need to multiply 3 by in order to get a product of 12?" The answer is 4. At that point we need to not only multiply the denominator by 4 but also the numerator by 4. Thus, we have multiplied the fraction by 4/4 (another name for the number 1) and we have not altered the value of the fraction. Instead, we have just given it a different name—in our example, we have renamed 2/3 to 8/12. There is a tendency to want to reduce that answer to the lowest terms (which will bring us right back to 2/3). However, remember that we are in the midst of a process. This conversion of 2/3 to 8/12 is one step in the addition process of two or more fractions.

EXAMPLE: Convert the fractions ½ and ⅓ to fractions with a LCD.

From our previous methods we can see the LCD is 6. Consider the fraction ½. We have a denominator of 2 and we wish to convert this to a fraction with a denominator of 6. What do we want to multiply 2 by in order to obtain the 6? We need to multiply by 3. So, we proceed to multiply the numerator and denominator by 3:

$$\frac{1 \times 3}{2 \times 3} = \frac{3}{6}$$

So, 3/6 is another name for 1/2 with a denominator of 6.

Consider ⅓. To get a denominator of 6 in this case we will need to multiply by 2 on both the top and the bottom.

$$\frac{1 \times 2}{3 \times 2} = \frac{2}{6}$$

With this fraction, another name for 1/3 becomes 2/6.

EXAMPLE: Convert the following fractions to those with an LCD:

$$\frac{1}{2}, \ \frac{1}{6}, \ \frac{2}{5}$$

The LCD of the fractions is 30.

$$\frac{1 \times 15}{2 \times 15} = \frac{15}{30}$$

$$\frac{1 \times 5}{6 \times 5} = \frac{5}{30}$$

$$\frac{2 \times 6}{5 \times 6} = \frac{12}{30}$$

It is a common mistake to think we have to multiply all three fractions by the same value—that is not the case. What we want all three fractions to have is the same denominator. We multiply each fraction by whatever value will convert the denominator to the LCD, remembering to multiply both numerator and denominator by that value so as not to alter the fraction's value.

PRACTICE EXERCISE 2.G

Convert each of the following groups of fractions to the same denominator. (These are the same fractions that you found the LCD for in Practice Exercise 2.F.)

1. $\frac{1}{2}, \ \frac{5}{6}$ 2. $\frac{1}{2}, \ \frac{2}{3}, \ \frac{3}{4}$ 3. $\frac{3}{4}, \ \frac{5}{8}, \ \frac{2}{3}$ 4. $\frac{1}{2}, \ \frac{1}{3}, \ \frac{2}{5}$ 5. $\frac{3}{8}, \ \frac{2}{3}, \ \frac{4}{5}$

Addition and Subtraction

We are now ready to begin to add and/or subtract fractions. The key is that fractions can only be added or subtracted once they have been converted to fractions with the same denominator. Then we simply add or subtract the numerators, keeping the same denominator.

KEY POINT

To add or subtract fractions:

1. Find the LCD.

2. Convert to fractions with the same denominator.

3. Add or subtract the numerators. The denominator remains the same.

4. Simplify to the lowest terms.

EXAMPLE: Add:

$$\frac{1}{2} + \frac{2}{3} + \frac{5}{6}$$

The LCD is 6. We can convert each fraction and keep the form of the original problem:

$$\frac{1}{2} \times \frac{3}{3} + \frac{2}{3} \times \frac{2}{2} + \frac{5}{6} =$$

$$\frac{3}{6} + \frac{4}{6} + \frac{5}{6} =$$

$$\frac{3+4+5}{6} = \frac{12}{6} = 2$$

We note that the last fraction in the problem had a denominator of 6, so it did not require any conversion. Also, we see in this problem when we simplified, we finished with a whole number.

When working with adding or subtracting mixed numbers, it is easy and consistent with our other operations on fractions to convert them to improper fractions.

EXAMPLE: Add:

$$3\frac{4}{5} + 2\frac{2}{3}$$

Converting to improper fractions, we have:

$$\frac{19}{5} + \frac{8}{3}$$

The LCD is 15.

$$\frac{19}{5} \times \frac{3}{3} + \frac{8}{3} \times \frac{5}{5} = \frac{57}{15} + \frac{40}{15} =$$

$$\frac{57+40}{15} = \frac{97}{15} = 6\frac{7}{15}$$

EXAMPLE: Subtract:

$$\frac{5}{6} - \frac{1}{4}$$

The LCD is 12.

$$\frac{5}{6} \times \frac{2}{2} - \frac{1}{4} \times \frac{3}{3} = \frac{10}{12} - \frac{3}{12} =$$

$$\frac{10-3}{12} = \frac{7}{12}$$

EXAMPLE: $3\frac{3}{4} - 2\frac{5}{6}$

The LCD is 12.

$$3\frac{3}{4} - 2\frac{5}{6} = \frac{15}{4} - \frac{17}{6} = \frac{15 \times 3}{4 \times 3} - \frac{17 \times 2}{6 \times 2} =$$

$$\frac{45}{12} - \frac{34}{12} = \frac{45-34}{12} = \frac{11}{12}$$

PRACTICE EXERCISE 2.H

Add and/or subtract the following:

1. $\frac{1}{2}+\frac{5}{6}=$ **2.** $\frac{3}{4}-\frac{1}{2}=$ **3.** $\frac{1}{2}+\frac{2}{3}+\frac{3}{4}=$ **4.** $2\frac{1}{2}-1\frac{2}{3}=$ **5.** $\frac{3}{4}+\frac{5}{8}-\frac{2}{3}=$ **6.** $1\frac{1}{2}+2\frac{1}{3}-3\frac{2}{5}=$

Comparing Fractions

Before we complete our arithmetic with fractions, it is important to consider the value of fractions. In other words, how does one fraction compare to another? The key to this problem is to consider fractions with the same denominator.

Consider how 1/3 compares to 2/3. From our practical experiences, we can readily agree that 1/3 is smaller than 2/3, or 1/3 < 2/3. So, we can see that if the fractions have the same denominator, all we need do is compare the numerators as if we were considering whole numbers.

EXAMPLE: Compare $\frac{5}{12}$ and $\frac{7}{12}$.

Since the denominators are the same, we compare the numerators. Since 5 < 7, we say:

$$\frac{5}{12}<\frac{7}{12}$$

Suppose that the denominators are not the same. What can we do? Again, we can get back to the previous type of problem if we find and convert the fractions to the same LCD.

EXAMPLE: Compare $\frac{5}{6}$ and $\frac{2}{3}$. The LCD is 6. Since $\frac{2\times2}{3\times2}=\frac{4}{6}$, we can now compare $\frac{5}{6}$ and $\frac{4}{6}$ to obtain $\frac{5}{6}>\frac{4}{6}$, so we can say $\frac{5}{6}>\frac{2}{3}$.

PRACTICE EXERCISE 2.I

Compare the following fractions and insert a >, <, or = sign.

1. $\frac{1}{2}$ — $\frac{5}{6}$ **2.** $\frac{2}{3}$ — $\frac{12}{18}$ **3.** $\frac{1}{5}$ — $\frac{1}{6}$ **4.** $\frac{10}{3}$ — $\frac{9}{5}$

> ### REMEMBER!
>
> Review on Fraction Operations
>
> #### To MULTIPLY
>
> 1. Multiply numerator × numerator and denominator × denominator.
> 2. Simplify.
>
> #### To DIVIDE
>
> 1. Change the problem to multiplication by multiplying the first fraction by the reciprocal of the second.
> 2. Multiply the two fractions and simplify.
>
> #### To ADD or SUBTRACT
>
> 1. Find the LCD of all the fractions.
> 2. Convert each fraction to the LCD.
> 3. Once all fractions have the LCD, add or subtract the numerators.
> 4. Simplify.

Uses of Fractions

With each chapter we are building not only knowledge of numbers, but also use of them in the real world. The allied health arena uses fractions in two systems of measurement. Fractional notation is used in both the apothecary and household systems. For this reason, any calculation or expression that results in a fraction in these systems should be expressed as one.

Household Measures

In Chapter 7, we will discuss the household system in detail. The purpose of the discussion here is to refresh your memory of the use of these numbers. Think back to the last time you were cooking, baking, or just watching somebody working in the kitchen. All the increments on the cup measure or the stick of butter or even the quart container are marked off in fractions (see Figure 2-1). Look at a medicine cup! Do you see markings for ½ ounce?

Apothecaries' Notation

Another place where we see fractions used is on packages of various allied health supplies. The most common of these are the labels on medications. Since the apothecaries' system (the oldest system of measurement) commonly uses fractions, older medications such as morphine, phenobarbital, codeine, and aspirin will often have fractions on their labels. The fraction is used to depict the amount of the drug measured in grains (gr) in this case, which is a unit of measure of the apothecaries' system (see Figure 2-2). For this reason, we will soon see that it will be necessary to make relationships between numbers expressed as fractions and those expressed as decimals. We will also learn how to convert between systems of measure.

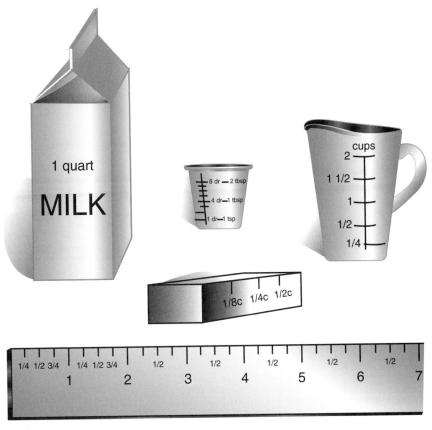

FIGURE 2-1

Measurement Tools Using Fractions

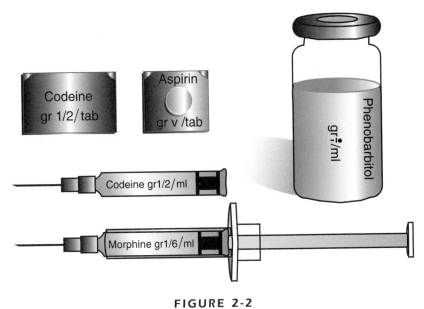

FIGURE 2-2

Apothecaries' Measures

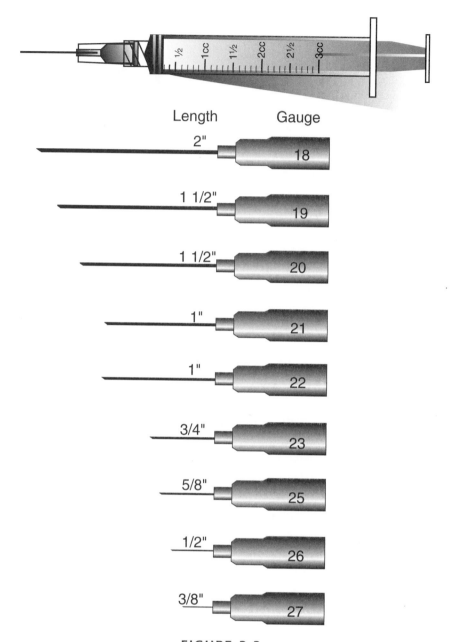

FIGURE 2-3
Syringe and Needles Measured with Fractions

Syringe Calibrations

In health care, fractions are used on syringes and needles to identify various measures of this equipment (see Figure 2-3). Many of the commonly used 3 cc syringes, for example, have the increments of cc marked with fractions.

Needle Size

Also, the lengths of needles used for injection are expressed as fractions. Often it is necessary to consider the length of a needle when preparing an injection. For example, if a patient is thin, with very little fat tissue (adipose tissue), and you are preparing a subcutaneous injection (sc)—one that will be delivered into the adipose tissue—you may want to choose between a 3/4-inch and 5/8-inch needle. Using our knowledge of fractions, how can we determine which is smaller?

Find the lowest common denominator and convert:

$$\frac{3}{4} = \frac{}{8}$$

$$\frac{3}{4} = \frac{6}{8} \qquad\qquad \frac{5}{8}$$

$$\frac{6}{8} > \frac{5}{8}$$

Therefore, the smaller needle is the 5/8-inch needle.

Sodium Chloride Percent Solutions

Lastly, intravenous solutions are referred to with fractions (see Figure 2-4). Most intravenous solutions contain percentages of various basic elements and compounds. Sodium chloride (NaCl) is the main component of most solutions. Normal saline (NS) is 0.9% NaCl. This common solution will be discussed in further detail later. It is similar in concentration to that of body fluids. So, $\frac{1}{2}$NS would be 0.45% NaCl.

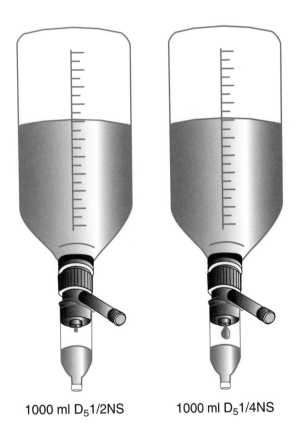

1000 ml D$_5$1/2NS   1000 ml D$_5$1/4NS

FIGURE 2-4
Fluids Named Using Fractions

LEARNING ACTIVITIES

1. Look at a 1 cup measure. List all the fractional measurements you find.

2. Look at a stick of butter. What fractional measures are indicated on the wrapper?

3. Look through your medicine cabinet. Look for the dosage, including the numerical quantity, of various drugs. What numbers expressed as fractions do you find?

4. If available from a nursing clinical laboratory, look at the markings on syringes and needles. What fractional measurements do you find?

5. After looking at various needle sizes in question 4, and with your knowledge of fractions, determine which is larger, ⅝ or ½? Find the lowest common denominator and convert.

CHAPTER REVIEW EXERCISES

1. Create improper fractions for the following mixed numbers:

   a. $3\frac{1}{2}$

   b. $1\frac{2}{3}$

   c. $5\frac{2}{7}$

2. Simplify the following fractions:

   a. $\frac{18}{27}$

   b. $\frac{8}{6}$

   c. $\frac{35}{25}$

   d. $\frac{12}{18}$

   e. $\frac{18}{12}$

   f. $\frac{250}{75}$

3. Find the LCD of the following groups of fractions:

   a. $\frac{1}{2}, \frac{3}{5}$

   b. $\frac{1}{4}, \frac{3}{8}, \frac{5}{3}$

   c. $\frac{1}{2}, \frac{1}{3}, \frac{1}{5}$

   d. $\frac{1}{2}, \frac{3}{4}, \frac{2}{5}$

4. Convert the following fractions to fractions with the same LCD:

   a. $\frac{1}{4}, \frac{3}{8}, \frac{5}{3}$

   b. $\frac{1}{2}, \frac{3}{4}, \frac{2}{5}$

5. Compare the following fractions and insert either a >, <, or = sign.

   a. $\frac{1}{2} \underline{\quad} \frac{1}{5}$

   b. $\frac{3}{7} \underline{\quad} \frac{5}{7}$

   c. $\frac{3}{4} \underline{\quad} \frac{9}{12}$

   d. $\frac{2}{3} \underline{\quad} \frac{5}{8}$

   e. $\frac{7}{6} \underline{\quad} \frac{12}{5}$

   f. $2\frac{1}{5} \underline{\quad} 2\frac{2}{7}$

6. Add, subtract, multiply, or divide the following groups of fractions as indicated:

   a. $\frac{1}{2} + \frac{1}{4} =$

   b. $\frac{4}{5} + \frac{8}{15} =$

   c. $1\frac{1}{8} + \frac{7}{12} =$

   d. $1\frac{3}{4} + 2\frac{1}{2} + 3\frac{1}{6} =$

   e. $\frac{12}{5} - \frac{2}{5} =$

   f. $\frac{13}{18} - \frac{4}{9} =$

   g. $1\frac{1}{2} - \frac{3}{4} =$

   h. $3\frac{1}{4} - 2\frac{5}{6} =$

   i. $\frac{1}{2} \times \frac{1}{4} =$

   j. $\frac{3}{5} \times \frac{2}{5} =$

k. $\dfrac{11}{10} \times \dfrac{8}{5} =$

l. $8\dfrac{1}{2} \times \dfrac{3}{4} =$

m. $\dfrac{2}{3} \times 3\dfrac{1}{2} \times \dfrac{5}{8} \times 12 =$

n. $\dfrac{7}{6} \div \dfrac{3}{5} =$

o. $\dfrac{5}{6} \div 15 =$

p. $3\dfrac{3}{4} \div 2\dfrac{1}{3} =$

CRITICAL THINKING

Interpret the following quantities and translate all symbols and abbreviations using Appendix 1:

1. $\overline{ss}$
2. tab
3. cc
4. sc
5. NaCl
6. NS
7. ½NS
8. ¼NS
9. ½ C
10. ¾ tsp
11. ½ tsp
12. ½ gal
13. $\overline{ss}$ ʒ
14. 2 tbsp
15. ½ qt
16. ½ pt
17. ¼ C
18. You are making four loaves of nut bread with the following recipe. Determine the amount of each measure you will use.

    ⅓ C butter

    ¾ C sugar

    2 eggs

    ¾ C milk

    2 C flour

    ½ tsp soda

    ½ tsp baking powder

    ½ tsp salt

    ½ C chopped nuts

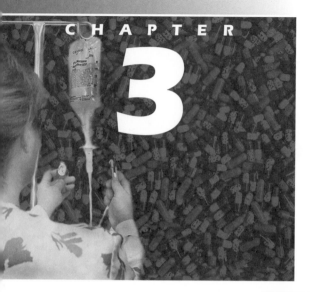

CHAPTER 3

Decimals

OBJECTIVES

Upon completion of this chapter, you will be able to:

- Describe place value.
- Perform operations on decimals.
- Convert between fractional and decimal forms of numbers.
- Apply decimal number forms to metric measurements.

Introduction

Evidence of a decimal system, the number system we use today, dates back to the third century B.C. in India. The system was formalized during the Middle Ages and is now referred to as the Hindu-Arabic system. This number structure and place values were brought to Europe and popularized during the early thirteenth century by Fibonacci in his *Liber Abaci* (Book of Counting). An Italian mathematician, Fibonacci brought the decimal system to Italy where roman numerals were still being used.

Decimals

Decimals, as they relate to health applications, primarily focus on scientific off-shoots of the metric system. Decimals are predominantly used in many of the applied areas including drug dosages.

What is a decimal? It is a combination of the digits 0 through 9 associated with a decimal point that separates the portion of the number that is not whole. The key to understanding decimals is to recognize that every digit in a decimal has a place value. Suppose we consider the decimal 347.568.

The portion to the left of the decimal is the whole number three hundred and forty-seven (347). If we think about what that means we recognize this number consists of three digits that each has value associated with its specific position. The 7 is in the first position as we move away from the decimal point. It is in the *one's* place and therefore its value is 7×1 or 7. Added to that 7 is the next value of 4, which is in the *ten's* place—a multiple of 10 beyond the previous one's place. It therefore has a value of 4×10 or 40. The next position is again a multiple of 10 beyond the last place ($10 \times$ ten's place) or the *hundred's* place. With a value of 3 in that place, we have 3×100 or 300. Therefore, the three places added are $300 + 40 + 7$ or 347.

Previously as we were moving away from the decimal point we were moving to the left and multiplying. As we reverse the process and start moving in the opposite direction, we would expect as we move to the right that we would divide successively by tens. As we move to the right of the decimal point, the first place in our example has a value of 5. It is in the one's/10 or tenth's place. Therefore, it has a value of $5 \times \frac{1}{10}$ or $\frac{5}{10}$. The next place value is divided by 10 again and the 6 is in the hundredth's place. Similarly, continue to divide by 10 and the 8 is in the thousandth's place. So, the portion of the number following the decimal point is the sum of $5/10 + 6/100 + 8/1,000$. If we use a common denominator of 1,000 to combine those numbers, we end up with $568/1,000$ or five hundred and sixty-eight one thousandths.

Typically, we read the numbers following the decimal point as if they were whole numbers and then append the place value of the last digit. So, if we considered the decimal 0.3248, we would name that as three thousand two hundred and forty-eight ten thousandths, as the last number (the 8) is in the ten thousandth's position.

Table 3-1 is a guide to place value.

TABLE 3-1 Place Value

millions	hundred thousands	ten thousands	thousands	hundreds	tens	ones	•	tenths	hundredths	thousandths	ten thousandths	hundred thousandths	millionths

PRACTICE EXERCISE 3.A

Name the place value underlined in each of following examples:

345.5678   *Answer:* The 6 is in the hundredth's place.

1. 132456.859   **2.** 347.8900   **3.** 0.00978   **4.** 6.02   **5.** 0.009

An important consideration in working with decimals is notation, especially since we will be applying decimal points. There is absolutely no difference in value for the decimals .5 and 0.5. However, there is a difference in notation. The second (the 0.5) has a zero in front of the decimal point. That zero is important and we will always leave our answers that are less than one with a leading zero in front of the decimal point. The reason is quite practical. For example, suppose we were administering a medication and were supposed to give one-half (five-tenths) gram. If that one-half value were written as .5, there is a chance the decimal might not be seen and suddenly we might give 5 grams—a gigantic and perhaps costly mistake! By placing the leading zero and having the one-half value written as 0.5 there is less chance for error. When we see that leading zero, we go looking for the decimal point, which leads us to a decimal value rather than a whole number.

Operations on Decimals

Two methods must be considered for operations on decimals. If we are using a calculator, then simply all the operations are at our fingertips with the aid of a manual. If using a calculator, we need to be especially careful of entering series of additions and multiplications (or divisions) according to the *order of operations* (we will need to check the manual to see if the calculator is programmed according to this or not). Most four-functioned calculators (those with just +, −, ×, ÷) are not. Most, if not all, scientific and graphing calculators are programmed this way. If you are simply performing one operation in a problem, this will not matter.

Many health professionals do not always have a calculator handy to do all problems. Therefore, we will consider the standard methods of working with decimals.

Addition

To consider addition of two or more decimals, it is easiest if we write the decimals vertically, lining each decimal point under the previous decimal point. The process then becomes one of simple addition, remembering to *carry* when a column of numbers adds up to more than 9.

EXAMPLE: Add 3.578 and 0.9 and 7.8897 and 4

Placing the numbers in vertical form, we have:

$$
\begin{array}{r}
{}_{2\ 1\ 1} \\
3.578 \\
0.9 \\
7.8897 \\
\underline{4\quad} \\
16.3677
\end{array}
$$

The small numbers above the problem represent the values that we are carrying since the previous column added to more than 9.

Notice that we lined all the decimal points under each other. Also, note the whole number 4 has an implied decimal point following it. We place that number under the whole numbers in our problem. Many find it useful to add extra zeros to some of the numbers to fill out all the columns as illustrated below:

$$
\begin{array}{r}
3.5780 \\
0.9000 \\
7.8897 \\
\underline{4.0000} \\
16.3677
\end{array}
$$

Subtraction

When we consider subtraction of decimals, again we wish to line up the decimal points. The process of subtraction begins as if we were subtracting two whole numbers once that decimal point is lined up. We also need to remember that if the top digit in our subtraction is less than the value below, we will need to *borrow* a one's digit from the previous column, now giving us a value in the current column that is larger than 9. This enables us to subtract the bottom value from the top, and we proceed to the next column. The notation for this, if you wish to write it down, can be a bit cumbersome. It is always valuable for us to check our answer by adding it back to the bottom number to see if it adds up to the original number we were subtracting from.

EXAMPLE: $1.246 - 0.353$

Writing in a column we have:

$$
\begin{array}{r}
1.246 \\
- \ 0.353 \\
\hline
\end{array}
$$

In the case of subtraction we will write the values borrowed above in the fairly standard notation.

$$
\begin{array}{r}
{}^{0\ {}^{1}1\ 1} \\
1.246 \\
- \ 0.353 \\
\hline
0.893
\end{array}
$$

EXAMPLE: Subtract 0.992 from 1.009.

$$
\begin{array}{r}
{}^{0\ \ 9\ 1} \\
1.009 \\
- \ 0.992 \\
\hline
0.017
\end{array}
$$

PRACTICE EXERCISE 3.B

Add or subtract the following decimals as indicated. You may wish to verify your results on a calculator.

1. $0.956 + 1.2379$

2. $1.347 + 0.56 + 23.008 + 6$

3. $3.256 - 1.009$

4. $5 - 0.375$

5. $1.347 + 2.50 - 3.750$

Multiplication

Multiplication of decimals does not require us to line up decimal points, although we may. The multiplication portion of a problem is an example, in essence, of simply multiplying two whole numbers—that is, ignoring the decimal points. However, to determine the value of the product (answer), we need to count the total number of decimal places following the decimal points in the entire problem. Again, as in the other operations we have considered, we set up the problems in a vertical manner.

EXAMPLE: How many decimal places will be in the product of
23.125×45.23?

Since there are three decimal places following the decimal
point in 23.125 and two places following the decimal point
in 45.23, there will be a total of 3 + 2 or 5 decimal places in
the product of the two numbers.

EXAMPLE: Multiply: 23.125×45.23. We begin by setting up the
problem vertically. Recall that there is no need to line up
the decimal points.

$$
\begin{array}{r}
23.125 \\
\times\ 45.23 \\
\hline
69375 \\
46250 \\
115625 \\
92500 \\
\hline
104594375 \rightarrow 1045.94375
\end{array}
$$

From our previous example, we needed five decimal places
beyond the decimal point, so we placed the decimal point
between the 5 and the 9.

EXAMPLE: Multiply 13.0×0.005.

$$
\begin{array}{r}
13.0 \\
\times\, 0.005 \\
\hline
650 \rightarrow 0.0650
\end{array}
$$

Notice that in this problem we needed to have four decimal
places following the decimal point. When we performed
the multiplication, we found there were only three numbers
in our product. Therefore, we needed to place a zero before
the 6 prior to inserting the decimal point. Also, we needed
to add the zero before the decimal point for clarity.

Division

As we begin to consider division of decimals, the main idea we need to recall is
that we may only divide by *whole* numbers. So, if we are dividing by a number
that has a decimal point with numbers to the right, we must convert that number
to a whole number by moving the decimal point an appropriate number of places
to the right. In order not to change the value of our answer, we correspondingly
must do the same to the number we are dividing. We move the decimal point by
multiplying each number by the same multiple of 10.

EXAMPLE: Divide 178.948 by 2.2. Setting up a typical division
problem, we write:

$$2.2\overline{)178.948}$$

Since 2.2 is not a whole number, we need to move the
decimal point one place to the right—multiply the number

by 10. In order not to change the value of the problem we need to do the same to 178.948. Therefore, we have converted the original problem to the following:

$$2.2\overline{)178.948} \rightarrow 22\overline{)1789.48}$$

We can now begin standard long division. The first step is to place the decimal point directly above its position in the decimal under the division sign. That helps us to have the correct value in terms of the decimal places in our answer.

$$22\overline{)1789.48}$$

Now we can begin the division process.

$$
\begin{array}{r}
81.34 \\
22\overline{)1789.48} \\
\underline{176} \\
29 \\
\underline{22} \\
74 \\
\underline{66} \\
88 \\
\underline{88} \\
0
\end{array}
$$

EXAMPLE: Divide 1 by 0.25.

$$0.025\overline{)1} \rightarrow 25\overline{)1000}$$

Notice that the whole number under the division has an implied decimal point following it. Therefore, when we need to move the decimal point three spaces to the right for the 0.025, we also have to add zeros following the 1. Now we can begin to divide.

$$
25\overline{)1000.} \rightarrow
\begin{array}{r}
40. \\
25\overline{)1000.} \\
\underline{100} \\
0
\end{array}
$$

Notice that we had to add a zero following the 4 in our answer, as the multiplication left no remainder in the rest of the problem and the 4 was in the ten's place.

So, our problem $1 \div 0.025 = 40$. Does that make sense? Since the division is the "opposite" operation of multiplication, we can multiply the 40×0.025 and we will see our answer is indeed 1.

PRACTICE EXERCISE 3.C

Multiply or divide the following as indicated:

1. 23.4×1.23 **2.** 3.4×0.004 **3.** 75×2.2 **4.** $176/2.2$ **5.** $3.4075/1.45$

Fractions vs. Decimals

In Chapter 2 we considered fractions. Fractions were one representation of numbers. Decimals are also another way to represent numbers. Since these are two different names for the same numbers, we can find a connection between them. In other words, how do we make a conversion between fractions and decimals?

One way is to recognize familiar forms—fractions that we commonly use in both their fractional and decimal form. For example, for many the fraction ½ and the decimal 0.5 are interchangeable. However, suppose the fraction is not common to us or we are not quite sure. The conversion from fractions to decimals can be made by simple division.

EXAMPLE:　Convert ¼ to its decimal equivalent.

The fraction ¼ means $1 \div 4$ and so the problem reduces to dividing 1 by 4 using long division.

$$
\begin{array}{r}
0.25 \\
4\overline{)1.00} \\
\underline{8} \\
20 \\
\underline{20} \\
0
\end{array}
$$

Therefore, the decimal equivalent of ¼ is 0.25. Notice that we did not move any decimal points in this problem, as we were dividing by a whole number.

EXAMPLE:　Convert ⅜ to its decimal equivalent.

$$
\begin{array}{r}
0.375 \\
8\overline{)3.000} \\
\underline{2\,4} \\
60 \\
\underline{56} \\
40 \\
\underline{40} \\
0
\end{array}
$$

The decimal equivalent of ⅜ is 0.375.

The question arises as to whether fractions when divided always divide evenly as in the last two examples. Let us consider the following example.

EXAMPLE:　Convert ⅔ to its decimal equivalent.

$$
\begin{array}{r}
0.666\ldots \\
3\overline{)2.000} \\
\underline{1\,8} \\
20 \\
\underline{18} \\
20 \\
\underline{18} \\
2
\end{array}
$$

As we can see, this decimal continues to have a quotient of 6 and a remainder of 2 each time we divide. That remainder will always continue and the fraction never divides evenly. To accurately represent this idea, we indicate having the 6 *repeat* by placing a bar over the number the first time it repeats.

Therefore, ⅔ has a decimal representation of

$$0.\overline{6}$$

Not all fractions that repeat do so in one digit. It may take several places for many common fractions to repeat. Also, the entire decimal portion may not repeat, but instead only a portion of the decimal may do so.

EXAMPLE: Convert 5/12 to its decimal representation.

$$
\begin{array}{r}
0.4166\ldots \rightarrow 0.41\overline{6} \\
12\overline{)5.0000} \\
\underline{4\,8} \\
20 \\
\underline{12} \\
80 \\
\underline{72} \\
80 \\
\underline{72} \\
8
\end{array}
$$

REMEMBER!
When converting from fractions to decimals, each result will either be a decimal that divides evenly (called a terminating decimal) or one that repeats (called a repeating decimal).

Conversion from decimal representation to fractional notation is rarely done in applied areas. We occasionally need to take a fraction in a practical situation and convert it to a decimal, but the reverse process is not often used. It is fairly easy to change terminating decimals to fractions. We would simply need to place the decimal disregarding the decimal point in the numerator of a fraction and divide by the value of the last decimal place—and simplify.

EXAMPLE: Convert 0.625 to fractional notation.

Since the last number in the decimal is in the thousand's place, we divide 625 by 1,000 or $0.625 = \frac{625}{1000}$

If we notice common factors of 125 in both the numerator and denominator (or successive factors of 5) we can simplify the fraction in the following way:

$$\frac{625}{1000} = \frac{5 \times 125}{8 \times 125} = \frac{5}{8}$$

So, the fractional representation of 0.625 is 5/8.

What if the decimal is repeating? The process to convert a repeating decimal back to a fraction is a bit more involved. It requires a series of algebraic equations, so we will not attempt it here. The manipulation required, besides the lack of a practical reason to do so, becomes the reason for not focusing on this conversion.

PRACTICE EXERCISE 3.D

1. Convert the following fractions to decimals:
   a. 3/4   b. 1/6   c. 3/8   d. 2/9   e. 5/3
2. Convert the following decimals to fractions:
   a. 0.33   b. 0.875

Importance of Units

If we asked you to consider the number 6, you might be thinking of the quantity, or what six looks like. But if we asked you to consider 6 pounds (6 lb), this should have a different meaning for you conceptually. You may be thinking of objects that weigh approximately this much. Now consider the quantity 6 kilograms (6 kg). What does 6 kg look like? Do you have a concept of what 6 kg would be? There are 2.2 lb for each 1 kg, so a pound is approximately half the size of 1 kg (see Figure 3-1). The units of measure, pounds and kilograms, have assigned meaning to the quantity. In the science and nursing community you will always see units with numbers, since the meaning of the entire quantity—value and units—is so important to the applied situation.

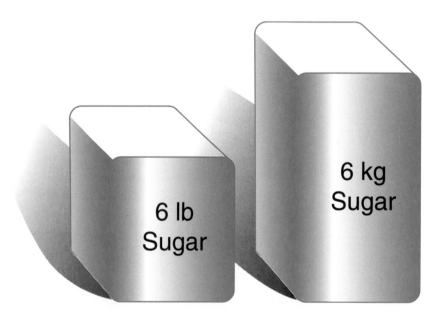

FIGURE 3-1
Six Pounds of Sugar vs. Six Kilograms of Sugar

EXAMPLE: If you were baking and needed to add flour, consider the importance of reviewing the recipe. If you read *two* of something should be added, it would make a big difference if it were 2 tablespoons or 2 cups.

As you proceed through this book, you will see a great deal of importance is placed on the units corresponding to numbers. The method of solving problems in Chapter 6, "Introduction to Dimensional Analysis," is based on the units of quantities.

LEARNING ACTIVITIES

The following activities are utilized to continue to build problem-solving skills in allied health situations. Some of the exercises utilize the metric system for examples. Decimals are commonly used with the metric system. You will see when we discuss this system that it is based on powers of 10. Therefore, the use of decimals makes conversions with this system easier.

1. A length of a needle is 3/8 inches. Convert to a decimal.

2. Which quantity is larger: 1.35 cc or 1.53 cc?

3. Which is larger: 0.06 g (gram) or 0.6 g?

4. The quantity of medication that is ordered to be given is ¼ g. Write the quantity in decimal form.

5. The amount of drug ordered to be given is 0.5 g. Express this quantity as a fraction. Reduce to the lowest terms.

CHAPTER REVIEW EXERCISES

1. Perform the following operations on decimals as indicated: Verify your answers on a calculator.

    a. $102.34 + 5.7304 + 0.789$

    b. $3.575 - 0.884$

    c. 2.5×3.45

    d. $176 \div 2.2$

    e. $100.0 + 32.56 + 82$

    f. $2 - 0.875$

    g. 3.0×1.0001

    h. $31.096 \div 0.23$

    i. $0.0075 + 0.750 + 0.075 + 7.5$

    j. $32.5 - 0.079$

    k. 55.2×2.2

    l. $29 \div 0.9$

    m. $123 \div 1.11$

    n. $12.5 + 0.725 - 3.56$

2. Convert the following fractions to decimals:

    a. 5/3

    b. 9/4

    c. 1/160

    d. 2/7

    e. 9/5

    f. 5/9

3. Convert the following fractions to decimals:

    a. 0.125

    b. 0.11

CRITICAL THINKING

1. Place the following numbers in increasing order:

   2.9007, 2.0907, 2.97, 2.907

2. Express ½NS as a decimal. Refer to Appendix 1.

3. A patient weighs 65.3 kg. Interpret the unit of measure.

4. What is the importance of assigning units to measurements? Give an example of when you needed to know the units of a quantity.

5. Which is smaller: 0.1 mg or 0.01 mg?

6. What is the importance of placing a zero to the left of a decimal, for example, 0.5? Give an example of when it would be important to express numbers this way.

7. A medication for injection is ordered. The volume to be administered is 0.75 cc. Express this decimal as a fraction. Reduce to the lowest terms.

8. The physician has ordered a patient to receive 0.125 mg (milligrams) of a medication. You are preparing to administer the drug. The tablet you find available for the patient is labeled as 0.25 mg. Compare the ordered amount with the available amount. Convert the two decimal numbers to fractions. Then find common denominators and compare. Which number is larger? How would you be able to administer the amount ordered? Will you need one half of the tablet or will you need two tablets?

9. This syringe shows increments of cc utilizing fractions. A medication for injection is determined to be given in a volume of 1.5 cc. Shade the syringe to fill it from the hub to the correct line.

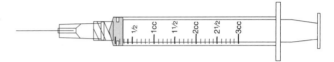

10. You are taking some measurements in chemistry lab. The mass of a beaker with water is 96.43 g. If the mass of the beaker is 30.02 g, then what is the mass of the water?

11. You and your friend ride bikes one afternoon. Your friend travels 3.4 km (kilometers) to get to your house, then the two of you ride 10.5 km. What is the total distance that your friend rode?

12. You have just traveled from New York to Maine. As you check the mileage recorded in your travel diary, you note that the total trip is recorded as 30.3 miles. Does this quantity seem to make sense?

Exponents and Scientific Notation

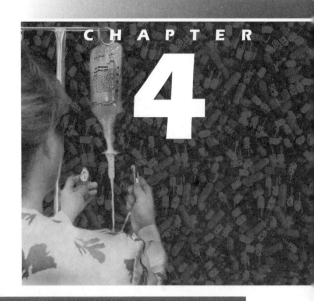

CHAPTER 4

OBJECTIVES

Upon completion of this chapter, you will be able to:

- Define an exponent.
- Perform operations on exponents.
- Place quantities in scientific notation.
- Multiply and divide numbers in scientific notation.
- Apply scientific notation to problems involving measurement.

Introduction

In the previous chapters we have discussed several different notations for numbers. We have considered fractional as well as decimal notation. There are many other types of notations for numbers. We will discuss exponents and scientific notation in this chapter.

Exponents

Many times in applied areas we consider repeated products of the same number, which is especially true of the number 10. Rather than write the same number several or even many times, we use a notation that represents the same idea. For example, suppose we consider the product $2 \times 2 \times 2$. We notice that the 2 is multiplied by itself three times. We identify this with the following notation:

$$2 \times 2 \times 2 \text{ is the same as } 2^3.$$

Note that 2 is called the *base* and 3 is called the *exponent*.

We often refer to 2^3 as *2 to the third power* or *2 raised to the third power*. Recognize that no matter how we speak of the quantity it still has a value of 8. It is a common mistake for us to refer to it as 6 because we are thinking about 2 being multiplied in conjunction with the number 3. We need to remember, however, that we are not multiplying 2 by 3, but instead are multiplying 2 by itself three times.

EXAMPLE: 10^5 means 10 multiplied by itself 5 times. So,
$10^5 = 10 \times 10 \times 10 \times 10 \times 10 = 100,000$.

Notice in this example that 10 is the base and 5 is the exponent. When 10 is the base, a shortcut to finding the value is for us to recognize that the number for the exponent is the number of zeros following 1. In this example we can see that our value turned out to be 1 followed by 5 zeros.

EXAMPLE: 3^1 means there is exactly one 3 in the problem and essentially no multiplication takes place. Therefore, $3^1 = 3$.

We can conclude from this problem that any base to the first power yields the base.

What about other powers? Occasionally we encounter working with zero as an exponent. Any base (other than 0) raised to the zero power always has a value of 1.

EXAMPLE: Find the value of 10^0.

Since we are raising 10 to the zero power, our answer must be 1. Recall, regardless of the base, any number raised to the zero power has a value of 1—it is another name for the number 1.

Negative exponents imply division by the base to a positive power. In other words, the reciprocal of the same base but now to a positive power.

EXAMPLE: Consider 4^{-2}. If we want to find the value of this quantity, we can rewrite the quantity as $1/4^2$. Since $4 \times 4 = 16 = 4^2$, $1/4^2 = 1/16$.

In our work with exponents, which is chiefly involved with scientific notation, we will not be evaluating a lot of different bases, but we do need to have an understanding of the basic notation.

PRACTICE EXERCISE 4.A

1. Write the following numbers in exponential notation as a product, for example, $5^2 = 5 \times 5$.
   a. 3^4 b. 4^3 c. 10^2 d. 10^{-2}

2. Find the value of each of the following numbers represented, for example, $5^2 = 5 \times 5 = 25$.
   a. 3^4 b. 4^3 c. 10^2 d. 10^{-2} e. 3^0

We will consider multiplying and dividing quantities involving exponents later in the chapter as we work with scientific notation.

Scientific Notation

What is scientific notation? Why do we need another notation? What does this have to do with exponents? All of these questions are important as we consider introducing scientific notation.

In science we encounter quantities that are extremely large or extremely small. Because of the numbers of zeros involved, whether as a large whole number or as a decimal, it is awkward as well as time-consuming to work with calculations on these numbers in that form. Therefore, we have a standardized form for considering those numbers. The notation standardized by the science community is called scientific notation.

Consider the large number 602,000,000,000,000,000,000,000. This quantity is used in chemistry to count a number of particles, for example atoms or molecules. This quantity is called a *mole*. As a dozen is always 12, a mole is always 602,000,000,000,000,000,000,000 particles. The number itself has a special name—it is called *Avogadro's number*. In scientific notation we write this same quantity as 6.02×10^{23} particles.

These two representations are of the same number—two names for the same quantity. It is important that we recognize the numbers have the same value. Certainly, we can see it is much shorter to write the number in the second format, although it may not look as familiar.

We notice that the first three digits of the number are the same. In the second representation we see that there is a decimal point after the 6 and then the 0 and the 2. The 6.02 is then followed by a "×" that indicates multiplication, or sometimes "·" is also used. Next we see the 6.02 is multiplied by 10^{23}. As we discussed, when considering 10 to some power—in this case 23—the value of that quantity is 1 followed by the number of zeros equal to the power—in this case, 1 followed by 23 zeros.

What happens when we multiply a decimal by a power of 10? Suppose we want to multiply 6.02 by 1,000. By using multiplication of decimals from Chapter 3, we arrive at

$$6.02 \times 1,000 = 6,020$$

We notice that multiplying by 1,000—1 followed by three zeros—moves the decimal point three spaces to the right. We want to notice as well that another form of 1,000 is 10^3. We can conclude, upon further investigation, that when multiplying by a power of 10, we move the decimal point to the right one space for each zero in the number or one space to the right for each positive number in the exponent.

If we go back to our example of 6.02×10^{23}, we see that we could find the value of the number by moving the decimal place in 6.02 twenty-three places to the right. As we think about this, we can see that it takes two spaces to get to the end of 6.02 and then we follow this by another 21 zeros, which is exactly our original number. Thus,

$$6.02 \times 10^{23} = 602,000,000,000,000,000,000,000$$

> **KEY POINT**
>
> Scientific notation simply places a given number so that there is exactly one nonzero number in front of the decimal point followed by an appropriate power of 10 to bring us back to the original value. The reason we multiply by a power of 10 is because that multiplication moves the decimal point back to the original value of the number as we noticed in our previous example.

> **REMEMBER!**
>
> To place a number in scientific notation:
>
> 1. Rewrite the number so that there is exactly one nonzero digit in front of the decimal point.
> 2. Multiply by 10 raised to a power to return to the original value.
>
> *Note:* Multiplying by 10 raised to a positive power moves the decimal point to the right. Multiplying by 10 to a negative power is actually dividing the number and therefore moving the decimal point to the left. It is important to recognize that we do *not* move the decimal point in the original number, but instead move the decimal point in the number we have just placed in the correct format to check that we have maintained the same value.

EXAMPLE: Place 5,003 in scientific notation.

The first nonzero digit is 5. So, we place it in front of the decimal point:

5.003

We see that in order to maintain the same value as the original number we have to move the decimal point three places to the right (a positive direction). Therefore, we multiply by 10^3. Thus:

$$5,003 = 5.003 \times 10^3$$

EXAMPLE: Place 0.0003224 in scientific notation.

The first nonzero digit is 3. We place 3 in front of the decimal point:

3.224

We see that in order to return to the original value of our number we have to move the decimal point four spaces to the left (a negative direction). Therefore, we multiply 3.224 by 10^{-4}:

$$0.0003224 = 3.224 \times 10^{-4}$$

As we practice more examples we notice a pattern appearing.

> **KEY POINT**
>
> If the original number is *larger than 10* to begin with, the exponent on the 10 will be *positive*.
>
> If the original number is *less than 1*, the exponent on the ten will be *negative*.
>
> If a number is more than 1 but less than 10, it is already in scientific notation.

PRACTICE EXERCISE 4.B

Place the following numbers in scientific notation:

1. 9,178   **2.** 917,800,000   **3.** 0.09178   **4.** 917.8

5. 0.0000009178   **6.** 9,178,000,000,000,000,000,000

7. What do the answers to problems 1–6 have in common? How do they differ?

Operations on Exponents and Scientific Notation

Multiplication

Since we will be working with numbers in scientific notation, we need to perform operations on them. We will not be adding or subtracting them because of the restrictions needed to do so (you need to have the same exponent on 10) and more importantly because it is not needed in the applications we will be considering. The first operation we will consider is multiplication. Suppose we wish to multiply the following numbers in scientific notation:

$$(1.2 \times 10^3) \times (3.2 \times 10^2)$$

Because this equation is one giant multiplication problem, we can split it into two parts. We can multiply the two decimals and then multiply the two powers of 10. We know how to multiply the decimals. What about the powers of 10? Let's leave our problem for a moment and see what happens when we multiply numbers with the same base.

Let us explore multiplying $10^2 \times 10^4$. We know,

$$10^2 = 10 \times 10 \text{ and } 10^4 = 10 \times 10 \times 10 \times 10$$

Therefore,

$$10^2 \times 10^4 = (10 \times 10) \times (10 \times 10 \times 10 \times 10) = 10^6$$

and

$$10^2 \times 10^4 = 10^6$$

If we look for a relationship between our original problem and our answer, we can see a pattern. It is a useful pattern because we certainly do not want to write out all the powers of 10 each time—that would be a waste of the notation. We recognize that since $2 + 4 = 6$, we can state:

KEY POINT

To multiply numbers with like bases, add the exponents!

Although our example involves only positive exponents, this concept also works for negative exponents as well as zero.

EXAMPLE: Multiply $2^5 \times 2^3$. Since the bases are the same (2), we merely add the exponents:

$$2^5 \times 2^3 = 2^{5+3} = 2^8$$

EXAMPLE: Multiply $10^6 \times 10^{-3}$. Again, we have like bases, so we can add the exponents. However, this time we have to recall how to add signed numbers from Chapter 1.

$$10^6 \times 10^{-3} = 10^{6+(-3)} = 10^3$$

PRACTICE EXERCISE 4.C

Multiply the following numbers with exponents:

1. $4^2 \times 4^3$ **2.** $10^4 \times 10^7$ **3.** $2^{-3} \times 2^4$ **4.** $10^{-5} \times 10^{-2}$ **5.** $10^1 \times 10^{-6}$ **6.** $10^3 \times 10^{-3}$

EXAMPLE: Let us now return to our previous problem:

$$(1.2 \times 10^3) \times (3.2 \times 10^2)$$

Multiplying the decimals,

$$1.2 \times 3.2 = 3.84$$

Multiplying the powers of 10,

$$10^3 \times 10^2 = 10^{3+2} = 10^5$$

Our product of these two numbers in scientific notation becomes:

$$(1.2 \times 10^3) \times (3.2 \times 10^2) = 3.84 \times 10^5$$

Before we proceed, we need to check that our decimal portion of our answer is in the proper from. In this case, 3.84 has exactly one digit before the decimal point. If it had more or less digits before the decimal point, we would continue to convert the final answer into the correct form for scientific notation.

EXAMPLE: Multiply $(2.5 \times 10^{-6}) \times (5.0 \times 10^8)$. We begin by multiplying the decimal portions:

$$2.5 \times 5.0 = 12.5$$

Multiplying the powers:

$$10^{-6} \times 10^8 = 10^{-6+8} = 10^2$$

So,

$$(2.5 \times 10^{-6}) \times (5.0 \times 10^8) = 12.5 \times 10^2$$

However, the 12.5 has two decimal digits before the decimal point and it can only have one in scientific notation. So, we will work with the 12.5 to place it in scientific notation:

$$12.5 = 1.25 \times 10^1$$

Recall we had to move the decimal place one space to the right in 1.25 to get the value back to 12.5. Therefore, the power on 10 needed to be a positive one.

So, putting the entire problem together:

$$12.5 \times 10^2 = (1.25 \times 10^1) \times 10^2$$

Now we need to combine the powers of 10:

$$= (1.25 \times 10^1) \times 10^2 = 1.25 \times 10^{1+2} = 1.25 \times 10^3$$

We can see that if the decimal is not in scientific notation following the multiplication of the decimals we can place that number in scientific notation and combine powers of 10.

PRACTICE EXERCISE 4.D

Multiply the following numbers in scientific notation. Make sure your result is in scientific notation.

1. $(1.2 \times 10^4) \times (3.4 \times 10^2)$ **2.** $(3.0 \times 10^3) \times (4.0 \times 10^6)$

3. $(9.8 \times 10^{-6}) \times (7.2 \times 10^2)$ **4.** $(3.00 \times 10^{-22}) \times (6.02 \times 10^{23})$

Division

Suppose rather than multiplying two numbers in scientific notation, we wish to divide them. Suppose our problem is the following:

$$\frac{5.00 \times 10^5}{2.0 \times 10^1}$$

As we can recognize from our previous work, it seems that we will divide the decimals and then divide the powers of 10. The decimal division is straightforward. However, how do we divide numbers with the same base? Let's consider a problem and explore the concept. Consider:

$$\frac{10^5}{10^2} = \frac{10 \times 10 \times 10 \times 10 \times 10}{10 \times 10}$$

Since we can cancel two of the tens in the numerator and denominator of the fraction, we see that we are left with three tens in the numerator multiplied together. Therefore:

$$\frac{10^5}{10^2} = \frac{10 \times 10 \times 10 \times 10 \times 10}{10 \times 10} = 10 \times 10 \times 10 = 10^3$$

If we try to look for a connection between the original exponents (5 and 2) and the resulting exponent 3, combined with our discovery of adding exponents when multiplying like bases, we recognize that $5 - 2 = 3$. Rather than adding exponents, we will now subtract.

KEY POINT

To divide numbers with like bases, subtract the exponents!

Again, although our example was based on positive exponents, the subtraction of exponents also works for negative and zero exponents.

EXAMPLE: Divide

$$\frac{10^6}{10^2}$$

Since we have like bases, we need only subtract the exponents:

$$\frac{10^6}{10^2} = 10^{6-2} = 10^4$$

EXAMPLE: Divide

$$\frac{10^{-2}}{10^5}$$

Again, we have to subtract exponents. The only difference with this problem is that it involves negative exponents. This requires that we again recall our work in Chapter 1.

$$\frac{10^{-2}}{10^5} = 10^{(-2)-5} = 10^{-7}$$

When working with negative exponents in the denominator, there is a tendency because the negative sign is present to think we are doing subtraction; however, we must remember to subtract whatever value is in the denominator from the value in the numerator.

EXAMPLE: Divide

$$\frac{10^2}{10^{-3}}$$

$$\frac{10^2}{10^{-3}} = 10^{2-(-3)} = 10^{2+(3)} = 10^5$$

PRACTICE EXERCISE 4.E

Divide the following numbers with exponents:

1. $\dfrac{4^3}{4^2}$ **2.** $\dfrac{10^4}{10^7}$ **3.** $\dfrac{2^{-3}}{2^4}$ **4.** $\dfrac{10^{-5}}{10^{-2}}$ **5.** $\dfrac{10^1}{10^{-6}}$ **6.** $\dfrac{10^3}{10^{-3}}$

EXAMPLE: Now that we can divide numbers with like bases, we can return to our problem:

$$\frac{5.00 \times 10^5}{2.0 \times 10^1}$$

We consider the division of decimals, $5.00 \div 2.0 = 2.5$, and we can consider the division of the powers of 10: $10^5 \div 10^1 = 10^{5-1} = 10^4$. As we put the problem back together we have:

$$\frac{5.00 \times 10^5}{2.0 \times 10^1} = 2.5 \times 10^4$$

We must be careful to check to see if our answer is in scientific notation. Since 2.5 has exactly one nonzero digit in front of the decimal point, we have an answer in the proper form. If our answer were not in the proper form, we would convert it.

EXAMPLE: Divide

$$\frac{1.2 \times 10^{-2}}{2.5 \times 10^{-4}}$$

First, we will divide the decimals:

$$1.2 \div 2.5 = 0.48$$

Recall, when dividing these decimals by long division, we must make sure the number we are dividing by is a whole number. Now we will divide the powers of 10:

$$\frac{10^{-2}}{10^{-4}} = 10^{-2-(-4)} = 10^{-2+(4)} = 10^2$$

Therefore,

$$\frac{1.2 \times 10^{-2}}{2.5 \times 10^{-4}} = 0.48 \times 10^2$$

However, our answer is not in scientific notation, as there is not one nonzero digit in front of the decimal point. Therefore, we must convert the 0.48 to scientific notation:

$$0.48 \times 10^2 = (4.8 \times 10^{-1}) \times 10^2 =$$

Recognize that in order to return 4.8 to its same value (0.48), we need to multiply 4.8 by 10^{-1} to move the decimal point back one space to the left—making it smaller. We can now work with the powers of 10.

$$(4.8 \times 10^{-1}) \times 10^2 = 4.8 \times 10^{-1+2} = 4.8 \times 10^1$$

We can conclude:

$$\frac{1.2 \times 10^{-2}}{2.5 \times 10^{-4}} = 4.8 \times 10^1$$

It is important to mention that when working with operations on scientific notation, once we have multiplied (or divided) the decimals, the value we obtain never changes—just the name. If it is not in scientific notation, we rewrite it, but we do not move the decimal point in the original number—only in the rewritten scientific notation version to return to the original value.

PRACTICE EXERCISE 4.F

Divide the following numbers in scientific notation. Make sure your result is in scientific notation.

1. $\dfrac{6.93 \times 10^6}{3.00 \times 10^2}$ 2. $\dfrac{1.52 \times 10^{-2}}{8.0 \times 10^5}$ 3. $\dfrac{6.02 \times 10^{23}}{8.75 \times 10^{25}}$ 4. $\dfrac{2.0 \times 10^5}{7.5 \times 10^{-5}}$

Applications of Exponents

Exponents and scientific notation are an intimate part of the health sciences. These number forms we will see every day. To illustrate the point, let us look at some basic chemistry concepts.

Matter

Matter is anything that takes up space and has mass. Mass is responsible for the weight of a body. Weight is the result of the earth's attraction for a body. As you study all the substances that the earth and all the occupants are made of, you will experience quantities that will not seem real because you cannot visualize them. But remember, these substances are there because of the definition of matter. Consider an electron! An electron is a very tiny piece of matter that revolves around the central core or the nucleus of an atom (see Figure 4-1). Atoms are the basic building blocks of all elements. The mass of an electron is 9.1096×10^{-28} grams. The unit of measure used here for the electron is the *gram*.

Do you think you can see electrons? No! What does this quantity look like?

0.00000000000000000000000000091096 grams

In comparison, hold two paper clips in your hand. Their mass is 1 gram. Scientific notation allows us to express quantities in a form that makes them easier to work with. The size of the electron is so minute that it makes it hard to imagine.

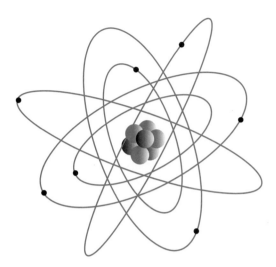

FIGURE 4-1

A carbon atom has a central nucleus of protons and neutrons with an electron cloud moving around the positively charged center.

If you were performing an experiment with atoms, such small substances and quantities could be quite inconvenient. For this reason, often we use larger amounts of substances, to make it easier to perform operations. A standard amount that is often used to simplify performing calculations on quantities of very small atoms of elements is one *mole* of the substance. The mole is the amount of substance that contains as many specified entities (molecules, atoms, ions, electrons, etc.) as there are atoms of carbon-12 in exactly 0.012 kg of that nuclide (nucleus), or 6.02×10^{23} particles. One mole has 6.02×10^{23} particles of a substance. One mole of hydrogen (H_2) contains 6.02×10^{23} H_2 molecules. One mole of e^- (electrons) has a mass of 5.49×10^{-4} g. Do these numbers seem more realistic? Throughout your health sciences many mathematic computations will be performed on numbers in scientific notation.

Look at these numbers in scientific notation:

KEY POINT

Speed of light = 3×10^{10} cm/sec

This quantity is expressed in units that identify a *rate,* which is a distance per time ratio. This quantity is 30,000,000,000 cm/sec (a bit more than 670 million miles per hour).

Mass of the earth = 6×10^{27} g

Consider the mammoth size of this number. This quantity is 6,000,000,000,000,000,000,000,000,000 g (about 13,200,000,000,000,000,000,000,000 pounds).

(From *CRC Handbook of Chemistry and Physics* by D.R. Lide (Ed.), 1990, Boston: CRC Press)

Laboratory Reports

Other uses of scientific notation are in the expression of various constituents of blood.

Look at the laboratory report shown in Figure 4-2. This report gives us the total white blood cell count (WBC) and the red blood cell count (RBC) for this individual. Note how, for convenience, the results are abbreviated on the laboratory report form. Under *normal value,* the normal range for each is expressed in scientific notation. The normal value range for WBC is $4.0–9.0 \times 10^3$, which means 4,000–9,000 WBC. In this case, the patient's value is 13.7, which is interpreted as 13.7×10^3 or 13,700 WBC, a value not in the normal range.

The normal range for the RBC value varies between men and women. For men the normal range is $4.5–5.7 \times 10^6$ or 4,500,000–5,700,000 RBC. In this example, the patient is male, and his laboratory report indicates a value of 4.23 or 4,230,000 RBC, which is a value lower than the normal range.

Measurements

Exponents help us to delineate units of measure when determining dimensions. We use them almost every day without even thinking! Consider finding the area of a box of computer paper (see Figure 4-3).

| 06/05 | Albany Medical Center | Interim Report |
| 10:29 | Clinical Laboratories | |

Name: Manning, John   Loc: D-6   Rm: D 601B   Age: 33Y   Sex: M
H#   : 85543   Dr: Palm, Gilbert
Acct   : 10648032

H33815   Coll: 06/05/99   06:30   Rec: 06/05/99   06:43   Phys:

Hemogram & Plat				Sta
WBC Count	*13.7	(4.0–9.0)	THO/CMM	
RBC Count	*4.23	(4.5–5.7)	MIL/CMM	
Hemoglobin	*12.8	(13.6–16.7)	GM/DL	
Hematocrit	*37.1	(40.0–49.0)	%	
MCV	87.7	(82.3–93.2)	U3	
MCH	30.4	(27.8–31.9)	UUG	
MCHC	34.6	(32.8–35.5)	GM%	
Red Cell Distribution	11.9		%	
Platelet Count	290	(130–350)	K/CMM	
Mean Platelet Vol	7.8		U3	
Percent Neut	65	(41–67)	%	
Percent Lymph	*23	(28–42)	%	
Percent Mono	*9	(4–8.5)	%	
Percent Eos	2	(0–5)	%	
Percent Baso	1	(0–1)	%	

FIGURE 4-2

Complete Blood Count Interim Laboratory Report

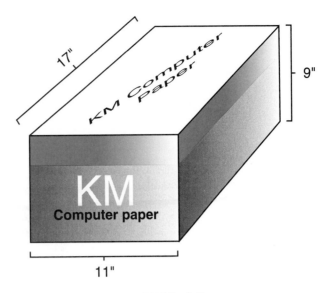

FIGURE 4-3
Box of Computer Paper

Area is the product of the length of the box multiplied by the width.

$$\text{Area (A)} = \text{Length (L)} \times \text{Width (W)}$$

What are the units of the quantities expressing the length and width? Be careful to find the units of measure accurately!

$$A = 17\,L \times 11\,W$$
$$= 17\,\text{in} \times 11\,\text{in}$$
$$= 187\,\text{in}^2$$

So, the area of the box is 187 in^2, or 187 *square* inches. It is important to recognize that there is a difference between inches and square inches. If you were buying a rug, a linear measurement of cut rug would not cover the surface of the floor. However, a square measure of rug would cover the floor of a room in the same manner that 187 in^2 indicates the whole surface of the top of the box.

Volume

Volume is another dimension. It is the product of three measurements.
Volume is defined as

$$\text{Volume (V)} = \text{Length (L)} \times \text{Width (W)} \times \text{Height (H)}$$
$$V = L \times W \times H$$
$$= 17\,\text{in} \times 11\,\text{in} \times 9\,\text{in} = 1{,}683\,\text{in}^3$$

Referring to the same box (Figure 4-3), the volume of the box is 1,683 in^3, or 1,683 *cubic* inches. Volume denotes what the container can hold. In this case, volume is all the space inside the box. It describes how much it can hold. Volume is three-dimensional. Again, it is from this relationship that we derive cubic cen-

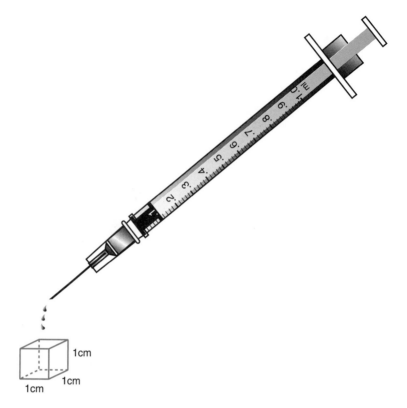

FIGURE 4-4
1 cm³ = 1 ml

timeters (cc) or milliliters (ml), a volume measurement that we use frequently in health care measurements. One milliliter of H_2O fills or takes up the space of one cubic centimeter (see Figure 4-4). It is from this relationship that we define volume measurements.

In health care we frequently use syringes. Syringes measure liquid volume. The barrel of the syringe is three-dimensional. Figure 4-4 shows the derived relationship of 1 cc and 1 ml as equivalents.

Based on the discussion so far, we have been asked to conceptualize relationships regarding mass measurements. We have also been given examples and discussions of the derivation of volume measurements. Let's take it one step further and discuss one more concept that requires a knowledge of exponents—density!

Density

Density is a mass per volume relationship. The units utilized to express this quantity are grams per cc.

Look at two 1,000 ml beakers and determine their mass. Fill each beaker with equal volumes of different substances. Fill one with water and the other with corn syrup. Determine the combined mass of each container and simplify the equation:

$$\text{Density} = \text{mass/volume}$$

$$= g/cm^3$$

Density of water = 253.5 g/100 ml

= 2.53 g/ml

Density of syrup = 280.5 g/100 ml

= 2.80 g/ml

What do we observe? As we already know, water is clear or transparent. The consistency of water is thin. Corn syrup, on the other hand, is slightly opaque. It is more difficult to look through and even pour. The consistency of syrup is thick and tends to pour in glops. It should not be surprising that when measuring the density of equal volumes of these two substances, the density of the corn syrup is more. Consider another example—cork and lead. These two substances have very different properties. If we have equal volumes of the two substances, their densities would reflect the same variation as the mass of these two objects.

LEARNING ACTIVITIES

1. A patient's laboratory report indicates the WBC value to be 13.5×10^3. Convert this number to a whole number. Determine if this number is within normal range.

2. A male patient's laboratory report indicates the RBC count to be 3.2×10^6. Convert this number to a whole number. Determine if this number is within normal range.

3. Find the area of the top of the box of photocopy paper shown here. Remember to include appropriate units on all quantities.

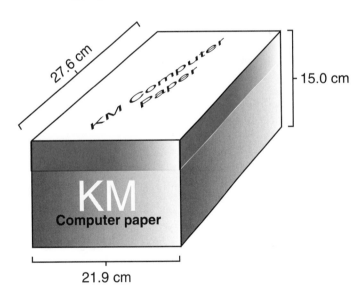

4. Find the volume of the box of photocopy paper. (Remember those units!)

5. A room has the dimensions of 8.0 feet by 6.5 feet. You want to approximate the amount of square feet of rug you will need to provide wall-to-wall coverage. How much rug will you need?

6. You wish to make a cement step at the end of your walkway. The dimensions of the step will be 24 in by 12 in by 3.0 in. What will be the volume of concrete needed to fill the space for the proposed step?

CHAPTER REVIEW EXERCISES

As you work through these exercises, note how your challenge to the problem-solving process is growing as your abilities also are growing.

1. Write the following products in exponent notation:

   a. $2 \times 2 \times 2 \times 2$

   b. 5×5

   c. 10

   d. $\dfrac{1}{10 \times 10 \times 10}$

2. Find the value of the following:

   a. 3^2

   b. 5^4

   c. 10^8

   d. 10^{-3}

   e. 3^0

3. Multiply:

   a. $10^2 \times 10^5$

   b. $5^2 \times 5^{-3}$

   c. $4^{-3} \times 4^{-2}$

   d. $10^6 \times 10^0$

4. Divide:

   a. $\dfrac{10^2}{10^5}$

   b. $\dfrac{5^2}{5^{-3}}$

   c. $\dfrac{4^{-3}}{4^{-2}}$

   d. $\dfrac{10^6}{10^0}$

5. Place the following numbers in scientific notation:

   a. 8,100,000

   b. 47,500

   c. 0.000092

   d. 0.76

   e. 8000

   f. 0.0000000061

6. Convert 1.550003×10^{-3} to a decimal not in scientific notation.

7. Convert 2.589988×10^6 to a decimal not in scientific notation.

8. Perform the following operations and place your answers in scientific notation:

   a. $(2.0 \times 10^{-3}) \times (2.2 \times 10^2)$

   b. $(3.0 \times 10^2) \times (4.00 \times 10^3)$

   c. $(2.1 \times 10^5) \times (6.0 \times 10^{-3})$

   d. $\dfrac{2.0 \times 10^5}{4.0 \times 10^2}$

   e. $\dfrac{6.02 \times 10^{23}}{2.00 \times 10^{-10}}$

   f. $20 \times (1.2 \times 10^{-5})$

   g. $(6.02 \times 10^{23}) \times (5.0 \times 10^{-2})$

   h. $\dfrac{6.02 \times 10^{23}}{1.4 \times 10^{25}}$

   i. $(3.0 \times 10^4) \times (4.5 \times 10^{-3})$

   j. $\dfrac{5.0 \times 10^{12}}{8 \times 10^{-2}}$

9. Perform the following operations and place your answers in scientific notation:

   a. $\dfrac{(3.0 \times 10^2) \times (1.0 \times 10^{-6})}{6 \times 10^3}$

   b. $\dfrac{(1.2 \times 10^6) \times (8.5 \times 10^{-2})}{2.4 \times 10^{-3}}$

   c. $\dfrac{(3.25 \times 10^2) \times (4.1 \times 10^{-1})}{4.52 \times 10^{-3}}$

   d. $\dfrac{(5.7 \times 10^2) \times (3.45 \times 10^5)}{3.0 \times 10^{-3}}$

CRITICAL THINKING

For questions 1–6, interpret the following abbreviations using Appendix 1.

1. CBC

2. cm

3. WBC

4. m^2

5. RBC

6. ml

7. Penicillin is often ordered in a unit of measure called *units,* which refers to the biologic activity of the drug. If a patient is prescribed 500,000 units of penicillin per dose, express this number in scientific notation.

8. Referring to question 7, if a bottle of penicillin has 6,000,000 units, how many doses of penicillin would you get from the bottle? Solve this problem with an equation using scientific notation. Then check your answer by solving the equation utilizing whole numbers. Can you see the advantage of shortening the numbers with scientific notation expression? Does your answer make sense?

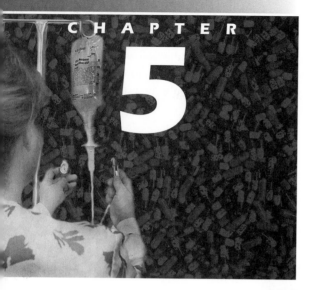

CHAPTER 5

Percents

OBJECTIVES

Upon completion of the chapter, you will be able to:

- Convert between decimal, percent, and ratio notations.
- Identify the parts of a solution.
- Interpret weight/volume, volume/volume, and weight/weight percent solutions.
- Interpret the concentrations of the major intravenous percent solutions.

Introduction

As we move toward more and more applications, consider another notation: another name for a quantity. Consider the percent notation: denoted %. Percent notation is common to everyday experience. We know what it means if there is a sale that is 50% off, that taxes may take 33% of our paycheck, etc. But, what does percent actually mean?

If we break apart the word *percent* into its two syllables we can begin to understand the concept. *Per* generally means a division and *cent* is from the Latin word for 100. So, when we encounter a percentage such as 50%, the % sign actually means to divide by 100 to find the value of the number. If we take 50 and divide by 100, we obtain 50/100, which is 0.50 when converted to its more familiar decimal form. Therefore, 50% is another name for the decimal 0.50, also known as ½.

Percents to Decimals

If we want to convert a percentage to its decimal form, we first need to drop the percent sign. In order not to change the value, we need to divide by 100. Dividing by 100 can be accomplished simply by moving the decimal point two spaces to the left within the given number.

KEY POINT

To convert from a percent to a decimal, we:

1. Drop the % sign

2. Divide by 100—move the decimal point two spaces to the left.

3. Place a zero in front of the decimal point for clarity.

EXAMPLE: Convert 27.5% to decimal form.

First, drop the % sign:

$27.5\% \rightarrow 27.5$

Next, divide by 100—move the decimal point two spaces to the left:

$27.5 \rightarrow .275$

Place the zero in front for clarity:

0.275

So, $27.5\% = 0.275$.

EXAMPLE: Convert 75% to its decimal form.

Following the same reasoning, drop the % sign first:

$75\% \rightarrow 75$

When moving the decimal point, recognize that one is not literally present because what is left is a whole number. However, recognize that because 75 is a whole number, it has an implied decimal point following the last digit. Therefore, place the decimal point and then move it two spaces to the left.

$75\% \rightarrow 75 \rightarrow 75. \rightarrow .75 \rightarrow 0.75$

Therefore,

$75\% = 0.75$

Becoming more comfortable with this process, you may find yourself moving from the percentage straight to the answer.

EXAMPLE: Convert 300% to its decimal form.

Since $300 = 300.$, dropping the % sign can move the decimal point two spaces to the left and obtain:

$300\% = 3.00 = 3$

Can you keep the two zeros following the decimal point if you wish? Although the zeros do not change the value of the number, within applied situations they do affect the precision of the number. We will discuss that later in the text in detail (see Chapter 19), but for now it is just best to drop them as indicated.

Occasionally, we encounter mixed numbers involved with percent signs. This most often happens when we consider bank interest, but does occur, as well, in working with solutions. When we encounter a mixed number percentage that we wish to convert, we first change the mixed number to an improper fraction. We then change the improper fraction to a decimal and finally change the decimal percentage back to its decimal form.

EXAMPLE: Convert $2\frac{1}{2}\%$ to its decimal form.

Since

$$2\frac{1}{2} = \frac{5}{2} = 2.5$$

then

$$2\frac{1}{2}\% = 2.5\% = 0.025$$

Therefore,

$$2\frac{1}{2}\% = 0.025$$

These particular conversions are useful when we are trying to work with an applied problem. Often a problem involving a percentage needs to be converted prior to doing any calculations.

Decimals to Percentages

We also have occasion to change a decimal to its percentage form. In order to complete this process, we need to reverse the previous process. In order to reverse a mathematical process, we need to reverse the order of the steps and change to the opposite operation. Therefore, in order to *convert a decimal to a percentage,* we first of all need to multiply by 100—the last step in our previous process was to divide by 100. To multiply by 100 we simply need to move the decimal place two spaces to the right. The very first thing we did in the previous problems was to drop the % sign. Therefore, the last step we will take in this process is to append the % sign.

KEY POINT

To convert from a decimal to a percentage, we:

1. Multiply by 100—move the decimal point two places to the right.

2. Append the % sign.

EXAMPLE: Convert 0.375 to a percent notation.

First, move the decimal point two spaces to the right:

0.375 → 37.5

Now we add on the % sign:

37.5%

So,

0.375 = 37.5%

EXAMPLE: Convert 0.1 to percent notation.

As we begin to move the decimal two spaces to the right, we notice that there is only one digit to the right of the decimal point. Therefore, we will have to add a zero to the digit so that we have indeed moved the decimal point two spaces:

0.1 → 0.10 → 10 → 10%

As we append the % sign we see that our result is

0.1 = 10%

EXAMPLE: Convert 1.50 to percent notation:

1.50 → 150 → 150%

Therefore,

1.50 = 150%

PRACTICE EXERCISE 5.A

1. Convert the following percentages to decimal notation:
   a. 62.5%   **b.** 1%   **c.** 25%   **d.** 0.9%   **e.** 175%   **f.** $1\frac{1}{2}$%

2. Convert the following decimals to percent notation:
   a. 0.65   **b.** 0.125   **c.** 0.333   **d.** 0.0045   **e.** 0.2   **f.** 1.4

Ratio Notation

In some applications, especially those involving solutions, we encounter another notation that is related to the percent notation. That notation is the ratio notation. This particular notation is typified by having two numbers separated by a colon, for example, 1:2. This 1:2 is referred to as a *one to two ratio*. For every one part of the first substance there are two parts of the second substance. It is often convenient to convert from this ratio notation to one involving percent notation. To make this conversion, we first need to recognize that this ratio notation with the colon can be easily translated to a fraction by placing the first number in the numerator and the number following the colon in the denominator. Therefore, a 1:2 ratio is another name for the fraction $\frac{1}{2}$. As a fraction we can convert it to its decimal notation and then to its percent notation.

KEY POINT

To convert from ratio to percent notation, we:

1. Replace the colon with a division sign.
2. Convert the fraction to decimal notation.
3. Convert the decimal to a percent.

EXAMPLE: Convert the ratio 1:5 to a percent notation.

We first convert 1:5 to the fraction 1/5. Dividing 1 by 5 as we did in Chapter 3 we obtain:

$$1/5 = 0.2$$

We can now convert 0.2 to percent notation by multiplying by 100 (decimal point two spaces to the right) and appending the % sign:

$$0.2 = 0.20 = 20\%$$

So, we can say the ratio 1:5 is the same as 20%.

EXAMPLE: Convert the ratio 1:1,000 to percent notation:

$$1:1,000 = 1/1,000 \rightarrow 1,000\overline{)1.000}$$
$$\begin{array}{r} 0.001 \\ 1\,000 \\ \hline 0 \end{array}$$

and changing to percent notation:

$$0.001 = 0.1\%$$

PRACTICE EXERCISE 5.B

Convert the following ratios to a percent notation:

1. 1:10   **2.** 1:4   **3.** 1:100   **4.** 1:250

Applying Percentages

We are now ready to consider some preliminary applications of percent. Often we are asked to take a percentage of a certain given quantity. When reading or considering such a problem it is important for us to interpret the *of* as a multiplication. The percentage needs to be converted to a decimal so that the multiplication can be completed.

EXAMPLE: Find 35% of 200.

We first convert the 35% to a decimal:

$$35\% = 0.35$$

To complete the problem, we need to multiply the 0.35 and the 200. Note that the phrase *of 200* was used in the initial problem.

$$0.35 \times 200 = 70$$

Does the answer 70 make sense to us? Well, 35% is about one third and 70 is approximately one third of 200, so 70 seems to be a reasonable answer.

EXAMPLE: Yesterday a patient received 1,500 ml of an intravenous (IV) fluid. Today you are asked to increase this amount by 25%. How much do you give the patient?

Our first thought, after rereading the problem several times, is to multiply the 1500 ml by 25%:

$$25\% = 0.25$$

So, $1{,}500 \text{ ml} \times 0.25 = 375 \text{ ml}$

Is 375 ml a reasonable amount to administer in this problem? As we reread the problem, we see that the patient received 1,500 ml yesterday and we are to *increase* that amount. It seems we have missed something if we give 375 ml—an amount that is a lot less. What does the 375 ml represent? It represents the amount of the increase, not the total amount. Therefore, we have to add the 375 ml to yesterday's amount.

$$
\begin{array}{r}
1{,}500 \text{ ml} \\
+ \quad 375 \text{ ml} \\
\hline
1{,}875 \text{ ml}
\end{array}
$$

The patient should receive 1,875 ml today.

REMEMBER!

To convert from a percent notation to a decimal:

1. Drop the % sign.
2. Divide by 100 (move the decimal point two spaces to the left).

To convert from a decimal to a percent notation:

1. Multiply by 100 (move the decimal point two spaces to the right).
2. Append the % sign.

To convert from ratio to percent notation:

1. Replace the colon with a division sign.
2. Convert the fraction to decimal notation.
3. Convert the decimal to a percent.

Solutions

At this point, we have looked at percentages from an arithmetic point of view. Now, let us learn how this concept is applied to solutions in the health sciences.

In modern nursing/health sciences many solutions of various types for many patient needs are available commercially (see Figure 5-1). The health care professional is responsible for understanding the product, the concentration of the solution being supplied, and how to administer the product.

Nutritional Solutions

There will be situations, however, where the solution that is prescribed may require preparation in the clinical and patient care areas. Depending on the environment, the clinical pharmacy staff will be responsible for the majority of solutions that require mixing close to the time of administration. But again, the professional needs to be able to describe what is being supplied.

EXAMPLE: A patient is prescribed total parenteral nutrition (TPN) or hyperalimentation. This is the administration of a nutritionally adequate hypertonic solution consisting of glucose, protein substances, minerals, and vitamins through a catheter into the central circulation. This type of solution can supply an individual with all the nutrients the body requires when the patient is unable to eat (see the Nutrition Order Sheet). The solution is ordered by the physician specifically for the individual patient. The concentrations and amounts of the various additives are quite variable. It is the nurse's responsibility, as it is with anything he or she delivers to the patient, to ensure that the amounts in the solution that are being supplied from the pharmacy correspond with what the physician ordered and is consistent with this patient's regime. The amount of dextrose and lipids added to the solution are usually ordered in percentages. You will need to interpret the label of the solution for accuracy.

Last but not least, there will be situations where it will be necessary for the bedside nurse as well as the chemistry laboratory worker to prepare percent solutions. Often formulas for feeding, irrigating solutions, antiseptic cleansing agents, chemicals for use both in hospital and outpatient settings will require preparation. In the community, often it is necessary to instruct families in the preparation of percent solutions to be used in the home setting.

Percent Solutions

What does percent (%) solution mean? The *percent refers to the part or substance per 100 parts of solution*. There are *X* number of parts in every 100 parts.

A solution is considered a uniform mixture. There are two parts to a solution. One part is the solute, which represents the smaller dissolved quantity. Often, but not always, the solute is a solid such as salt, sugar, or a dry, pure chemical. But a solute can also be a 100% concentrated liquid chemical. For this reason, often the units of the solute are expressed in a dry weight measure such as grams.

The other part of the solution is the solvent. The solvent is the substance that does the dissolving and represents the larger quantity. It may also be referred to as the diluent. Most often the diluent or solvent is water, but it may also be normal saline.

ALBANY MEDICAL CENTER HOSPITAL
ADULT
PARENTERAL NUTRITION ORDER SHEET

Order has 24-hr. automatic stop unless specified here: X _____ days.

Standard start time for ordered solution is 1700

Standard multivitamins/ trace elements added daily, selenium after 14 days-

For listing of added amounts see AMCH Formulary

Infusion rate will vary with volume, infuse at rate on label

ALLERGIES:

_125689_   _D - 501_

_MR 2346895_

Pack, Mary

DOB 06/24/1967   Sex F

ATT John MD, Susan B 340

PATIENT IDENTIFICATION PLATE

A. STANDARD DEXTROSE-AMINO ACID SOLUTIONS (Amount supplied per day)

Circle mode of delivery and check box for desired solution

APPROXIMATE   STANDARD   ELECTROLYTES

(Label on solution bag may vary slightly from concentrations listed below)

TOTAL PROT/DEX	PROTEIN	DEX	MINIMUM	RATE GIVEN OVER	Na	K	Ca	Mg	Cl	P	Ac
KCAL	G	G	VOLUME (L)	24 HOURS	mEq	mEq	mEq	mEq	mEq	mmol	mEq
PERIPHERAL/CENTRAL SOLUTION											
☐ 500	50	90	1.5	63 ml/hr	60	55	10	9	60	25	92
CENTRAL / PICC SOLUTIONS											
☐ 1000	75	200	1.5	63 ml/hr	60	55	10	9	60	25	125
☐ 1250	75	280	1.5	63 ml/hr	60	55	10	9	60	25	125
☐ 1500	75	350	1.5	63 ml/hr	60	55	10	9	60	25	125
☐ 1750	75	425	2	83 ml/hr	60	55	10	9	60	25	125
☒ 2000	75	500	2	83 ml/hr	60	55	10	9	60	25	125
☐ Other: _____ g _____ g			Order rate and volume in Section D		60	55	10	9	*	25	*
			"Standard electrolytes" defined as:		60	55	10	9	*	25	*

(* Chloride and Acetate will vary with amount of protein ordered)

B. NON-STANDARD DEXTROSE-AMINO ACID SOLUTIONS (order electrolytes, additives, volume/rate and fat emulsion in sections C.,D.,E.)

Central   ☐   (a) Protein _____ g/day

(b) Dextrose _____ g/day (maximum dextrose concentration = 350 g/L)

Peripheral   ☐   (a) Protein _____ g/day

(b) Dextrose   ☐   5% (50 g/L)   ☐   7.5% (75 g/L)

C. ELECTROLYTE OPTIONS AND OTHER ADDITIVES   **(CHECK ONE:)**

☐   **NO Electrolytes or Additives**   (nothing added to dextrose, amino acids, vitamins and trace minerals solution)

☐   **GIVE ONLY electrolytes and additives listed below**   (no standard electrolytes added to solution)

☒   **ADD electrolytes and additives listed below to STANDARD electrolytes as defined above in section A.**

OPTIONAL ADDITIVES (designate amount to be added per day) (Note: Cl and Ac will vary with amount of protein ordered)

Sodium Chloride _30_ mEq	Sodium Phosphate* _____ mEq	Sodium Acetate _____ mEq
Potassium chloride _____ mEq	Potassium phosphate* _10_ mEq	Potassium Acetate _____ mEq
Magnesium (sulfate) _5_ mEq	Calcium(gluconate) _5_ mEq	Vitamin K _____ mg
Human insulin _____ units	Other: _Pepcid 40mg Zn 10mg B12 1mg_	

*(1mEqNaPO4 = 23mgP = 0.75mMP and 1mEq KPO4 = 21mgP = 0.68mMP)

D. VOLUME / RATE OPTIONS   Dextrose/Amino Acid solution dispensed in minimum volume or volume specified below whichever is greater.

For specific volume needs, please check volume desired/day: NURSING: Infusion rate will vary with volume, infuse at hourly rate on label

☐ 1L (42ml/hr)   ☐ 1.5 L (63ml/hr)   ☐ 2 L (83ml/hr)   ☐ 3 L (125ml/hr)   ☒ _2.0_ L   ☐ Minimum Volume

Dextrose/Amino Acid solution infused over 24 hours unless specified below:

Cycle _____ Liters over _____ hours (always titrate rate upward over first hour, titrate rate down during last hour)

E. FAT EMULSION: (No fats dispensed unless dose specified below)

20 g ☐   50 g ☐   70 g ☐   100 g ☒   Other: _____ g

(20% 100 ml = 200 kcal)   (20% 250 ml= 500 kcal)   (20% 350 ml= 700 kcal)   (20% 500 ml=1000 kcal)

Infuse fats over 10 hours UNLESS specified otherwise: Infuse fats over _____ hours = _50_ ml per hour

(recommended maximum infusion rate for 20% fat emulsion is 50ml/hour)

Date Ordered	Time Ordered	Time Posted	Order must be received in pharmacy by 1200	
			Physician Signature: _Susan JohnM_	pager # _12/6_

90621 6/95 T

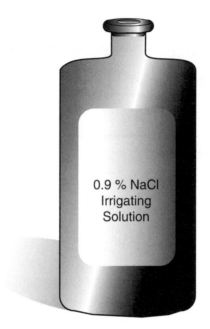

FIGURE 5-1
Normal Saline Irrigating Solution

EXAMPLE: A very highly concentrated solution will have a large or small amount of solute?

large

The percentage of a solution tells the strength of the solution:

$$\frac{35 \text{ grams salt}}{100 \text{ ml solution}} \qquad \frac{10 \text{ grams salt}}{100 \text{ ml solution}}$$

A 35% salt solution is more highly concentrated than a 10% salt solution. These relationships express the concentrations of a solution.

KEY POINT

A concentration is equal to

$$\frac{\text{amount of solute (mass or volume)}}{\text{total volume of solution (mass or volume)}}$$

If you are still having trouble with this concept, take a 6 ounce cup of water and add 3 tablespoons of sugar. Take another 6 ounces in a second cup of water and add 1/2 cup of sugar. The solution in the second cup becomes so thick that it is even difficult to dissolve. In this situation the solute is sugar. The cup with more sugar makes a more concentrated solution.

In a 2% salt solution, the salt makes up 2 parts of the total 100 parts. The remaining 98 parts or 98% is, in this case, water. Recall all the arithmetic ways to interpret 2%:

$$2\% = 0.02 = \frac{2}{100} = \frac{1}{50} = 1:50$$

In this example, recall the use of ratios. Often in health care a solution is referred to in terms of ratios.

EXAMPLE: Prepare the following irrigating solution as a 2:3 concentration of H_2O_2 (hydrogen peroxide).

Interpreting the concentration required as a percentage:

$$2:3 = \frac{2}{3} = 3\overline{)2.000}^{0.666} = 0.67 = 67\%$$

What has been asked for is a 67% H_2O_2 solution. For every 2 parts of H_2O_2 you will add 1 part of H_2O. Let's say you wanted to prepare 1 liter of this 67% solution. How much of the liter will be H_2O_2 (the solute)? (*Note:* 1 liter = 1,000 cc.)

$$0.67 \times 1,000 \text{ cc} = 670 \text{ cc will be } H_2O_2$$

How much of the liter will be H_2O?

If the total amount to be made is 1,000 cc and 670 cc is the H_2O_2, then

$$1,000 \text{ cc} - 670 \text{ cc} = 330 \text{ cc } H_2O$$

Note that in this case, the solute does make up the larger quantity. The value of the percentage reflects the concentration of the solute.

Many health professionals will confess to finding percent concentrations and solutions a very challenging concept. Stop and look around you at everyday solutions: air, soft drinks, plasma, isopropyl alcohol, orange juice.

REMEMBER!

A solution is a uniform mixture of two or more substances, meaning that the solute is dissolved in the solvent.

Substances such as orange juice, tomato juice, milk of magnesia, and other antacids have solid particles in them that are not dissolved. For this reason, the implications of preparing suspensions requires shaking the container to mix the contents to as uniform a consistency as possible before using.

Types of Percent Concentrations

Why are solutions expressed in so many ways? The concentration of a solution means the amount of solute (mass or volume) divided by the total amount of solution (mass or volume). Each concentration that you encounter requires interpreting the relationship of the units expressed in terms of a percent. When interpreting the meaning of each type of percent, stop and ask yourself if your answer makes sense. Do the numbers and percentages reflect the situation you are being asked to interpret?

EXAMPLE: Weight (wt) per weight percent solution:

$$\% \text{ W/W} = \frac{\text{wt of solute (g)}}{\text{wt of solution (g)}}$$

a. What is the percent weight for weight concentration of a solution containing 25.0 grams of glucose in 250.0 grams of solution?

$$\frac{25.0 \text{ g}}{250.0 \text{ g}} = 250.0\overline{)25.0} = 0.1 = 10.0\%$$

The solution is a 10.0% W/W solution.

b. How much solvent (water) is in the solution?

250.0 g – 25.0 g = 225.0 g water

EXAMPLE: Volume (vol) per volume percent solution:

$$\% \text{ V/V} = \frac{\text{vol of solute (ml)}}{\text{vol of solution (ml)}}$$

a. Prepare a 1:10 dilution of sodium hypochlorite. Make 1,000 ml of solution. What is the percentage of solution you have been asked to prepare?

$$1:10 = \frac{1}{10} = 0.1 = 10\%$$

The solution is a 10% V/V solution.

b. How much solute (sodium hypochlorite) will you need?

0.1 × 1,000 ml = 100 ml represents the part or solute (sodium hypochlorite)

c. How much diluent (water) will you need?

1,000 ml – 100 ml = 900 ml represents the diluent (water)

Sodium hypochlorite is the active ingredient found in household bleach, cleaners, and disinfectants. The concentration prepared in this example is the percentage that is recommended by the Centers for Disease Control and Prevention for cleaning areas contaminated with large amounts of blood including porous surfaces. Health care providers must act as if the blood of every person were infected and therefore infectious. This approach to patient care is referred to by the CDC as *universal precautions,* and is intended to prevent percutaneous and mucous membrane exposure of health care workers to bloodborne pathogens.

EXAMPLE: Weight per volume percent solution:

$$\% \text{ W/V} = \frac{\text{wt of solute (g)}}{\text{vol of solution (ml)}}$$

a. What is the percent weight for volume concentration of a solution made by dissolving 16.2 grams of potassium chloride (KCl) in 842 ml of solution?

$$842\overline{)16.200000} = 0.01923 = 1.92\%$$

b. What is the percent weight for volume concentration of a solution of dextrose that is 50 grams per 100 ml?

$$100\overline{)50.00} = 0.50 = 50\%$$

EXAMPLE: Suppose we have a 35% W/V solution. Rewrite the percent notation of this solution so that it is in fractional form.

Recall that the % sign meant divide by 100. In every W/V solution there is a specific weight of a substance (solute) dissolved in a certain amount of solution. We can first divide the 35 by 100, but rather than placing it in decimal form, let us leave it in fractional form:

$$35\% = \frac{35}{100}$$

Using the idea that 1 g = 1 ml, we can say that this particular weight per volume solution can be identified as:

$$\frac{35}{100} \rightarrow \frac{35 \text{ g}}{100 \text{ ml}}$$

Therefore, a 35% W/V solution means that there are 35 g of solute dissolved in every 100 ml of solution.

EXAMPLE: $\text{mg }\% = \dfrac{\text{mg of solute}}{\text{deciliters of solution}}$

$$= \text{mg}/\text{dl}$$

$$= \text{mg}/100 \text{ ml}$$

$$= \text{mg }\%$$

Many laboratory results are reported in mg/dl. (See bottom of Adult Tube Feeding Order Form.) A deciliter is equivalent to 100 ml. Some laboratory chemistry results are reported in mg/100 ml. Blood cholesterol, triglycerides, creatinine, calcium, and bilirubin are reported in mg/dl or percent (%), that is, cholesterol blood level of 225 mg/dl or 0.225 mg%.

Intravenous Therapy Solutions

Intravenous therapy solutions used in acute patient care areas to maintain or replace body fluids and electrolytes are percent solutions. Their concentrations are referred to either as a fraction, a decimal, or by percent. These solutions may have a variety of components including but not limited to sodium chloride (NaCl) and dextrose. The purpose of utilizing various concentrations of solutions is to produce a specific effect on the fluid compartments of the body. At times, it is desirable to give a concentration of solution into the vessels that is higher than that in the body cells and tissues, to cause body fluids to shift out of the body

ALBANY MEDICAL CENTER HOSPITAL

ADULT TUBE FEEDING
ORDERING FORM
ORDERS MUST BE RECEIVED IN FOOD
AND NUTRITION SERVICES BY 1200
Attention Nursing: For new Orders after 1200, refer to the
Materials Management Quick Reference Guide

MR 2346542

Fame, John
DoB 02/25/1970   Sex M
ATT Brown, Michael 350

Patient Identification Plate

A.   TYPE OF TUBE FOR INSERTION:
☒ Small-bore weighted feeding tube OR_____

B.   SELECT TYPE OF PRODUCT NEEDED: *See Reverse for indications
☒ **STANDARD FORMULA (1.0 Kcal/ml)**   Osmolite
☐ Low Protein   ☐ Fluid Restricted (2.0 Kcal/ml)
☐ High Protein   ☐ Partially Hydrolyzed
☐ Fiber Enriched   ☐ Other _____

C.   ADMINISTRATION AND RATE OF INFUSION:

** A New Order Form must be completed daily until final volume is reached.
** Please Check Mode of Tube Feeding Desired AND Select One Rate/ Volume Per Day

☒ **CONTINUOUS FEEDING**

☒ **DAY ONE:** Start feeding at 25 ml/hr full strength. Increase 20 ml/hr q 8 hrs (1080 ml/day 1)
OR until reach _65_ ml/hr.   **Order discontinued after 24 hours**

☐ **OTHER** _____
☒ **DAY TWO:** Advance feeding by 20 ml/hr q 8 hrs (2520ml/day 2)
OR until reach _125_ ml/hr.   **Order discontinued after 24 hours**
☐ **FINAL RATE/VOLUME:** Continue feeding at _____ml/hr., over _____hrs., and _____ml/day.
☐ Flush tube with 30 ml sterile water q 4 hours OR _____q shift.

☐ **BOLUS FEEDING:** NG/G tube Only. Bolus rate not to exceed 100 ml over 5 minutes.
☐ **FIRST DAY:** Start feeding 120 ml/feeding at full strength q 3 hours between 0600 to
2200 OR _____. Advance by 120 ml/feeding to maximum of
360 ml/feeding OR _____.Order discontinued after 24 hours.
☐ **OTHER RATE/VOLUME:** _____
☐ **FINAL RATE/VOLUME:** _____ml/feeding, _____ml/day, and _____ feedings/day.
☐ Flush tube with 50 ml sterile water or _____before and after each feeding.

D.   ☐ DISCONTINUE TUBE FEEDING.

E.   MONITORING AND PLACEMENT STANDARD ORDERS:

** Check Box Only if Non Standard Options Desired

Chest X-ray after insertion to verify placement of small bore weighted feeding tube (MD must complete
requisition).
Dietitian consult.
Check residuals per Nursing protocol. Notify MD for persistent residuals > 200 ml, cramping, distention,
nausea, vomiting, diarrhea, OR ☐ Other_____
Record weight on Monday, Wednesday, and Friday.
Monitor Input/ Output for 7 days.
Daily Profile I and PO4 X 3 days. Fingerstick glucose q shift X 2 days, continue if glucose > 240 mg/dl.

☐ Baseline CBC with differential, Profile II, and Mg + + (if not documented within past 72 hours).
☐ Other Labs _____

Michael Brown	11/18	12²⁰
PHYSICIAN SIGNATURE	**DATE**	**TIME**

95688 11/94 T

Adult Tube Feeding Ordering Form

TABLE 5-1 Weight Per Volume Solutions

Solution	Solute/Solvent	% Solution
sodium chloride 0.9% or 0.9% NaCl or normal saline (NS)	0.9 g NaCl per 100 ml H_2O	0.9% NaCl
sodium chloride 0.45% or 1/2 strength NS	0.45 g NaCl per 100 ml H_2O	0.45% NaCl
sodium chloride 0.2% or 1/4 strength NS	0.2 g NaCl per 100 ml H_2O	0.2% NaCl
dextrose and NS	5 g dextrose and 0.9 g NaCl per 100 ml H_2O	5% dextrose and 0.9% NaCl
dextrose and 1/2 strength NS	5 g dextrose and 0.45 g NaCl per 100 ml H_2O	5% dextrose and 0.45 g NaCl
dextrose and 1/4 strength NS	5 g dextrose and 0.2 g NaCl per 100 ml H_2O	5% dextrose and 0.2% NaCl

tissues and into the vessels of circulation. Thus, the concentration has a medical and/or physiologic purpose with a desired outcome for the patient.

Some solutions whose purpose is to replace body fluids do not cause changes or shifts in body fluids. Because these solutions do not cause shifts in fluid they are referred to as normal to the body. This means the concentration of the solution is isotonic or has the same concentration as body fluids. An isotonic saline (NaCl) solution has a concentration of 0.9% NaCl. This solution is called normal saline.

Considering your knowledge of percent solutions, study Table 5-1. Note the expressions for the different concentrations of solutions, as well as the examples of combination solutions. These percent solutions are weight per volume solutions. Note their expression in terms of amount of solute per amount of solvent.

LEARNING ACTIVITIES

1. What is the percent concentration of normal saline?

2. What is the amount of solute (in grams) and solvent (in milliliters) in 1,000 ml of normal saline?

3. You wish to make 1,000 ml of ½ strength normal saline (0.45% salt).

   a. How much salt will you need?

   b. How much water will you need?

4. You need 500 ml of a 20% bleach (sodium hypochlorite) solution.

   a. How much bleach will you need?

   b. How much water will you need as a solvent?

5. Suppose you have a 60% weight per volume solution. Rewrite the percentage in fractional form labeling the units involved.

CHAPTER REVIEW EXERCISES

1. Convert the following to percentages:
   a. 0.272
   b. 0.009
   c. 0.7
   d. 0.0001
   e. 1.32
   f. 2½

2. Convert the following to decimals:
   a. 13.2%
   b. 0.045%
   c. 10%
   d. 168%

   e. 100%
   f. 0.7%

3. Convert the following ratios to percentages:
   a. 1:4
   b. 1:8
   c. 1:500
   d. 1:10,000

4. Find 10% of 1,000.

5. Find 0.9% of 250.

6. Find 25% of 132.8.

7. Find 20% of 50%.

CRITICAL THINKING

1. Water volume increases 9% when it freezes. If you begin with 500 cm^3 of water that is then frozen, how much will the volume of ice increase? What will be the total volume of the ice?

2. A patient is placed on a strict diet and is told to lose 45 pounds. The patient loses 36 pounds over a period of 3 months. What percent of the weight-loss goal has the patient met?

3. Prepare 1,000 ml of a 40% cresol solution. Cresol is a pure or 100% drug. How much cresol will you need to prepare the solution? How much solvent will you need?

4. How many ounces of glycerin are there in 30 ounces of a 60% solution of glycerin?

5. If you were preparing 250 ml of a 0.9% solution of salt for a gargle, how much salt is needed?

6. Mary Smith has been receiving intravenous fluids for 5 days. A nasogastric tube was inserted and 250 ml

of 50% Ensure solution was ordered q4h × 6 (every 4 hours for 6 times). Calculate how much Ensure and water is needed to make 250 ml of a 50% solution. How much Ensure do you need? How much water do you need?

7. A sample of 5% dextrose (glucose) and water solution has a mass of 152.4 g. How much dextrose is present? How much solvent (water) is present?

8. A 2:250 saline solution is used as a gargle for a sore throat. Is this isotonic? Why or why not?

9. How much 3.0% W/V solution can be made from 38.6 g of NaOH?

10. Prepare 4,000 ml of 2% Betadine solution. The amount of solute to be used is unknown. The amount of finished solution desired is 4,000 ml. How much Betadine is needed to make the solution? How much water is needed?

Introduction to Dimensional Analysis

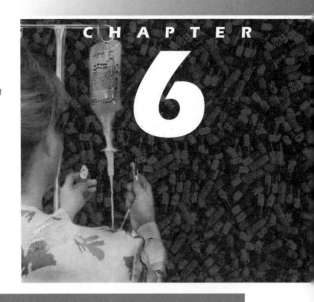

CHAPTER 6

OBJECTIVES

Upon completion of this chapter, you will be able to:

- Write conversion factors as fractions.
- Explain dimensional analysis.
- Solve conversion equations with one or more conversion factors.
- Recognize the significance of units assigned to numbers.
- Evaluate the results of your computations for value and label appropriateness.

Introduction

Now that you are finished with introductory material regarding arithmetic, are you ready to begin more applied problems? Before we can continue, we need to introduce the method to be used for the rest of the book.

Almost all of the problems you will encounter in the nursing/health science area are a matter of conversion from one unit to another. Whether you are converting from an amount of drug to the number of tablets to give, a patient's weight to his or her medication dosage, or the volume of intravenous fluid to the drops per minute of an infusion, and so forth, the calculation can be completed more easily with a multiplication of conversion factors. This process, called dimensional analysis, is the focus of this chapter. The name itself is a bit overwhelming; fortunately, the method is not.

> **KEY POINT**
>
> A conversion factor includes a value (a number) and a label (the units).

> **KEY POINT**
>
> Dimensional analysis is the multiplication of a series of fractions in which the numerator and denominator contain related conversion factors.

Conversion Factors

Suppose we consider the relationship that there are 12 inches in a foot (12 inches = 1 foot). That relationship provides a connection between the two measures: inches and feet. This represents a conversion factor. Conversion factors can be represented in fractional form. We may say that there are 12 inches per foot. The *per* implies division and we can write that statement in the following way:

$$\frac{12 \text{ inches}}{1 \text{ foot}}$$

You will notice that not only did we write the value in both the top and the bottom of the fraction, but we also wrote the units associated with those values—a critical part of dimensional analysis. It is important to recognize that we can also represent this same relationship in another way: 1 foot per 12 inches. In this case, we could represent the fraction as:

$$\frac{1 \text{ foot}}{12 \text{ inches}}$$

This represents two different forms of the same conversion factor. We notice that the fractions according to the values in the numerator and denominator have a different value (1/12 is not the same as 12/1). However, both fractions represent the same conversion factor. We can tell the difference between the two easily by referring to the units listed in the top and the bottom.

PRACTICE EXERCISE 6.A

Write the following conversion factors in two fractional forms:

1. 3 feet = 1 yard

2. 16 ounces = 1 pound

3. 5,280 feet = 1 mile

4. 60 minutes = 1 hour

The Method of Dimensional Analysis

Now that we have considered conversion factors, we can begin to piece them together in a systematic way to make our conversion. In this chapter, we will begin with examples that some of us could complete in our head without dimensional analysis, as they are common and are within our daily experience. We use them to illustrate the method with which we are working to introduce us to dimensional analysis.

Let us convert 12 yards to feet. We know there is a connection between the two units: 1 yd = 3 ft. We will use that conversion factor to complete the process.

$$\frac{12 \text{ yards}}{1} \times \frac{3 \text{ feet}}{1 \text{ yard}} = 36 \text{ feet}$$

So, 12 yards converts to 36 feet. We notice that we began with the given quantity and then we used the conversion factor that we had previously mentioned. The question is how do we know to represent the 1 yd = 3 ft as:

$$\frac{3 \text{ feet}}{1 \text{ yard}} \text{ or } \frac{1 \text{ yard}}{3 \text{ feet}}$$

Let us consider the equation that led to our answer. We notice that the units we began with (the *numerator* of the first fraction) were in yards. Therefore, if we place yards in the *denominator* of the next fraction, those two units have canceled and we are left with the unit of feet, which is our goal. Therefore, our selection of what goes on top and bottom of the fraction is based on what units we wish to eliminate (cancel).

It is important to notice that we made our first quantity (12 yd) into a fraction simply by placing it over 1. We also should not leave this first example thinking that each conversion we will attempt will be this short. In this particular problem, there was exactly one conversion factor making the connection between the units given and the units we desired in our answer. This made the problem easier. The method continues in the same manner for multiple conversion factors and is not difficult—just longer.

Strategy for Dimensional Analysis

Let us consider a strategy for dimensional analysis:

KEY POINT:

1. Identify.

   After considering the given conversion or reading the given problem several times, we need to identify two quantities: *units given* and *units of answer*.

2. Make a plan.

   How do I get there? That is, how do I get from the units given to the units of the answer? Is there a single conversion factor that will take me from one directly to the other? Are there multiple conversion factors I must consider? In making my plan, I want to make the shortest route possible. Many times there are several ways to get to the answer, but one is either the shortest or the most efficient. If we live on the East Coast, it is not necessary or efficient to go to Paris in order to get to Chicago!

3. Start with the units given.

4. Arrange the conversion factor(s).

   Systematically arrange your conversion factors so that the units of your answer are the only units remaining after canceling.

   $$\frac{\text{units given}}{1} \times \frac{\text{other unit}}{\text{units given}} \times \frac{\text{units of answer}}{\text{other unit}} = \text{units of answer}$$

5. Perform arithmetic.

6. Verify the answer.

   Does the answer make sense relative to what you may have estimated in the beginning? Does the answer make sense from a practical standpoint? This often depends on the specific type of application you are considering.

Single Conversion Factors

EXAMPLE: Convert 3 pounds to ounces.

Units given: pounds

Units of answer: ounces

Is there a single, or multiple conversion factors that will take us from pounds to ounces? There is a single common conversion factor:

16 ounces (oz) = 1 pound (lb)

This conversion factor, as always, might be written two ways:

(A)$\frac{16 \text{ oz}}{1 \text{ lb}}$ or (B)$\frac{1 \text{ lb}}{16 \text{ oz}}$

Beginning with the units given

$$\frac{3 \text{ lb}}{1} \times \frac{?}{?}$$

we see that we wish to have lb in the next denominator so that unit will cancel:

$$\frac{3 \text{ lb}}{1} \times \frac{}{\text{lb}}$$

Since we want lb on the bottom, we see that we will use conversion factor (A) from above with ounces on top:

$$\frac{3 \text{ lb}}{1} \times \frac{16 \text{ oz}}{1 \text{ lb}} =$$

Now we can cancel the lb and we are left with oz in the numerator, which is the units of our answer. We can proceed to do the arithmetic. We can recall that what we are essentially doing here in terms of arithmetic is multiplication of fractions. Thus, we can be on the lookout for canceling within the numbers as we multiply. In this problem that will not occur because there are all ones in the denominators:

$$\frac{3 \text{ lb}}{1} \times \frac{16 \text{ oz}}{1 \text{ lb}} = 48 \text{ oz}$$

As we check our answer, it makes sense that the answer should be larger and the value checks correctly.

Multiple Conversion Factors

EXAMPLE: Convert 3 days to minutes.

Units given: days

Units of answer: minutes

There is not a single step or conversion factor that is familiar that will take us from days to minutes. However, there is a conversion factor from days to hours and a second from hours to minutes. So, in this problem we will use two conversion factors:

$$1 \text{ day} = 24 \text{ hours}$$

$$1 \text{ hour} = 60 \text{ minutes}$$

Let us begin by setting up our equation with our units given:

$$\frac{3 \text{ days}}{1}$$

We see that we will need to set up our first conversion factor so that days will cancel in the denominator. Therefore:

$$\frac{3 \text{ days}}{1} \times \frac{24 \text{ hours}}{1 \text{ day}}$$

We are not finished because the units left in our expression are not the units of our answer. We also do not stop to calculate each step, as it is easier if we wait until the end equation. We need to use our second conversion factor with hours in the next denominator:

$$\frac{3 \text{ days}}{1} \times \frac{24 \text{ hours}}{1 \text{ day}} \times \frac{60 \text{ minutes}}{1 \text{ hour}} = 4,320 \text{ minutes}$$

This particular equation was easy, as there were all ones in the denominator of the fraction. That is not always the case. Because of all the ones, again there was no opportunity to cancel.

Again, as far as the value of our answer, we would expect it to be fairly large intuitively.

Let us consider an example that does not have all ones in the denominators of the fractions.

EXAMPLE: Convert 420 hours to weeks.

Units given: hours

Units of answer: weeks

Conversion factors: 24 hours = 1 day

7 days = 1 week

$$\frac{420 \text{ hours}}{1} \times \frac{1 \text{ day}}{24 \text{ hours}} \times \frac{1 \text{ week}}{7 \text{ days}} = \frac{420 \text{ weeks}}{168}$$

$$= 2\,\tfrac{1}{2} \text{ weeks (or 2.5 weeks)}$$

You will notice in the preceding version of this problem that we did not cancel and the result is that we had a fraction that did not look too friendly. Let us consider the equation again with some canceling.

$$\frac{\overset{5}{\cancel{\overset{\cancel{60}}{420}}} \text{ hours}}{1} \times \frac{1 \text{ day}}{\underset{2}{\cancel{24}} \text{ hours}} \times \frac{1 \text{ week}}{\cancel{7} \text{ days}} = \frac{5 \text{ weeks}}{2} = 2\,\tfrac{1}{2} \text{ weeks}$$

Applied Conversion Factors

The problems we will be considering in future chapters will be based on conversions between systems of measurement, as well as many applications to medication orders, and so forth. As an introduction to those areas, let us consider a problem that is applied. For now the conversion factors will be given; in future chapters we will use conversion factors from a card of factors (see tear-out conversion card).

EXAMPLE: The normal level of glucose in the bloodstream is 65 mg/dl (milligrams per deciliter). How much glucose is present in the bloodstream of a person whose blood capacity is 7 liters?

The 65 mg/dl is not a standard conversion factor, but it is one when considering levels of glucose as described in the problem. In order to complete this problem, we also need to know that there are 10 deciliters in every liter.

Units given: liters

Units of answer: milligrams

$$\frac{7\,L}{1} \times \frac{10\,dl}{1\,L} \times \frac{65\,mg}{1\,dl} = 4{,}550 \text{ mg of glucose}$$

Given our setup of the problem, we can see that the arithmetic in this case is merely one of multiplying; no canceling is needed or is possible. The difficulty with working with applied problems is analyzing the situation to know what is given and what we are looking for. This comes through a combination of several readings of the problem, as well as recognizing some key phrases such as *how much glucose*. Glucose is a solid and therefore must be measured by some unit of mass (or weight), so we are able to determine that what we want regarding glucose is mg. Also, we need to develop the ability to recognize that this question is simply a *conversion from liters of blood to milligrams of glucose* using the necessary conversion factors.

REMEMBER!

In using dimensional analysis to solve a problem:

1. Identify units given and units of answer.
2. Make a plan.
3. Start with units given.
4. Arrange conversion factor(s).
5. Perform arithmetic.
6. Verify answer.

Accuracy in Problem Solving

Developing an expertise with dimensional analysis comes very quickly once you have the concept. If you have previously learned other methods of calculating medication orders or other allied health applications, leaving the former method aside, it will soon be apparent that plugging in numbers with their units allows for very little error in the configuration of the equation. However, what will always be with you as a nurse or allied health professional is the need to check your work. Does your answer make sense? This needs to be an integral part of the problem-solving process. In the practice examples performed so far in this chapter, when converting feet to inches you knew the quantity you would end up with would be a greater number because the quantity of inches in 1 foot is a larger number. What happens with problems or calculations in which the relationship between units is not so easily determined? You need to stop and ask: *Does my answer make sense?*

The Three Checks

In nursing/health sciences there is very little room for error. The patient or client's well-being is at hand with the interventions we provide. When preparing to administer anything to a patient in the health care system, check the information three times. If you were bringing a patient his lunch tray, for example, refer to the Key Point box that follows.

> **KEY POINT**
>
> 1. Check the name, room number, and nutrition order on the requisition with the food as you pick up the tray, and prepare to walk to the patient's room.
>
> 2. Check the name and room number on the patient's door, over or on his bed, and his identification bracelet with the information on the requisition slip. Deliver the tray to the bedside table.
>
> 3. Check a third time the nutrition requisition slip against the patient's identification bracelet.

It is with the same degree of caution that all health care orders and calculations need to be checked.

Equivalent Units

One of the most common measurement relationships we use in health care is 1 ounce = 30 cc. If a patient is required to drink $1\frac{1}{2}$ liters of liquid as preparation for an ultrasound test, usually as the patient is prepared he is instructed in terms he can understand. Typically he would be instructed to drink approximately 6 glasses of fluid. Using the equivalent of 1 glass = 1 cup, the conversion from the order for $1\frac{1}{2}$ liters to glasses is arrived at by:

$$\frac{1\frac{1}{2} \text{ liters}}{1} \times \frac{1,000 \text{ cc}}{1 \text{ liter}} \times \frac{1 \text{ oz}}{30 \text{ cc}} \times \frac{1 \text{ cup}}{8 \text{ oz}} = 6\frac{1}{4} \text{ cups}$$

which is approximately 6 cups.

Note when solving this situation as an equation, relationships have been made between each one of the equivalents that will lead to the desired units of measure. There is more than one equivalent utilizing the same units of measure. The key is to choose the equivalents that will lead to the unit of measure that has been requested.

LEARNING ACTIVITIES

1. A patient drank 6 ounces of orange juice. Convert this amount to cc.

2. The nursing implication for administering a medication recommends diluting the medication in 10 ounces of distilled water. How many cups of distilled water will you measure?

CHAPTER REVIEW EXERCISES

Make the following conversions using the conversion factors listed below. Be sure to write out your dimensional analysis equation.

1 lb = 16 oz	1 min = 60 sec
	1 hr = 60 min
1 yd = 3 ft	1 day = 24 hr
	1 week = 7 days
1 ft = 12 in	1 yr = 52 wk

1. Convert 3 lb to ounces.
2. Convert 5 ft to inches.
3. Convert 2 days to hours.
4. Convert 240 sec to minutes.
5. Convert 130 wk to years.
6. Convert 2.5 hr to minutes.
7. Convert 5 yd to feet.
8. Convert 80 in to feet.
9. Convert 3½ min to seconds.

   (*Hint:* Change 3½ to either an improper fraction or a decimal.)
10. Convert 270 min to hours.
11. Convert 256 oz to pounds.
12. Convert 10 yd to inches.
13. Convert 75 ft to yards.
14. Convert 144 hr to days.
15. Convert 17 wk to days.
16. Convert 3 hr to seconds.
17. Convert 60 hr to minutes.
18. Convert 2 wk to minutes.
19. Convert 13,104 hr to years.
20. Convert 4 wk to seconds.

CRITICAL THINKING

For questions 1–9, interpret the following abbreviations using Appendix 1.

1. h
2. min
3. q
4. q.d.
5. q.h.
6. TPN
7. U
8. sol
9. q.o.d.
10. Mr. Jack has returned to his room following diagnostic tests throughout the morning. He is just in time for lunch. His physician has prescribed a full liquid lunch postexam.

    4 ℥ sherbet

    1 glass (8 ℥) of water

    ½ glass of orange juice

    ½ cup of soup

    a. What key points would you incorporate as you serve his lunch tray?

    b. Convert each liquid of Mr. Jack's intake for lunch to cc.

    c. Calculate Mr. Jack's total liquid intake for lunch.

    d. Enter the total in the appropriate space on the "Intake and Output Record."

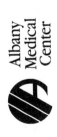

Albany
Medical
Center

INTAKE AND OUTPUT

Date: _____

PATIENT IDENTIFICATION PLATE

LEFT IN BAG

0700 #	SOLUTION/RATE	AMT.	1500 #	SOLUTION/RATE	AMT.	2300 #	SOLUTION/RATE	AMT.

INTAKE

TIME	FEEDINGS	SOL. #	INF.	SOL. #	INF.	SOL. #	INF.	SOL. #	INF.	COMMENTS
TOTAL										

OUTPUT

						INTIALS

SIGNATURE _____   INITIALS/STATUS _____

9535 1 0/90

93

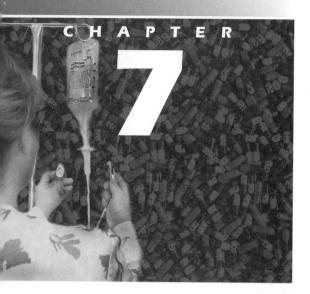

7

Household Measurement System

Upon completion of this chapter, you will be able to:

- Apply the principles of dimensional analysis to the household measurement system.

- Solve conversion equations within the household measurement system.

- Recognize the appropriateness of answers to equations within a familiar measurement system.

- Evaluate the results of your computations for quantity and label appropriateness.

Introduction

One of the best ways to practice the new computation skills is to utilize this skill on a measurement system that is familiar to you. Quarts (qt), cups (C), ounces (oz or ℥), tablespoons (tbs or T), teaspoons (tsp or t), inches (in), and feet (ft) are units that we encounter in everyday life. When solving equations that require converting from one unit of measure to another within a system such as the household system, it is easy to verify your answer because you already have a concept of what your answer should look like.

In this chapter, we will present all the units of measure for the household system that could have application to nursing/health sciences. To make this topic as realistic as possible, most of the relationships we have chosen to discuss are usually encountered in day-to-day activities. Approximate equivalents may differ from one reference to another. The quantities we are utilizing to define conversion factors we have found to be most consistent across disciplines.

Household System of Measure

Do you already have a concept of the size of the various measures in the household system? Whether you are measuring an ounce of medication for a patient or adding milk to your favorite recipe at home, the units of the household system represent the same quantity (see Table 7-1).

The only exception to this is the glass measurement. Often, this particular unit of measure is not included in a table of measurements because the quantity it represents is defined by the institution in which you are working. It can mean

TABLE 7-1 Household System of Measure

60 drops (gtt)	=	1 teaspoon (tsp or t)
3 teaspoons	=	1 tablespoon (tbs or T)
2 tablespoons	=	1 ounce (oz or ℥)
8 ounces	=	1 cup (C)
2 cups	=	1 pint (pt)
2 pints	=	1 quart (qt)
4 quarts	=	1 gallon (gal)
12 inches (in or ″)	=	1 foot (ft or ′)
36 inches	=	1 yard (yd)

6 or 8 ounces. When we ask for a glass of milk at home, we are also asking for an amount that is nonspecific. You do not know if you will be given a 4 ounce or 16 ounce glass of milk (see Figure 7-1).

The drop is not a very exact quantity. Depending on the size of the dropper, the size of a drop can be very different. The Latin word for drop is *gutta*. The abbreviation for the drop comes from this root, gtt. Today most droppers are calibrated so that the quantity can be accurately measured (Figure 7-2). More frequently, the dropper is used to measure fractions of a milliliter rather than numbers of drops. Droppers when packaged with medication are designed for that specific medication.

What does a teaspoon look like? A measured teaspoon looks similar to the teaspoon that is part of the place setting at breakfast or lunch; however, it is not a specifically measured quantity. But it is the same as the vanilla you measured for your favorite dessert recipe. The relationship of drops to teaspoons will be discussed in Chapter 8.

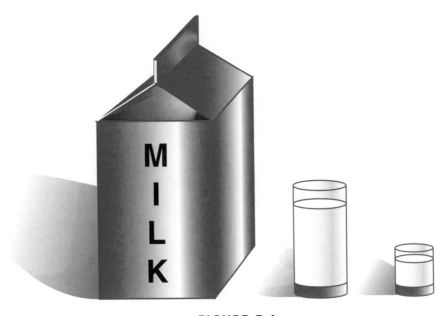

FIGURE 7-1
What does a glass of milk really mean?

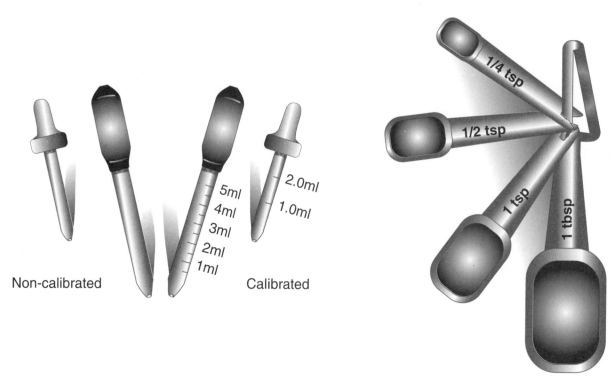

FIGURE 7-2

Household Measuring Devices

How about a tablespoon? What does this quantity look like? What is the difference between a teaspoon and a tablespoon? It takes 3 teaspoons to make 1 tablespoon: 3 t = 1 T (Figure 7-3).

How many tablespoons are in 1 ounce? Utilizing a 1 ounce medicine cup, look at the relationship between these units. One tablespoon fills half of the cup. Two tablespoons is equivalent to 1 ounce: 2T = 1 ʒ . Looking at Figure 7-4, how many teaspoons are in 1 ounce? If 3 t = 1 T, and 2 T = 1 ʒ , then in 1 ʒ there are

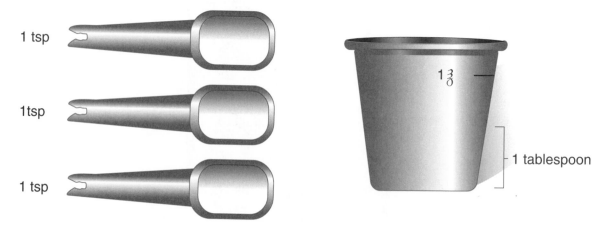

FIGURE 7-3

3 tsp = 1 T

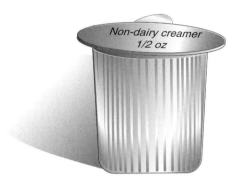

FIGURE 7-4

¹/₂ oz Nondairy Creamers

6 t. Does this make sense? If you need more assistance to make the relationships solid, turn to the "Learning Activities" in this chapter.

What is the quantity of a commercial nondairy creamer used to lighten coffee? The next time you are out for coffee, read the lid. Most are 1 ʒ . You will find some that are only a ¹/₂ ounce.

How much milk was in the single-serving carton you purchased in the cafeteria for lunch? The size of this container is 8 ounces, 1 cup, or ¹/₂ pint. Look at some of the other examples in Figure 7-5. A can of soda holds 12 ounces. Twelve ounces is more than 1 cup, but less than 2 cups. The thin-necked soda bottle has a capacity of 1 quart or 2 pints. A family-size cardboard carton of milk holds ¹/₂ gallon or 2 quarts. The large plastic milk container measures 1 gallon or 4 quarts.

Whether we are building concepts of quantities or solving conversion equations, making relationships with known quantities assists us to better grasp the ideas. We will be more likely to recognize inconsistencies when working through the evaluation step and asking if the answer makes sense.

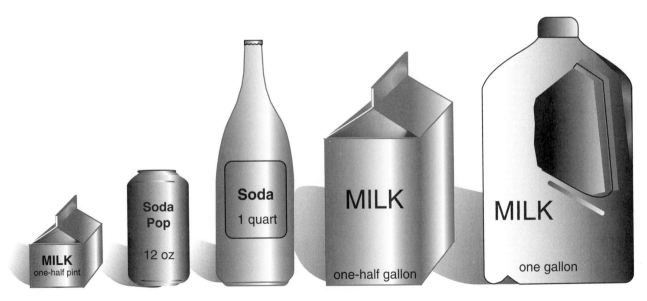

FIGURE 7-5

Are you able to name the household quantity that each of these common containers holds?

PRACTICE EXERCISE 7.A

Solve the following exercises using dimensional analysis equations and conversion factors given in Table 7-1. After you complete the exercises compare your work with the explanations provided below.

1. 2 C = ___ oz   **2.** 2 C = ___ T   **3.** 2½ gal = ___ oz   **4.** 216 t = ___ C

EXAMPLE: Convert 2 cups to ounces.

Units given: cups

Units of answer: ounces

Using our conversion card, we can determine that there is a direct connection between the two units we are working with—namely 1 cup = 8 ounces. This will help us to easily set up the equation.

Starting with the units given:

$$\frac{2 \text{ cups}}{1} \times \frac{8 \text{ ounces}}{1 \text{ cup}} = 16 \text{ ounces.}$$

Recall from the last chapter the reason why we set up equations this way—the conversion factor has ounces in the numerator and cups in the denominator so that cups will cancel. This process allows us to have our remaining answer in ounces—our goal in this problem.

Before leaving this problem we should check to see that our answer makes sense. From our practical knowledge of the household system, 16 ounces certainly seems reasonable for two cups.

EXAMPLE: Convert 2 cups to tablespoons.

Units given: cups

Units of answer: tablespoons

Referring to Figure 7-2, we observe there is not a direct conversion between cups and tablespoons. However, there is a conversion between cups and ounces, and a second conversion factor between tablespoons and ounces. Therefore, we need these two conversion factors to reach the units of the answer:

1 cup = 8 ounces

1 ounce = 2 tablespoons

Setting up our problem we start with the units given:

$$\frac{2 \text{ cups}}{1} \times \frac{8 \text{ ounces}}{1 \text{ cup}} \times ?$$

We have positioned the first conversion factor so that cups will cancel. However, this problem requires two conversion factors. With one conversion factor, the current unit of our answer would be ounces—not the units of our answer. To complete the problem, we place the unit ounces in the denominator of the third fraction.

$$\frac{2 \text{ cups}}{1} \times \frac{8 \text{ ounces}}{1 \text{ cup}} \times \frac{2 \text{ tablespoons}}{1 \text{ ounce}} = 32 \text{ T}$$

We notice that all the conversion factors in the bottom of each fraction have a value of one. This means that there is no opportunity to cancel any values—only units. This will not always be the case as we will see in future examples.

Also, it will become less time consuming as we start to use the standard abbreviations for units.

$$\frac{2 \text{ C}}{1} \times \frac{8 ℥}{1 \text{ C}} \times \frac{2 \text{ T}}{1 ℥} = 32 \text{ T}$$

EXAMPLE: Convert 2½ gallons to ounces.

Units given: gallons

Units of answer: ounces

Using Figure 7-2, choose the following conversion factors:

1 gallon = 4 quarts

1 quart = 2 pints

1 pint = 2 cups

1 cup = 8 ounces

As we start to set up this problem, we recognize that we have to convert the 2½ to either an improper fraction or a decimal. The use of a decimal here is probably easiest since it is one-half and we can easily convert—2½ = 2.5. We do need to be careful however as answers within the household system do not generally have decimal answers. Therefore, if our answer has a decimal we will have to convert back to a fractional format. Setting up our equation:

$$\frac{2.5 \text{ gal}}{1} \times \frac{4 \text{ qts}}{1 \text{ gal}} \times \frac{2 \text{ pts}}{1 \text{ qt}} \times \frac{2 \text{ C}}{1 \text{ pt}} \times \frac{8 ℥}{1 \text{ C}} = 320 ℥.$$

EXAMPLE: Convert 216 teaspoons to cups.

Units given: teaspoons

Units of answer: cups

We will use several conversion factors once again as we consult Figure 7-2.

3 t = 1 T

2 T = 1 ℥

8 ℥ = 1 C

Setting up our equation:

$$\frac{216 \text{ t}}{1} \times \frac{1 \text{ T}}{3 \text{ t}} \times \frac{1 ℥}{2 \text{ T}} \times \frac{1 \text{ C}}{8 ℥} =$$

We can cancel several of our factors:

$$\frac{\overset{9}{\cancel{\overset{72}{\cancel{216}}}} \text{ t}}{1} \times \frac{1 \text{ T}}{\cancel{3} \text{ t}} \times \frac{1 ℥}{2 \text{ T}} \times \frac{1 \text{ C}}{\underset{1}{\cancel{8}} ℥} = \frac{9}{2} = 4\tfrac{1}{2} \text{ C}$$

In this equation the denominators were not all 1s, which allowed us to cancel some common factors. Ultimately, this made the calculations easier to complete. If we had not realized the possibility of canceling in this problem our end result would have been the same, but instead of dividing 216 by 48 we have simplified the division to 9/2.

LEARNING ACTIVITIES

The more "real" your learning is, the easier it will be to remember concepts. Some suggested learning activities to assist with studying the household system follow:

1. Open the drawer or cupboard in your kitchen at home that has all the measuring devices. Find the following:

   • measuring spoons

   • measuring devices for medications (hollow spoons/pediatric)

   • 1 ounce medication measuring cup

   • measuring cups

   • quart and half-gallon containers

2. Using water, take time to conceptualize the quantity of one unit of measure it would take to fill another larger-size quantity/container.

   a. For example, fill a 1 teaspoon measure three times and empty it into a 1 ounce measuring cup. How full is the cup? Now pour this amount into a cup measure. How full is the cup measure?

   b. Pour the 3 teaspoons already measured back into the 1 ounce measuring cup. Fill a 1 tablespoon measure with water. Add the tablespoon to the 1 ounce measure. How full is the cup?

   c. How many 1 ounce measuring cups would it take to fill the quart measure? If unsure, give it a try. Keep filling the 1 ounce measure and pouring it into the quart measure until full.

3. Referring to Figure 7-5, after having gained a better concept of quantities, which of the kitchen containers is most similar to the intravenous solution pictured previously? (See Figure 2-4 as needed.)

4. You purchase a package of Kool-Aid. The instructions say to add 1 cup of sugar to the contents of the package and fill with water to a level of 2 quarts (actually this constitutes a w/v solution). Shake vigorously.

   a. You have misplaced your measuring cup and can only find a ½ teaspoon measure. How many ½ teaspoons of sugar will you need of sugar?

   b. You have purchased paper cups that hold 5 ounces. How many of the cups will you be able to completely fill?

   c. There is a knock on the door and there are 15 thirsty children wanting Kool-Aid. How much will each child receive if all are to receive an equal amount? How much will each child get if they all receive an equal amount after you save 8 ounces for yourself?

5. You need to give 7 mg of a drug. The drug comes in a concentration of 42 mg per ounce (42 mg/ʒ). How many teaspoons will you administer? Solve this example with an equation, then ask yourself if the answer makes sense. This example could be solved easily in your head. Check your written mathematic computation to see that your answer makes sense.

CHAPTER REVIEW EXERCISES

Convert the following quantities within the household system of measurement. Be careful to show your equation and label your answer. Make sure you check to see that the value of your answer makes sense.

1. 1½ T = _____ t
2. 12 ʒ = _____ C
3. 4 T = _____ ʒ
4. 3 qt = _____ pt
5. Convert 3 cups to:
   a. ounces
   b. tablespoons
   c. teaspoons
6. Convert 144 T to:
   a. t
   b. ʒ

   c. C
   d. qt
7. Convert 1½ gallons to:
   a. qt
   b. pt
   c. C
   d. t
8. Convert 1,200 t to:
   a. T
   b. C
   c. qt
   d. pt

CRITICAL THINKING

1. You need to give 5 mg of a drug. The drug is supplied in a concentration of 30 mg per ounce. How many teaspoons will you give? Does your answer make sense?

2. You have directions to administer 1 teaspoon of a medication. The bottle contains 8 ounces. How many teaspoons are in this bottle?

3. A prescribed medication has a concentration of 50 mg per ounce. If you need to administer 25 mg, how many tablespoons will you give?

4. A particular wound soak requires that you add 32 ounces of sterile water. You purchase 1 gallon of sterile water. How many soaks can you prepare?

5. A large container of a common stock solution contains 1 gallon of a liquid. You are to use 8 ounces of the liquid each day. How many days will it last?

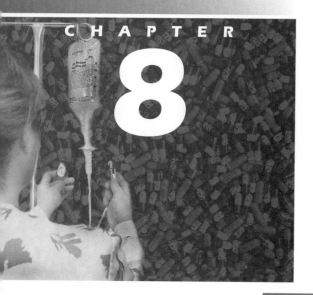

CHAPTER 8

Apothecaries' Measurement System

OBJECTIVES

Upon completion of this chapter, you will be able to:

- Write roman numerals.
- Interpret the roman numeral number system.
- Write apothecaries' symbols.
- Explain the relationship of apothecaries' units.
- Solve conversion equations within the apothecaries' measurement system.
- Solve conversion equations between the apothecaries' and household measurement system.
- Recognize the expression of quantities and units in the roman numeral and apothecaries' forms.
- Evaluate the results of your computations for value and label appropriateness.

Introduction

The apothecaries' system of measurement is an ancient system that was formalized in France during the sixteenth century. The word *apothecary* comes from the Greek word for pharmacist, and refers to one who mixes and dispenses medicine. Figure 8-1 is a mortar and pestle, the historical symbol for an apothecary.

Ancient medical professionals used this system of measurement. It was brought to the United States from England during the years of early colonization. Units for weight and volume exist only in this system. The apothecaries' system of measurement is based on the unit of weight known as the grain (gr) (Figure 8-2). The abbreviation is usually gr so that the unit is not confused with the metric unit of grams (g). Each grain is approximately 1/2 inch long and less than 1/8 inch in diameter—similar in size to one piece of rice. The grain literally refers to a grain of wheat. The millet grain was used as the weight to balance the scale for weighing quantities of wheat.

Units of Weight

There are some inherent problems with this system of measurement. A system based on grains of wheat, a nonuniform mass, allows for more approximations than exact values. In today's nursing/health science environment, systems of

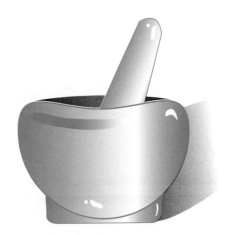

FIGURE 8-1
Mortar and Pestle

measurement are required to be extremely precise. We have become a highly sophisticated and scientific society. It is also necessary to measure amounts that are one million times smaller than the grain, which is impossible in the apothecaries' system. Therefore, this system is not desirable and is in the process of being phased out. The majority of mass measurements for medications, which are the major use of this system, are now given in metric units. The majority of apothecary unit applications are with older drugs that were historically measured using this system, or with oral liquid volumes of medication. Medications such as codeine, aspirin, and phenobarbital often have both an apothecary and metric equivalent on the label (Figure 8-3).

After the grain, the next unit of apothecary weight utilized for medication dosages is the dram (dr or ʒ). The dram is derived from the dracma, which is a

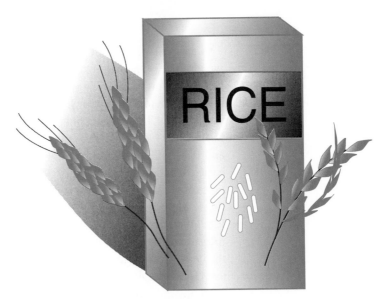

FIGURE 8-2
The Grain

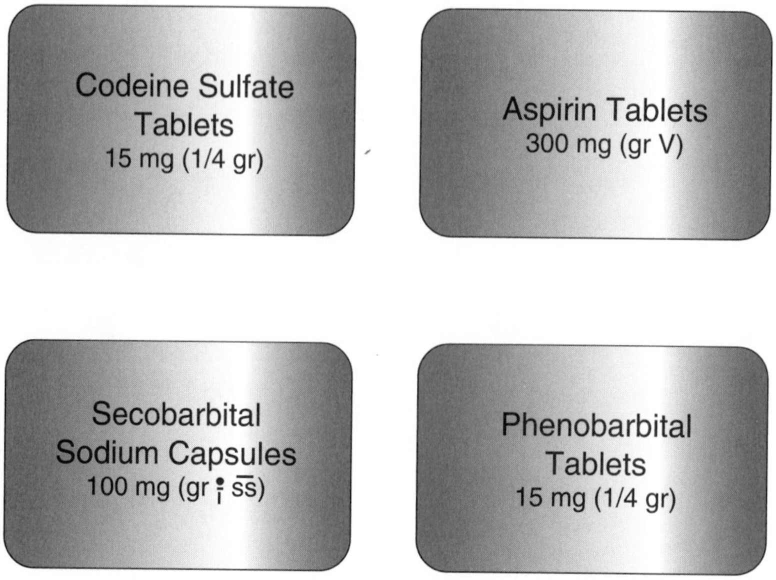

FIGURE 8-3

Medications Measured in Both the Apothecaries' and Metric Systems

silver coin that is supposed to weigh approximately the same as 1 dram. It takes 60 grains to make 1 dram. Figure 8-4 illustrates the relationship between the grain and the dram.

Next comes the ounce (oz or ℥). It is equivalent to the household ounce. However the symbol used to represent the apothecaries' ounce is an elongated "z". It takes 8 drams to make 1 ounce. (Refer to Figure 8-4.) Last is the pound. It takes 16 ounces to make 1 pound in the apothecaries' system, the same as the household measurement. This measure, whether in the household or apothecaries' system, is referred to as the Avoirdupois or English pound.

Units of Volume

The units of volume of the apothecaries' system are parallel to the units of weight. The basic unit of volume is the minim (℔ or m_x). *Minim* is derived from the Latin word meaning minimum. It is abbreviated as [m_x], or ℔. The minim is equivalent to the drop (gtt). In proportion, the minim and drop are the same size as the grain. The volume units of measure are parallel to the weight measures. Minims are frequently used to accurately measure volumes that are between 0.1 and 0.2 milliliters. Minim calibrations on the syringe are more prominent and easier to follow than one hundredths of a milliliter. Referring to Figure 8-5, it takes 60 minims or drops to make 1 fluid dram (fd or f℥). The fluid dram is similar to the weight unit of 1 dram. Likewise, 8 fluid drams make 1 fluid ounce. Fluid drams are more frequently used with medication orders than the dram as a measure of weight. An order for an oral liquid medication also may not express the quantity of drams as fluid drams but only as drams. In this case, the quantity and type of medication to be prepared is derived from the context of the order, for example, milk of magnesia ℥ ii.

Because of the similarity between the basic units of the apothecaries' system, the amount to memorize can be decreased. Referring to Table 8-1, if you are

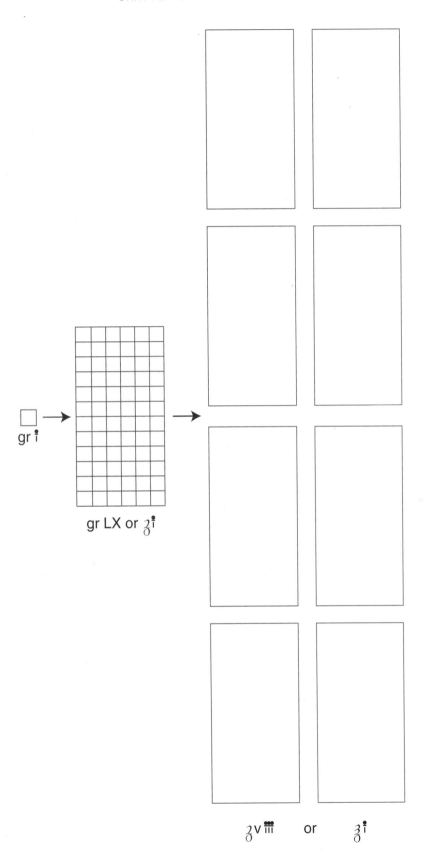

FIGURE 8-4
Relationship of the Grain, Dram, and Ounce

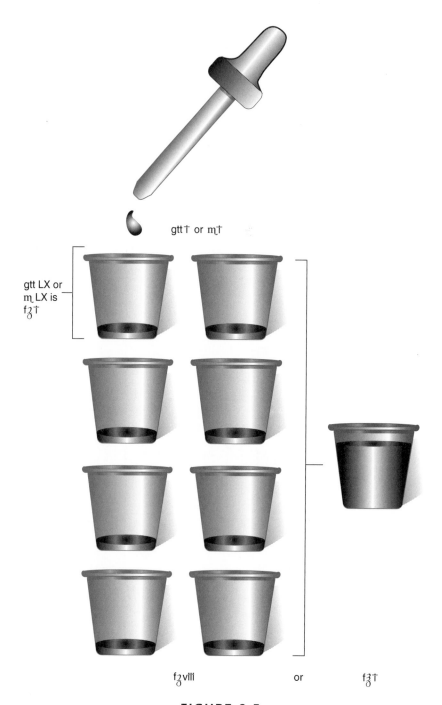

FIGURE 8-5

Relationship of the Drop/Minim, Dram, and Ounce

asked how many fluid drams are in 1 ounce, the answer is 8 fluid drams. The quantity of the answer is the same whether you are discussing weight or volume measures. If you are asked how many grains are in 1 dram, the answer is 60 grains. Again, the quantity of the answer, 60, is the same whether you are asked to answer grains, minims, or number of drops in 1 dram.

TABLE 8-1 The Apothecary System

Weight	Equivalent	Volume
1 grain (gr)		1 minim (♍ m$_x$) or 1 drop (gtt)
60 grains	1 dram (dr or ꒯)	60 minims
8 drams (dr or ꒯)	1 ounce (oz or ꒯)	8 fluid drams (fd or f꒯)

Apothecaries' Notation

Notation for the apothecaries' system varies from that of the other systems of measurement because of the age of the system. Apothecaries' units and quantities may be expressed with two different methods. If the apothecaries' units are expressed first, as historically they were, the quantity follows expressed as roman numerals. The second method is a result of updating the system. Since the apothecaries' system is in the process of being replaced, the notation has also lost importance and consistency. The expressions that are more likely to be used are Arabic numbers followed by the apothecaries' symbols.

The dram ꒯ and ounce ꒯ notation are quite unique and can also be confusing. One way to recall the difference in symbols is to recognize the number of humps or zigzags in the elongated z. The dram has two humps and the ounce has three. The dram is also a smaller quantity than the ounce.

KEY POINT

When the unit of measure is followed by the quantity, roman numerals are used to express the amount. When the unit of measure is preceded by the quantity, Arabic numbers are used.

60 gr = dr or ꒯ I

80 dr or ꒯ = oz or ꒯ X

32 oz or ꒯ = lb II

Roman Numerals

In modern times, we commonly think of roman numerals as a system of recording numbers used at the end of a movie or television show with the credits to indicate the year of production. However, roman numerals are sometimes found in medication prescriptions.

When thinking about any number system, it is important to remember that the number system in question is merely one way to represent a group of numbers. It is basically another name for those numbers, but the value or amount remains the same. The roman numeral system is a system that we refer to as additive. The values are added together to form the entire number—in a way similar to our own Hindu-Arabic system. The symbol and position of the numbers is the

TABLE 8-2 Values for Roman Numerals

Roman Numeral	Value
i or I	one
v or V	five
x or X	ten
L	fifty
C	hundred
D	five hundred
M	one thousand

key to working with roman numerals. The basic values in this system are given in Table 8-2.

Numbers larger than 100 are rarely used in the nursing/health sciences. Notice that some of the smaller numbers can be written either as capital or lowercase letters. Consistency is important. It is also significant to understand that what we are presenting here is not simply an exercise in roman numerals, but how to communicate the amount of a drug order. Understanding roman numerals in the context of their use is the key.

Rules for Roman Numerals

KEY POINT

Rule 1. A roman numeral that is repeated adds value as we read and move to the right.

EXAMPLE: iii is 1 + 1 + 1 or 3. It is worth noting that this could be represented as III and would have the same value. Often in nursing/health sciences, you will see a bar written over the group of roman numerals for emphasis and clarity. So, you might see:

iii as $\overline{\text{iii}}$

KEY POINT

Rule 2. A roman numeral of lesser value following one of greater value is added.

EXAMPLE: xviii. In this example there are lesser values following greater values. Therefore, we need to add the values associated with each value:

xviii = 10 + 5 + 1 + 1 + 1 = 18

> **KEY POINT**
>
> Rule 3. A roman numeral of greater value following one of lesser value is subtracted.

EXAMPLE: xxxix. The first three values are repeated. As we move from left to right, we add the values. The next numeral is a one followed by a ten, so we subtract the one from the ten:

$$xxxix = 10 + 10 + 10 + (10 - 1) =$$
$$10 + 10 + 10 + 9 = 39$$

For examples of roman numerals in the apothecaries' system, see Table 8-3.

> **KEY POINT**
>
> Rule 4. Never use more than three symbols in a row of the same numeral.

EXAMPLE: Forty is not represented as XXXX. A shorter representation is XL. Notice that ten preceding fifty indicates that there is a subtraction of ten from fifty or a value of forty.

> **KEY POINT**
>
> Rule 5. Generally, we use the largest and fewest numerals possible to represent a number. However, in preceding larger numbers with smaller numbers, only the increments closest in value to the larger numbers may be subtracted.
>
> • Ones may be subtracted from fives and tens only.
>
> • Tens may be subtracted from fifties and hundreds only.
>
> • Hundreds may be subtracted from five hundreds and one thousands only.

EXAMPLE: The number ninety-nine may not be represented by IC. Although admittedly shorter, we may not subtract a one from a hundred. What must represent ninety plus nine is XCIX.

TABLE 8-3 Apothecaries' System of Measure

gr 1	=	ℳ 1
gr LX	=	1 dr or ʒ
ʒ VIII or dr	=	1 ʒ or oz
f ʒ I	=	8 f ʒ
oz or ʒ XVI	=	1 lb

Nursing/Health Science Applications of Roman Numerals

Although the roman numeral system uses only whole numbers, in the nursing/health science arena, there are situations when fractional quantities are needed. Fractions are not usually used with roman numerals, with the exception of one half. One half is represented as:

$$\frac{1}{2} = \overline{ss}.$$

One half is the only fraction that has a special representation. It is derived from the word *semi*. Decimal numbers are not used with the apothecaries' system.

EXAMPLE: Convert $4\frac{1}{2}$ to roman numerals.

We first represent the four as iv and append the symbol for $\frac{1}{2}$. So,

$$4\frac{1}{2} = \text{ivss or more commonly as } \overline{\text{ivss}}.$$

Recall that the bar over the entire number is merely for clarity. Without the bar, a one (i) could easily be confused with the letter i. Most often we will see the number one represented as:

$$\overline{i}$$

EXAMPLE: Convert 5 drops to minims.

Since 1 drop (gtt) is the equivalent of 1 minim (ℳ), we can write:

$$\frac{5 \text{ gtt}}{1} \times \frac{1 \text{ ℳ}}{1 \text{ gtt}} = 5 \text{ ℳ}$$

EXAMPLE: Convert 3 f ʒ to f ʒ.

Units given: f ʒ

Units of answer: f ʒ

We see that there are 8 fluid drams to 1 fluid ounce, so we can make our conversion in one step:

$$\frac{3 \text{ f ʒ}}{1} \times \frac{8 \text{ f ʒ}}{1 \text{ f ʒ}} = 24 \text{ f ʒ}$$

We may represent the answer in Arabic numerals or we may represent it in roman numerals. If the choice is made (or perhaps implied from the question as it was asked in roman numerals) that we should answer in roman numerals, then the general convention is to write the unit label first with the roman numerals following. Consequently, we can represent this answer as follows:

$$24 \, f\text{℥} = f\text{℥} \, xxiv = f\text{℥} \, \overline{xxiv}$$

We can recognize the original problem and conversion as well as:

$$f\text{℥} \, \overline{\overline{iii}} = f\text{℥} \, \overline{xxiv}$$

EXAMPLE: Convert gr CCXL to ounces.

Units given: grains

Units of answer: ounces

We first look to establish our route in this problem. This often becomes a bit more difficult in the apothecaries' system because we are less comfortable with it than say the household or even metric system. Checking our conversion card, we recognize that there is a connection between grains and drams and then drams and ounces. Accordingly, we can with our two conversion factors make the transition from grains to ounces.

Before we begin our dimensional analysis equation, we need to convert our roman numeral back to an Arabic numeral for ease of calculation. Therefore, we convert CCXL to 240.

$$\frac{240 \text{ gr}}{1} \times \frac{1 \, \text{ʒ}}{60 \text{ gr}} \times \frac{1 \, \text{℥}}{8 \, \text{ʒ}} =$$

Canceling common factors, we have:

$$\frac{\overset{\overset{1}{\cancel{4}}}{\cancel{240} \text{ gr}}}{1} \times \frac{1 \, \text{ʒ}}{\cancel{60} \text{ gr}} \times \frac{1 \, \text{℥}}{\underset{2}{\cancel{8}} \, \text{ʒ}} = \tfrac{1}{2} \, \text{℥} \text{ or } \text{℥} \, \overline{ss}$$

PRACTICE EXERCISE 8.A

1. Convert the following Arabic numerals to roman numerals:

   a. 24   **b.** 27   **c.** 1½   **d.** 48   **e.** 180   **f.** 1996

2. Convert the following roman numerals to Arabic numerals:

   a. XXXIX   **b.** iii   **c.** LXXVIII   **d.** XCVIII   **e.** iiss   **f.** MCDXCII

The apothecaries' system can seem very unique because the units of this system are not encountered unless you are exposed to the application with medications. To assist with the learning process, recall the similarities between the mass and volume measurements. The units are parallel. The grain, minim, and drop are approximate equivalents. The following activities will assist you in learning the system. For these activities you will need a dropper, a small handful of rice, a medicine cup, and water.

1. Place 1 drop of water from the dropper in the medicine cup. Note the amount of space it takes up. How many minims are in the cup? _____

2. How many pieces of rice do you need to have a quantity parallel in measure to the 1 drop of water placed in the cup in question 1? _____

3. Place 60 drops of water in the medicine cup. Count out 60 pieces of rice and set them aside. How many fluid drams of water do you have?

   _____

   How many drams of rice do you have? _____

   What generalization can you make about these two quantities?

   _____

4. How many drams would it take to fill the medicine cup from question 3?

   _____

   Using another medicine cup, fill it to the dram line the number of times you need to fill the first medicine cup. Express the number of ounces you have in notation utilizing roman numerals. _____

5. If there are 8 ℥ in 1 ounce and 60 gr in 1 ℥, how many grains are in 1 ounce? Set up a dimensional analysis equation. _____

6. Express the answer to question 5 with roman numeral notation.

   _____

   You can easily see that the roman numeral expression in the nursing/health science area today could be very awkward.

7. When you go home today, look in your medication cupboard at the labels on medication bottles. Report the concentration or mass of drug per volume for three medications besides aspirin. Specifically look for the apothecary units on the aspirin bottle. You will not find apothecary units on newer medications such as Tylenol.

As we move into some applications of the apothecaries' system, we first need to discuss the use of these units in medication orders. When medication prescriptions are ordered by physicians, a mass or volume of a medication is ordered, for example, aspirin gr X q4h prn (aspirin grains ten every four hours as needed), milk of magnesia ℥ i po q4h prn (milk of magnesia ounces one by mouth every four hours as needed), or atropine sulfate gr 1/160 IM 1h pre-op (atropine sulfate grains 1/160 intramuscular one hour before surgery). Most frequently a relationship will need to be made between the mass of drug ordered and the volume of drug prepared for administration. Medications are solutions. The amount of drug or mass per volume is described in the information on the label. For example, morphine gr 1/6 per 1 ml, tells us that there are 1/6 grains of morphine, the mass of medication or solute, in each one milliliter of volume or the solvent in which it is contained.

If you were going to prepare to give the aspirin that was ordered, again checking the label of this medication, the label tells us there is aspirin gr V per each 1 tablet. In every tablet there are grains 5 of medication. This concept is important to understand so that you can problem solve what is being requested in each order.

KEY POINT

Consider the following as you solve examples:

1. What is the question asking?

2. What is the volume or concentration you have been supplied with?

3. What is the mass or weight of the drug ordered?

4. What is the form the drug has been provided in?

5. Will you be calculating the mass as well as the volume?

CHAPTER REVIEW EXERCISES

1. Convert the following to roman numerals:

   a. 2

   b. 24

   c. 18

   d. 29

   e. 45

   f. 1½

   g. 149

   h. 240

   i. 9½

   j. 499

2. Convert the following roman numerals to Arabic numerals:

   a. iv

   b. xix

   c. ss

   d. XLVIII

   e. iiss

   f. XCI

   g. CXI

   h. CCCXLIV

   i. CCXCIX

   j. MCMXCIV

In the following conversions be sure to show your conversion equation. It continues to be important to build your skill in setting up and solving these types of dimensional analysis equations.

3. Convert 12 ʒ to:

   a. ℥

   b. ♏

   c. gr

4. Convert gr CCXL to:

   a. ℥

   b. ʒ

5. Convert ℥ s̄s̄ to:

   a. ʒ

   b. gr

   c. ♏

6. Convert ʒ ⅲ to:

   a. gr

   b. ℥

   c. gtt

7. 180 gr = ʒ _____

8. ʒ xxiv = ℥ _____

9. ♏ xc = f ʒ _____

10. f ℥ x= f ʒ _____

CRITICAL THINKING

1. You make a calculation and find you need to prepare ℥ ss of a drug. How many minims is ℥ ss equal to? Draw up the amount calculated in a 3 cc syringe.

2. You are looking at a medication label for codeine tablets. Each tablet has gr 1/4 of codeine. An order reads to give codeine gr 1/2 po q3h prn. How many tablets will you give every three hours if needed?

3. You need to administer gtt X of an oral medication. For ease with preparation, draw this amount up in a sample syringe. What calibrations on the syringe below can you use to calculate the amount to draw up? Shade the picture below to show the amount to prepare.

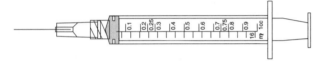

4. A patient has a standing order for aspirin gr X as needed. Referring to the figure below answer the following questions:

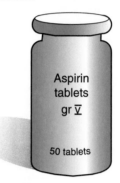

Aspirin tablets gr V̄

50 tablets

a. How many tablets should be administered?

b. How many doses are in this container?

Metric International (SI) System

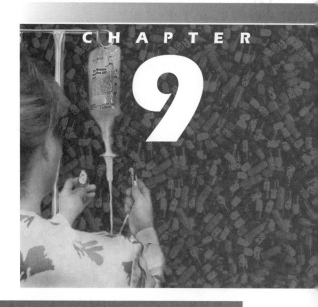

OBJECTIVES

Upon completion of this chapter, you will be able to:

- Recognize the value of prefixes and suffixes used in the metric system.
- Identify the relationship between metric linear units.
- Interpret the origin of metric volume units.
- Explain the relationship of metric mass units.
- Explain the relationship between metric units of weight and volume.
- Apply the meaning of metric quantities and units to learning activities.
- Evaluate your computations for value and label appropriateness.

Introduction

The metric system (also known as SI, from the French for Système International) is the system of weights and measures most often used by nursing/health science professionals. The metric system was invented in France during the late nineteenth century. It was not until 1960 that a standard system of abbreviations was adopted, referred to as the International System of Units. The metric system is the official system of measurement of many countries and is used exclusively in the scientific community. The predominance of this system occurs for many reasons. The base units on which the system is built in the nursing/health science arena are the meter (length), the gram (mass), and the liter (volume). Each amount measured in each area has the basic unit in its name: meter for length, gram for mass, and liter for volume. It is a decimal system, with each prefix representing multiples of 10. This makes the system easy to use.

The metric system can also accurately measure extreme quantities of medications or volumes of fluids. Whether we need to measure 1,000 ml of an intravenous solution or a microgram of a chemotherapy drug (an amount that is one millionth the size of a milliliter), the metric system is most able to deal with these amounts. Imagine if we wanted to accurately measure the same chemotherapy drug in either the household or apothecaries' system. Trying to measure in either system would be virtually impossible.

Table 9-1 lists prefixes, their relationship to the base units, and examples of metric measurements. The prefixes are used to change the meaning of the units

TABLE 9-1

Prefix	Meaning	Examples
kilo-	multiply by 1,000	1,000 g (gram) = 1 kg (kilogram)
hecto-	multiply by 100	100 m (meter) = 1 hm (hectometer)
deka-	multiply by 10	10 m (meter) = 1 dam (dekameter)
deci-	multiply by 1/10 (or 0.1) (divide by 10)	0.1 L (liter) = 1 dl (deciliter)
centi-	multiply by 1/100 (or 0.01) (divide by 100)	0.01 m (meter) = 1 cm (centimeter)
milli-	multiply by 1/1,000 (or 0.001) (divide by 1,000)	0.001 L (liter) = 1 ml (milliliter)
micro-	multiply by 1/1,000,000 (or 0.000001) (divide by 1,000,000)	0.000001 g (gram) = 1 mcg or μg (microgram)

in increments of 10. The prefixes alter the meaning of the base unit and make it smaller or larger. A decimeter (dm) is one tenth of a meter; therefore, there are 10 decimeters in a meter. A centimeter (cm) is one hundredth of a meter; therefore, there are 100 centimeters in 1 meter. Some examples have been provided to illustrate how the prefix changes the base unit.

PRACTICE EXERCISE 9.A

Using Table 9-1, answer the following:

1. Suppose we have 1 kilogram (kg). Is the kilogram larger or smaller than 1 gram (g)?
2. Is a milliliter (ml) larger or smaller than a liter (L)?
3. A centimeter (cm) is smaller than a meter (m). How many times smaller is it? How many centimeters in 1 meter?
4. A milligram (mg) is smaller than a gram (g). How many milligrams are there in 1 gram?
5. How many micrograms (μg) are there in 1 gram?

The abbreviations in the metric/SI system were made standard in 1960. That is, gram is always g, liter is always L, and meter is always m. They were standardized so that there would be less confusion with other units still in existence. For example, if we were to use gr for gram, there would be no way to distinguish it from the grain within the apothecaries' system. A word of caution, however, with respect to the microgram. In its printed form (on medication labels, etc.) it is common to see μg. We should be careful of writing this form by hand as it can easily be confused with mg for milligram. Therefore, microgram will most often be written as mcg. Table 9-2 lists the measurements in the metric system.

TABLE 9-2 Metric System of Measurements

Linear measure

1 meter (m)	=	10 decimeters (dm)
1 meter	=	100 centimeters (cm)
1 meter	=	1,000 millimeters (mm)
10 meters	=	1 dekameter (dam)
100 meters	=	1 hectometer (hm)
1,000 meters	=	1 kilometer (km)

Volume measure

1 liter (L)	=	10 deciliters (dl)
1 liter	=	100 centiliters (cl)
1 liter	=	1,000 milliliters (ml)
10 liters	=	1 dekaliter (dl)
100 liters	=	1 kiloliter (kl)

Mass measure

1 gram (g)	=	10 decigrams (dg)
1 gram	=	100 centigrams (cg)
1 gram	=	1,000 milligrams (mg)
10 grams	=	1 dekagram (dg)
100 grams	=	1 hectogram (hg)
1000 grams	=	1 kilogram (kg)
0.000001 gram	=	1 microgram (mcg or μg)

The Meter: Unit of Length

The fundamental unit of the metric system is the meter. It is the unit from which measures of weight and volume are derived. A meter is a linear measure that looks about the size of a yardstick. It is approximately 3 inches longer than 1 yard. Although basic calculations in nursing/health sciences do not often include the use of length, a patient's height is recorded in linear measure. The height may be recorded in feet and inches, meters, or centimeters. Most often the height is converted to meters or centimeters before the measure can be used in calculations.

Having a concept of the size of base units is important. Consider the basic conversion factor between the meter and inches: 1 meter (m) = 39.37 inches (in). If a patient is 2.0 meters tall, he or she is well over 6 feet tall. If a patient is 6 feet tall, he or she is a little less than 2 meters tall (actually 1.83 m). (Refer to Chapter 10 for more discussion of the relationship of metric measures of length to household measures.)

Look at a meter stick. The printed numbers on a typical meter stick are centimeters (see Figure 9-1). A millimeter (mm) is one thousandth of a meter; therefore, there are 1,000 millimeters on a meter stick. The smallest lines printed on the meter stick are millimeters. A sphygmomanometer or blood pressure cuff is a device that measures arterial pressure of the body vasculature. The units that accompany a blood pressure reading are millimeters of mercury or mm of Hg. The blood pressure reading is determined by how high or low the column of mercury becomes before distinguishing the arterial pulse.

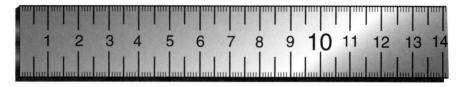

FIGURE 9-1
Fundamental Unit of the Metric System: The Meter

EXAMPLE: A patient is 175 cm tall. How tall is the patient in meters?

Units given: cm

Units of answer: m

Since there are 100 cm in 1 m, we can write:

$$\frac{175 \text{ cm}}{1} \times \frac{1 \text{ m}}{100 \text{ cm}} = 1.75 \text{ m}$$

Therefore, 175 cm converts to 1.75 m, or less than 2 meters.

EXAMPLE: A pair of crutches is designed to be used by people who are no taller than 6½ feet. Can the person in the previous example use these crutches?

Since a meter is a bit more than 3 ft, a person 2 meters tall would be more than 6 ft tall. The above patient is less than 2 meters tall, so the crutches could be used.

The Liter: Unit of Volume

The base unit for volume is the liter. When trying to visualize the liter (L), think of the size as similar to a quart. A quart is the size of a cardboard carton of milk. (Careful, not a half-gallon!) Remember the old-fashioned quart glass soda bottle? A quart is also the quantity made when a 12 ounce frozen container of orange juice is reconstituted. While not exact, for the purposes of conversion between metric and household, we use this approximation regularly. A typical continuous intravenous solution is in a container that is 1 liter (see Figure 9-2).

EXAMPLE: A patient is to receive 1,500 ml of fluid. How many liters will the patient receive?

Units given: ml

Units of answer: L

$$\frac{1,500 \text{ ml}}{1} \times \frac{1 \text{ L}}{1,000 \text{ ml}} = 1.5 \text{ L}$$

Therefore, the patient will receive 1.5 liters of fluid.

In nursing/health sciences we measure volumes in liters or cubic centimeters, although most any accounting of fluid volumes related to patients is referred to in total amounts of milliliters or cubic centimeters.

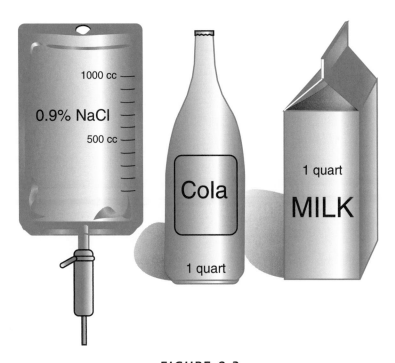

FIGURE 9-2

Basic Unit for Volume: The Liter (Similar to these measures)

EXAMPLE: A patient received 1 unit (500 cc) of whole blood. How many liters did the patient receive?

In this example we need to recall that 1 cc = 1 ml. Using that conversion factor with the connection between milliliters and liters, we have:

Units given: cc

Units of answer: L

$$\frac{500 \text{ cc}}{1} \times \frac{1 \text{ ml}}{1 \text{ cc}} \times \frac{1 \text{ L}}{1,000 \text{ ml}} = 0.5 \text{ L}$$

The patient received 0.5 L or ½ liter.

Derivation of Volume

Often we use millimeters and cubic centimeters interchangeably. The derivation that supports this is explained in Figure 9-3. The volume of a liter is that which could be contained in a cube measuring 1 decimeter on all sides. A decimeter is 10 centimeters. Look at the meter stick. It has 10 decimeters. Using Figure 9-3 and the meter stick, picture the size of a 1 decimeter cube. A 1 decimeter cube is 1 decimeter on each side: length, width, and height. Measurements of an object that include length, width, and height are cubic measures. A cubic measurement is a volume measure. Length (L), multiplied by height (H), and multiplied by width (W), is equal to a volume (V) measure: $L \times H \times W = V$. Considering the units for volume, multiplying the units of the three sides, you have three times the units or a cubic measure: $1 \text{ dm} \times 1 \text{ dm} \times 1 \text{ dm} = 1 \text{ dm}^3$. If the volume of a liter is that which can be contained in a 1 decimeter cube, then the relationship is made

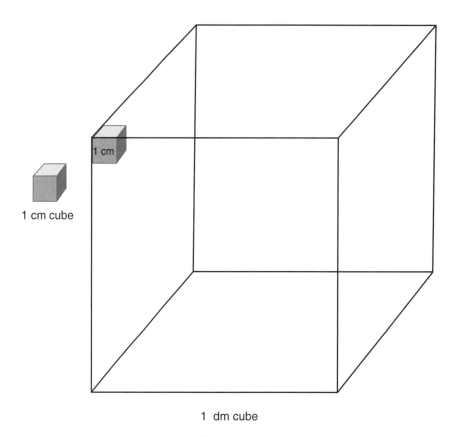

1 cm

1 cm cube

1 dm cube

FIGURE 9-3

The volume of 1 liter can be contained in 1 decimeter; 1 milliliter takes the space of $1/_{1,000}$ of a decimeter or 1 cubic centimeter.

that 1 milliliter takes the space of one thousandth of a decimeter or 1 cubic centimeter. It is due to this volume relationship that we are able to interchange milliliters and cubic centimeters. Thus, we can say it is correct to refer to fluid volume measurements with cubic centimeter (cc) units rather than milliliters (ml). Refer to the Key Points that summarize this concept.

KEY POINT

$$1,000 \text{ cm}^3 = 1,000 \text{ cc}$$

$$1,000 \text{ cc} = 1 \text{ L (liter)} = 1,000 \text{ ml}$$

$$1 \text{ cm}^3 = 1 \text{ cc} = 1 \text{ ml}$$

EXAMPLE: A patient received 1.5 liters of intravenous fluid. This needs to be recorded on the intake and output record in cc units of measure. Convert the quantity to cc.

Units given: L

Units of answer: cc

We need to convert 1.5 liters into cc:

$$\frac{1.5 \text{ liters}}{1} \times \frac{1,000 \text{ cc}}{1 \text{ liter}} = 1,500 \text{ cc}$$

EXAMPLE: Suppose we need to fill a 1 liter container and all we have on hand is a 5 ml (1 teaspoon) scoop. How many times would we have to pour the full 5 ml scoop in order to fill the container?

Units given: L

Units of answer: scoop

We need to convert 1 liter into (5 ml) scoops:

$$\frac{1 \text{ L}}{1} \times \frac{1,000 \text{ ml}}{1 \text{ L}} \times \frac{1 \text{ scoop}}{5 \text{ ml}} = 200 \text{ scoops}$$

Therefore, we would have to scoop 200 times in order to fill the 1 liter container. This example is very extreme; however, it illustrates the difference in the quantities.

Metric volumes are measured in volumetric glassware. These containers are designed to measure volumes with a high degree of accuracy. There are graduated cylinders, pipettes, burettes, flasks, and syringes, to name a few. When reading a column of fluid in one of these containers, it is important to determine the quantity by reading at the bottom of the meniscus. Figure 9-4 shows a reading of a column of medication in a graduated cylinder. Note the concave shape at the top

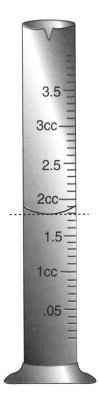

FIGURE 9-4
Read at the meniscus for all volumetric devices.

of the column. The quantity is determined by reading at the lowest point in the curve, which is the meniscus. The reading in this example is 1.8 cc. Syringe volumes are read by meniscus in the same manner.

The Gram: Unit of Mass

Mass is the amount of matter an object contains. Weight is the result of the gravitational pull on a mass. In a scientific laboratory these terms are used with consideration for their literal meaning. In nursing/health science you will see the terms used interchangeably. The base unit for mass in the metric system is the gram. A gram is about the size of two paper clips (Figure 9-5). Hold two paper clips in your hand. How does a gram compare to a kilogram? It takes 1,000 grams to make 1 kilogram (kg). The prefix *kilo* means 1,000. On the other hand, 1 milligram (mg) is equal to one thousandth of a gram and 1 microgram (mcg or μg) is equal to one millionth of a gram. These extremes of measure assist in measuring specific needs of patients.

The relationship to the household system that is usually used is 1 kilogram = 2.2 pounds. An easy way to remember the relationship between a pound and a kilogram is to think about your own weight. Most people do not like to share their body weight with others when expressed in pounds; however, if they can give a quantity in kilograms, it sounds better. For example, I would rather tell you I weigh about 52 kg than 115 lb. Thus, a kilogram is heavier than a pound.

EXAMPLE: A patient weighs 76.2 kg (168 lb). Express this weight in grams.

Units given: kg

Units of answer: g

Since the gram is a smaller unit of measure, we expect the patient's weight in grams to be a much larger value. Using the conversion factor that 1 kilogram = 1,000 grams, we have:

$$\frac{76.2 \text{ kg}}{1} \times \frac{1,000 \text{ g}}{1 \text{ kg}} = 76,200 \text{ g}$$

A patient weighing 76.2 kg weighs 76,200 grams.

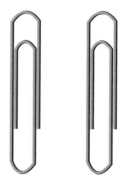

FIGURE 9-5

What is the size of a gram? About the size of two paper clips.

EXAMPLE: How many milligrams are contained in 2.4 g? How many micrograms?

Units given: g

Units of answer: mg, mcg

To convert grams to milligrams, we use the conversion factor 1 gram = 1,000 milligrams.

$$\frac{2.4\ \text{g}}{1} \times \frac{1{,}000\ \text{mg}}{1\ \text{g}} = 2{,}400\ \text{mg}$$

To convert grams to micrograms, we use the same conversion factor for milligrams and then continue with 1 mg = 1,000 mcg.

$$\frac{2.4\ \text{g}}{1} \times \frac{1{,}000\ \text{mg}}{1\ \text{g}} \times \frac{1{,}000\ \text{mcg}}{1\ \text{mg}} = 2{,}400{,}000\ \text{mcg}$$

We can once again see that a microgram is a very small unit of measure in that there are more than 2 million micrograms in just 2.4 grams of a substance.

EXAMPLE: A newborn weighs 3,250 g. An order for medication involves kilograms. How much does the newborn weigh in kilograms?

Units given: g

Units of answer: kg

$$\frac{3{,}250\ \text{g}}{1} \times \frac{1\ \text{kg}}{1{,}000\ \text{g}} = 3.25\ \text{kg}$$

The baby weighs 3.25 kg (which is a little over 7 pounds).

EXAMPLE: A newborn's diaper is weighed before and after it is used. The diaper weighs 32.0 g before and 38.5 g wet. Using the connection that 1 g = 1 ml, how many ml of fluid did the baby excrete?

The difference in the weight of the diaper is:

$$38.5\ \text{g} - 32.0\ \text{g} = 6.5\ \text{g}$$

Units given: g

Units of answer: ml

$$\frac{6.5\ \text{g}}{1} \times \frac{1\ \text{ml}}{1\ \text{g}} = 6.5\ \text{ml}$$

The baby excreted 6.5 ml of fluid, or slightly more than a teaspoon.

The Relationship Between Linear, Volume, and Mass Measures of the Metric System

The nursing/health science community functions in patient care areas, utilizing many units of value, quantities, and approximations that are based on scientific findings but require flexible interpretation. The variation in individuals, available products, and the real-life situation rather than the controlled laboratory experiment require health professionals to utilize measurement equivalents that are not used in a controlled scientific laboratory.

If we could fill a 1 centimeter cube, like the one pictured in Figure 9-3, with water at a temperature of 4.5 degrees Centigrade, we would find the mass of the water to be 1 gram. The mass of the water remains 1 gram even at temperatures of 20 degrees to 22 degrees Centigrade. Because of this relationship we are able to indicate that 1 cc H_2O = 1 ml H_2O = 1 g (see Figure 9-6). The 1 gram to 1 cubic centimeter relationship is used throughout nursing/health science.

Since 1 cubic centimeter containing 1 milliliter of water has a mass of 1 gram, the relationship can also be made that 1,000 milliliters or 1 liter has a mass of 1,000 grams or 1 kilogram.

KEY POINT

$$1 \text{ cc } H_2O = 1 \text{ ml } H_2O = 1 \text{ g}$$

For example, when calculations are done to determine the amount of fluid that is removed from a patient's abdomen during chronic ambulatory peritoneal dialysis (CAPD), the bag of removed fluid is placed on the hook of a spring scale to determine the volume of fluid. The scale has measurements in increments of ½ gram. To arrive at a volume measure in cubic centimeters, the relationship is used that 1 gram = 1 cubic centimeter.

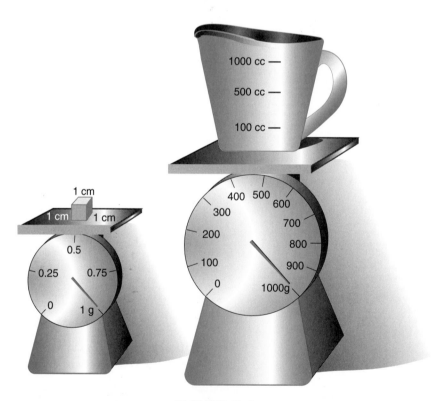

FIGURE 9-6
Relationship Between Metric Units of Weight and Volume

EXAMPLE: Prepare 250 ml of a 0.60% NaCl solution for nose drops. How much salt will be required?

Units given: ml

Units of answer: g (of salt)

(Recall that this would be an example of a weight/volume solution. We are being asked for a solid amount of salt.)

Recall that 0.60% implies $\rightarrow \dfrac{0.60\ g}{100\ ml}$

Therefore, setting up our equation we have:

$$\frac{250\ ml}{1} \times \frac{0.60\ g}{100\ ml} = 1.5\ g$$

So, we would need 1.5 g of salt for this solution. Does our amount make sense? Well, 0.60% is less than 1%, which in grams (since 1 g = 1 ml) would be 2.5. It will be slightly higher than one half this amount, since 0.6 is slightly more than 0.5. Therefore, our value seems reasonable.

PRACTICE EXERCISE 9.B

Using Table 9-2, convert the following:

1. 1 m = _____ cm

2. 1,000 ml = _____ L

3. 1 kg = _____ g

4. 1,000 mcg = _____ mg

5. 1 g = _____ mg

6. 1 L = _____ dl

Problem Solving Revisited

Utilizing the quantities of the metric system and your ability to solve equations, any relationship within the system can be made. A mechanism for checking your computations is based on the system identified in Chapter 6: section on "Accuracy in Problem Solving." Ask yourself when you have arrived at the answer if the answer makes sense in regard to the quantity of the answer.

KEY POINT

When converting within the metric system and computing:

- from a larger (L) to a smaller (S) value, the decimal point will be moved from the left (L) to the right (R).

Likewise, when solving an equation and moving:

- from a smaller (S) to a larger (L) value, the decimal point will be moved from the right (R) to the left (L).

Note how the "L" is on the same side for both applications of this acronym:

- larger (L) to smaller (S)

  left (L) to right (R)

- smaller (S) to larger (L)

  right (R) to left (L)

EXAMPLE: Recall the previous examples.

EXAMPLE: A patient is 175 cm tall. How tall is the patient in meters?

Units given: cm

Units of answer: m   Answer: 1.75 m

When solving an equation and moving from a smaller (S) to a larger (L) value, the decimal point will be moved from the right (R) to the left (L).

EXAMPLE: A patient weighs 76.2 kg. Express this weight in grams.

Units given: kg

Units of answer: g

Answer: 76,200 grams

When converting in the metric system from a larger (L) to a smaller (S) value, the decimal point will be moved from the left (L) to the right (R).

PRACTICE EXERCISE 9.C

Make the following metric conversions. Check your answer by also indicating if the conversion was from larger to smaller (L–S) or smaller to larger (S–L).

1. 0.9 g = _____ mg _____

2. 0.003 g = _____ mg _____

3. 200 mg = _____ g _____

4. 1,500 mg = _____ g _____

LEARNING ACTIVITIES

The learning activities for the metric system of measurement are designed to assist the learner to have a hands-on concept of what the units and quantities are like in size. These activities require a number of teaching aids that assist with the learning.

REMEMBER!

Linear measurements are one dimension (length).

1. Utilizing a meter stick, answer the following questions:

a. What units of measure do the numbers on the meter stick represent?

_____

b. What are the smallest units of measure on the meter stick?

_____

c. How many centimeters (cm) are on the meter stick? _____

d. How many millimeters (mm) are on the meter stick? _____

e. How many millimeters (mm) are in 1 centimeter? _____

2. Measure the length and width of your desk in centimeters. Convert the measures to meters.

   Length of desk _____ cm _____ m

   Width of desk _____ cm _____ m

REMEMBER!

Volume measurements are the amount of space occupied by three-dimensional objects.

---

3. Examine a graduated cylinder. What do the smallest lines or increments on the container measure? _____

4. Examine a variety of sizes of syringes: 1 cc, 3 cc, 5 cc, 10 cc, 20 cc, and 50 cc. Which syringe would hold the contents of a liquid medicine cup used to measure single-dose oral medications? _____

REMEMBER!

Mass measurements are the amount of matter that objects contain.

---

5. Using a balance scale, determine the mass of a 100 ml beaker.

   _____

6. Using a 20 cc syringe, measure 20 cc of water and add to the beaker in problem 5. What is the mass of the water alone? _____

CHAPTER REVIEW EXERCISES

Convert the following quantities using metric equivalents. Show your conversion equation using dimensional analysis.

1. 343 cm = _____ m

2. 1.3 kg = _____ g

3. 250 ml = _____ cc

4. 1,250 ml = _____ L

5. 2.4 m = _____ mm

6. 75 mg = _____ g

7. 2.7 L = _____ ml

8. 5,000 mcg = _____ mg

9. 1.35 m = _____ mm

10. 1.5 g = _____ mg

11. 500 m = _____ km

12. 5 L = _____ cc

13. 20 g = _____ mcg

CRITICAL THINKING

Show your calculation for each of the exercises below.

1. If a medication is supplied as 0.5 g in each tablet and you need to administer 0.25 g, how many tablets will you give?

2. A medication is supplied as 500 mg in each tablet.

The amount that was ordered to be given was 0.5 g. Before you can administer the tablet, what unit does the drug order need to be expressed in?

3. For problem 2, how many tablets will you give?

4. Read the label below. How much medication is in this vial? Provide your answer in mass units.

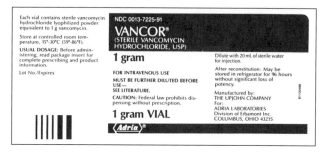

5. Below is a common oral antibiotic medication. What is the mass of medication per volume of solution when reconstituted?

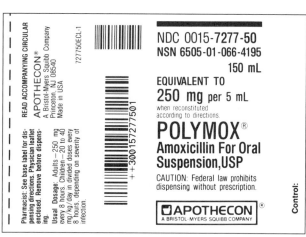

6. Suppose that we weigh a beaker partially full of water. After subtracting out the mass of the beaker, we find that there are 125 g of water. How many ml of water was in the beaker?

7. Suppose we have 9 grams of sodium chloride (NaCl) dissolved in a solution of 1 L. What is the strength (measured in a percentage) of this solution? What is another name for this solution?

Relationship of the Measurement Systems

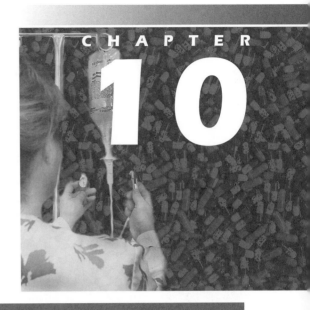

C H A P T E R

10

OBJECTIVES

Upon completion of this chapter, you will be able to:

- Describe the equivalents between the household, apothecaries', and metric systems.
- Recognize the inconsistencies when calculating between systems.
- Utilize the conversion card throughout the learning process.
- Convert between the apothecaries', household, and metric systems.

Introduction

The previous chapters have prepared you for the task that is at hand now. Clinical situations in which calculations are necessary require moving between all the systems of measurement. Conversions of quantities occur, for example, when calculating medication dosages, measuring intake and output, and finding the density of a solution. The treatment recommended for a patient, and therefore a dosage, may vary as much as each individual. Prescribed therapy is designed for the individual patient.

Conversions Between Systems

When calculating between the systems, the conversion factors that are used are not absolute. These relationships are considered approximate equivalents because it is impractical to make them equivalent to each other. The relationships between the systems that have been established enhance and promote the ease of movement between the systems. Choosing the most direct route through a calculation is desirable. You will observe many inconsistencies. It is for this reason that we will recommend a system for choosing conversion factors for a given calculation. Limiting the tendency to go back and forth between systems will favor as little variation in the final answer as possible. For example, do not convert from apothecary to metric and back to apothecary, or from apothecary to metric and then to the household system.

The biggest variations are seen between the apothecaries' system and the other systems because the apothecaries' system is so inaccurate. The mass of the units was developed and changed each year based on the current wheat crop. The relationship of the apothecaries' system to the household system is closer than the relationship between the apothecaries' and metric systems. This will be evident in the examples provided.

The examples and situations encountered when calculating between the measurement systems in the nursing/health science world are complex. This diversity occurs because of the variety of people, situations, and available products in a given clinical situation.

When many medications were first formally developed, the measurement systems employed were the apothecaries' and household systems. In more recent years, the measurement system used for most all medication development has been the metric system. Likewise, the physicians and other health care professionals prescribing the medications have also historically ordered medications and other treatments in the system most popular for the times. Current practice most often utilizes the metric system. However, physicians may still be found using the apothecaries' and household systems when ordering older medications. The move toward more standardization and acceptance of the metric system has decreased the amount of prescription ordering and available products in the apothecaries' and household systems, but these systems have not been completely eliminated.

EXAMPLE: Morphine gr 1/8 sc q3h prn.

This order may be prescribed with apothecary units or with metric units. Most morphine is supplied with both the apothecary and metric equivalents on the label.

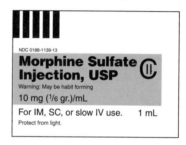

Your job is to ensure that the prescribed mass of the drug, whether it be grains or milligrams, is accurately calculated and prepared to be given by volume. The previous order was to administer the medication subcutaneously (sc). The responsibility of the nurse is to know how much volume needs to be drawn up into the syringe to be administered as a subcutaneous injection. A calculation needs to be made for the volume of medication to be administered.

The increasing shift of patient care to the community and to home care has increased the number of preparations that must be adapted for the understanding of the family member who is often the health care provider in the home setting. For the convenience of the layperson, many prescriptions are given in household measures to make it easier for medications and other treatments to be measured and administered in the home.

Conversions between systems are necessary because of the disparity between the system in which the prescribed treatment is ordered and how the medication is supplied and dispensed. A physician, when ordering a medication or treatment, may not be aware of the supply of the drug the pharmacy has available. This often occurs when a specific trade-name drug is filled with a generic equivalent.

Conversions Between the Apothecaries' and Household Systems

There are some aspects of the apothecaries' and household systems that make them fairly compatible. For instance, a drop is a drop! Whether you are referring to an apothecary or household drop, they are the same. The relationship of the ounce and the pound also remains the same.

EXAMPLE: Convert 5 minims to drops.

Since 1 drop (gtt) is the equivalent of 1 minim ($\mathbb{m}$):

$$\frac{5 \; \mathbb{m}}{1} \times \frac{1 \text{ gtt}}{1 \; \mathbb{m}} = 5 \text{ gtt}$$

EXAMPLE: Convert 3 f℥ to fʒ.

Units given: f℥

Units of answer: fʒ

From the conversion card, we can see that there are 8 fluid drams to 1 fluid ounce, so we can make the conversion in one step:

$$\frac{3 \text{ f℥}}{1} \times \frac{8 \text{ fʒ}}{1 \text{ f℥}} = 24 \text{ fʒ}$$

The answer may be represented in an Arabic numeral or roman numeral. When the choice is made, consider if the question was asked in a roman numeral. Suppose it was. Then we should answer in a roman numeral. The general convention is to write the unit label first with the roman numeral following. Consequently, we can represent this answer as follows:

$$24 \text{ fʒ} = \text{fʒ xxiv} = \text{fʒ } \overline{\text{xxiv}}$$

We recognize the original problem and conversion as:

$$\text{f℥ } \overline{\overline{\text{iii}}} = \text{fʒ } \overline{\text{xxiv}}$$

EXAMPLE: Convert gr CCXL to ounces.

Units given: grains

Units of answer: ounces

First establish the route to take for solving this problem. Often the difficulty with the apothecaries' system comes from less familiarity than with the household or metric system. Checking the conversion card, recognize that there is a connection between grains and drams and then drams and ounces. Therefore, we can make the transition with two conversion factors from grains to ounces.

Before we begin the dimensional analysis equation, convert the roman numeral back to an Arabic numeral for ease of calculation. Therefore, convert CCXL to 240.

$$\frac{240 \text{ gr}}{1} \times \frac{1 \text{ ʒ}}{60 \text{ gr}} \times \frac{1 \text{ ℥}}{8 \text{ ʒ}} =$$

Canceling common factors, we have:

$$\frac{\overset{1}{\cancel{240}} \text{ gr}}{1} \times \frac{1 \text{ ʒ}}{\cancel{60} \text{ gr}} \times \frac{1 \text{ ℥}}{\underset{2}{\cancel{8}} \text{ ʒ}} = \tfrac{1}{2} \text{ ℥ or ℥ } \overline{ss}.$$

The inconsistencies between these two systems occur in the relationship of the dram and the teaspoon to the ounce. On one hand, the dram and teaspoon are recognized as being approximately equivalent, but on the other hand, there are 8 drams in 1 ounce and 6 teaspoons to 1 ounce (Figure 10-1). So when calculating these units, be careful not to skew your answer by choosing a route for calculation that will cause this inconsistency to affect your answer.

Does 1 dram equal 1 teaspoon? Let us consider the following problem:

EXAMPLE: A. A 1 quart antacid preparation contains how many 2 teaspoon doses?

Units given: quarts

Units of answer: doses

Using the conversion card, observe that there is a connection between quarts and ounces, ounces and tablespoons, tablespoons and teaspoons, and lastly in the example between teaspoons and doses.

$$\frac{1 \text{ qt}}{1} \times \frac{32 \text{ ℥}}{1 \text{ qt}} \times \frac{\overset{1}{\cancel{2}} \text{ T}}{1 \text{ ℥}} \times \frac{3 \text{ t}}{1 \text{ T}} \times \frac{1 \text{ dose}}{\underset{1}{\cancel{2} \text{ t}}} = 96 \text{ doses}$$

B. A 1 quart antacid preparation contains how many 2 dram doses?

Units given: quarts

Units of answer: doses

Again, by consulting the conversion card, the necessary connections can be made. In this problem we can make our way from quarts to drams by going through ounces.

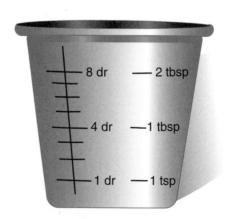

FIGURE 10-1

Relationship of Apothecaries' and Household Measures

The final connection, from drams to doses, can be made in the example:

$$\frac{1 \text{ qt}}{1} \times \frac{32\ \text{℥}}{1 \text{ qt}} \times \frac{8\ \text{ʒ}}{1\ \text{℥}} \times \frac{1 \text{ dose}}{2\ \text{ʒ}} = 128 \text{ doses}$$

C. How do the answers compare in parts A and B?

We can obviously see that there is a sizable difference in the number of doses in these two examples. We could certainly conclude that a dram does not equal a teaspoon. In this example, the difference was magnified because of the several conversion factors needed to solve the problems. If in fact we look closely at the conversion card and look for an answer within the metric system, the difference is that a dram is equal to 4 ml and a teaspoon is equal to 5 ml. The actual answer to the original question, comparing a dram and a teaspoon, is that they are approximately equal. In this problem we saw the approximation exaggerated. We should be careful, because of the inaccuracy, in using this conversion factor too extensively or in problems that require more than one conversion factor. The same holds true for the metric conversion. The 4 ml conversion factor is also quite approximate and not equal.

PRACTICE EXERCISE 10.A

1. 12 ʒ = _____ C
2. 5 C = _____ ʒ
3. ʒ 4 = _____ tsp
4. ♏ CLXXX = _____ tsp
5. f℥ CXXVIII = _____ pt
6. fʒ LXIV = _____ qt
7. fʒ XXXII = _____ C
8. ʒ iii = _____ T
9. ℥ iii = _____ t
10. ℥ ii = _____ T

Conversions Between the Apothecaries' and Metric Systems

A parallel relationship between the apothecaries' and metric system that makes some of the quantities easy to remember is that of the grain and drop. Recall that the grain, minim, and drop are equivalent in quantity. In the same way that it takes 15 grains to approximately equal 1 gram, it takes 15 drops to be approximately equivalent to 1 cubic centimeter. Recall from Chapter 8 that we referenced the grain as being similar in size to one piece of rice. Picture or actually count 15 pieces of rice and hold them in your hand. This amount is approximately equivalent to 1 gram (Figure 10-2). The drop or minim can be dropped one at a time until 15 drops equal 1 cubic centimeter.

REMEMBER!
1 gtt = 1 ♏ = 1 gr
1 cc = 1 ml = 1 g
15 gtt = 1 cc   15 gr = 1 g

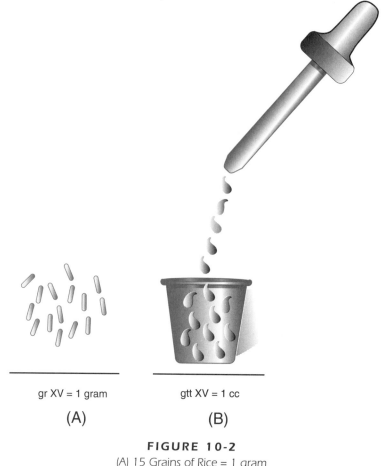

gr XV = 1 gram

(A)

gtt XV = 1 cc

(B)

FIGURE 10-2
(A) 15 Grains of Rice = 1 gram
(B) 15 Drops = 1 cc

The grain to milligram relationship has always been an interesting one. Many people find the grain difficult to substantiate, most likely because the relationship to metric changes. The harvested grain, which is what the measure was based on, is not a precise or accurate measure. Thus, the relationship of the milligram to the grain has been as few as 60 milligrams and as many as 65 milligrams. Reference can be found to 60, 62, 64, and 65 mg per 1 grain. Most often 60 mg is used as the equivalent to 1 grain.

REMEMBER!

60 mg = gr I = 1 gr

An advantage of the metric system is the convenience of measuring quantities less than 1 grain. It takes 60 mg to make 1 grain.

Occasionally you will see a preoperative order for *atropine gr 1/150 IM 1 h pre-op.* Look at how cumbersome a fraction of this size can be. The metric system provides a means of measuring medications that makes calculations much easier to complete. If the order reads *atropine 0.4 mg IM 1 h pre-op,* would you agree the mass of the drug appears to be a quantity that is easier to calculate? Table 10-1 illustrates many of the common conversion equivalents.

TABLE 10-1 Conversion Equivalents

Apothecary	Household	Metric
Volume		
1 minim (℔)	1 drop (gtt)	
15 minims		1 ml
1 fluid dram (f ℈)	1 teaspoon	
1 fluid dram (f ℈)		4 ml
	1 teaspoon	5 ml
½ fluid ounce (f ℥)	1 tablespoon	
8 fluid drams	1 fluid ounce	30 ml
8 fluid ounces	1 cup	
Mass		
8 drams	1 ounce	
1 grain		60–65 mg
15 grains		1 gram = 1,000 mg

EXAMPLE: Convert gr 1/150 to mg.

Units given: grains

Units of answer: milligrams

$$\frac{\frac{1}{150 \text{ gr}}}{1} \times \frac{60 \text{ mg}}{1 \text{ gr}} =$$

$$\frac{1}{150} \times \frac{60 \text{ mg}}{1} = \frac{60 \text{ mg}}{150} = \frac{3 \text{ mg}}{5} = 0.4 \text{ mg}$$

PRACTICE EXERCISE 10.B

1. ℔ XXX = _____ ml

2. ℈ ii = _____ ml

3. ℥ viii = _____ ml

4. gr X = _____ mg

5. gr XXX = _____ g

6. gr ½ = _____ mg

7. gr LX = _____ g

8. ℈ viii = _____ cc

9. ℥ i = _____ cc

10. ℔ XII = _____ cc

Conversions Between the Household and Metric Measurement Systems

Household and metric relationships are made more and more every day. Most people will experience these relationships as a result of comparing and reading labels in the grocery store.

A few years ago, people went to buy a quart of soda. Now, the advertisements promote the sale price on the liter bottle. Most all food containers have both a household and metric equivalent printed on the label. Referring to Figure 10-3, you can see the relationship between many of the equivalents of these two systems. A teaspoon is 5 cc. The best way to visualize this is to look at a medication cup that has measures for the teaspoon as well as cubic centimeters. A kitchen spoon may or may not actually be an accurate teaspoon equivalent to 5

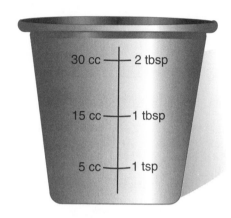

FIGURE 10-3
Relationship of Household and Metric Measures

cc. Again, on the medication cup increments show that 1 tablespoon is equal to 15 cc, which is also ½ ounce. The kitchen tablespoon may or may not be an accurate 15 cc. As discussed earlier, it takes 2 tablespoons to equal 1 ounce. One ounce is equivalent to 30 cc. This amount is the size of the medicine cup.

The cup measure varies with how institutions interpret this amount. If you are referring to an 8 ounce cup, then this is 240 cc. But many institutions refer to their cup of soup or carton of milk as 250 cc. It actually depends on how the quantity has been determined. If asked how many cc in ½ pint, the calculation is based on 1 pint that equals 500 cc. The answer is 250 cc. If asked how many cc in 8 ounces, the calculation is based on 1 ℥ = 30 cc, and the answer is 240 cc. This example demonstrates why it is important to take the direct calculation route that is intended. A difference of 10 cc is not critical in all situations, but potentially a discrepancy such as this one can add up over time.

Within the nursing/allied health community, the need to convert between the household and metric system is commonly for convenience in home care situations. Many patients and family members may not be comfortable with specific units of the metric system, so conversion to household equivalents is helpful for measuring medications or parenteral and enteral fluids.

EXAMPLE: Suppose a patient's family needs to make 2 gallons of a foot soak solution to have available for a series of treatments. If the patient is to use 1 liter per soak, how many soaks has the solution been prepared for?

Units given: gallons

Units of answer: soaks

Using the conversion factors between gallons, quarts, and liters, we have

$$\frac{2 \text{ gal}}{1} \times \frac{4 \text{ qt}}{1 \text{ gal}} \times \frac{1 \text{ L}}{1 \text{ qt}} \times \frac{1 \text{ soak}}{1 \text{ L}} = 8 \text{ soaks}$$

Therefore, with 2 gallons of the foot soak solution, the patient will have enough prepared for 8 treatments.

EXAMPLE: A patient is asked to drink 5 cups of a liquid prior to an ultrasound. You need to account for the volume on the I&O (input and output) sheet. How many cc did the patient drink?

Units given: cups

Units of answer: cc

After setting up the equation, we can multiply across (since the denominators are all ones). We obtain

$$\frac{5 \text{ C}}{1} \times \frac{8 \text{ ʒ}}{1 \text{ C}} \times \frac{30 \text{ ml}}{1 \text{ ʒ}} \times \frac{1 \text{ cc}}{1 \text{ ml}} = 1{,}200 \text{ cc}$$

EXAMPLE: A doctor's order indicates that a child is to have 10 ml of a cough medication at home. How many teaspoons should the parent be instructed to administer?

Units given: ml

Units of answer: tsp

Utilizing the conversion card, notice a direct connection between milliliters and teaspoons:

$$\frac{10 \text{ ml}}{1} \times \frac{1 \text{ tsp}}{5 \text{ ml}} = 2 \text{ tsp}$$

Therefore, the child should receive 2 teaspoons of medication.

PRACTICE EXERCISE 10.C

1. 2 tsp = _____ cc

2. 8 ʒ = _____ cc

3. 2 qt = _____ L

4. 4 pt = _____ ml

5. ½ tsp = _____ ml

6. ½ cup = _____ ml

7. 4 ʒ = _____ ml

8. 1 tbsp = _____ ml

9. 2 cups = _____ L

10. 4 pt = _____ L

Body Weight Conversions

Another situation in which it is necessary to convert between household and metric is for calculations based on body weight. While most people know what their weight is measured in pounds, few people in the Unites States have any idea how many kilograms they weigh. This conversion is important since many medication dosages are based on body mass. The amount of medication to be given is determined in units that consider the mass of drug per mass of the patient, or mg/kg. The main conversion factor is 1 kg = 2.2 lb. Since it takes 2.2 pounds to make 1 kilogram, our weight in pounds is more than twice what it is in kilograms. A person who weighs 176 lb has a mass of 80 kg.

REMEMBER!
1 kg = 2.2 lb

PRACTICE EXERCISE 10.D

Convert the following weights using the conversion factor: 1 kg = 2.2 lb. Show your equation.

1. Convert 100 kg to pounds.
2. Convert 100 lb to kilograms.
3. Which is larger, 100 kg or 100 lb? Why?
4. Convert 143 lb to kilograms.
5. Convert 195 lb to kilograms.

Rounding

When performing many of the calculations and conversions, it is important to recall the rules for rounding and to think critically when they are appropriate and not appropriate to use.

> **KEY POINT**
>
> When rounding to a specific place value, if the next value is 5 or higher, round the preceding value up. If the next place value is 4 or less, drop the value to the right.

EXAMPLE: Round 184.65 lb to the nearest whole pound.

Since the next place value beyond the whole number place value is 6, we round up the previous value—4—to 5. Therefore, our answer becomes 185 lb.

EXAMPLE: Round 0.4345 ml to the nearest tenth of a milliliter.

Since the first place beyond the tenth's place is 3, we simply drop the 3 and all place values to the right. Therefore, our answer is 0.4 ml.

The choice as to round or not to round is a critical thought question whose answer is based on the particular situation. If we were taking a patient history, it might be all right to round a patient's weight to the nearest kilogram after conversion from pounds. However, if we wanted to calculate a drug order based on body weight, it might be inappropriate to round. If a physician's order when calculated came to 1.25 tablets for a single dose, consideration would have to be given to the type of drug and how it is supplied before any rounding decisions could be responsibly made. An example of where rounding is commonly used is in calculating the number of drops per minute at which an IV solution should be set. It is common in this situation to round to the nearest whole number.

PRACTICE EXERCISE 10.E

Round the following values as indicated.

1. Round 87.89 kg to the nearest kilogram.

2. Round 87.89 kg to the nearest tenth of a kilogram.

3. Round 0.07325 ml to the nearest tenth of a milliliter.

4. Round 0.07325 ml to the nearest hundredth of a milliliter.

5. Round 22.2 drops to the nearest drop.

6. Round 66.6 drops to the nearest drop.

Calculating Rate

Each day we drive a car and recognize the speed on the speedometer is indicated in both miles per hour (mph) and kilometers per hour (kph). These are measurements of rate. Rate is any unit of measure divided by time. Since the prefix *kilo* means multiply by 1,000, a kilometer is 1,000 meters (1 km = 1,000 m).

EXAMPLE: Suppose you have a digital readout on your speedometer that gives a reading in kilometers per hour. You are traveling 80 km/hr on a road that has a speed limit of 55 mph. Are you going too fast?

Units given: km/hr (kph)

Units of answer: mi/hr (mph)

While the question at first seems to be straightforward, we do not have a conversion factor for kilometers and miles. It seems a bit unreasonable to convert to meters and then to inches and then to feet and finally to miles! We can use other references! A standard dictionary with a metric table indicates that:

$$1 \text{ km} = 0.62 \text{ mi}$$

In this dimensional analysis situation, there are units of measure in both the numerator and denominator. Often, you will wish to convert both of these units. However, in this example the hour units are both in the denominator of the units given and the units of the answer. The only units to convert are kilometers to miles:

$$\frac{80 \text{ km}}{1 \text{ hr}} \times \frac{0.62 \text{ mi}}{1 \text{ km}}$$

Notice that kilometers is placed in the denominator of the second fraction so that the units will cancel and we are left with miles in the numerator and hours in the denominator, thus giving us the units of the answer, miles per hour (mph).

$$\frac{80 \text{ km}}{1 \text{ hr}} \times \frac{0.62 \text{ mi}}{1 \text{ km}} = \frac{49.6 \text{ mi}}{1 \text{ hr}} = 49.6 \text{ mph}$$

Therefore, 80 kph is approximately 50 mph and we are not exceeding the speed limit.

PRACTICE EXERCISE 10.F

Determine the answer to the following questions by solving dimensional analysis calculations.

1. If you had to measure 2 gallons of water using a pint-size container, how many times would you need to fill the pint container?

2. A patient is told to drink 1,500 ml of fluid every day. You advise the patient to drink how many cups of fluid per day?

3. You make a calculation and find you need to prepare ℥ ss̄ of a drug. How many minims would you prepare? How many cc does this equal?

4. An order reads to give ʒ IV. How many teaspoons would you advise the mother to give?

5. You need to pour ʒ VIII of a medication. How many ounces is this quantity?

6. You need to give gtt XXX of a drug orally. A syringe will be helpful in order to measure this amount. How far will you fill the syringe and how many cc will this equal?

7. The metric system has the precision to measure fine quantities. A mass of 1 grain would contain how many micrograms?

8. A 3 liter container of liquid contains how many ounces?

9. Which is heavier, a kilogram or a pound?

LEARNING ACTIVITIES

The following activities are designed to assist you in developing a working knowledge of the relationship of the measurement systems. Use a 1 ounce medication cup for Learning Activities 1–3.

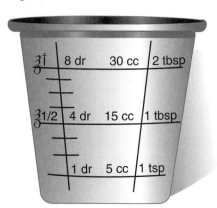

1. Fill a medication cup with water to the 1 teaspoon marking. Place the cup on a flat surface and observe other measurements equal to this amount of fluid.

   a. By observation, how many cc are in the cup?

   b. Does the level of the water come below or above the line for 1 dram ʒ i?

   c. How many teaspoons would you need to make 1 tablespoon (1 tbsp)?

2. Fill the medication cup with water to the 1 tablespoon marking. Place the cup on a flat surface and observe other measurements equal to this amount of fluid.

   a. By observation, how many cc are in the cup?

   b. By observation, how many ʒ are in the cup?

    c. By observation, how many tsp are in the cup?

    d. By observation, how many ʒ are in the cup? How many tablespoons would you need to fill the cup?

3. Fill the medication cup with water. Place the cup on a flat surface and observe other measurements equal to this amount of fluid.

    a. By observation, how many cc are in the cup?

    b. By observation, how many ʒ are in the cup?

    c. By observation, how many tsp are in the cup?

    d. By observation, how many tbsp are in the cup?

    e. By observation, how many ʒ are in the cup?

For questions 4–7, you will need a dropper, water, a handful of rice, and a medication cup.

4. Using the relationship that a piece of rice is similar in mass to an apothecary grain, count out 15 pieces of rice. What similar metric quantity is this?

5. Now count out 60 pieces of rice. What similar apothecary quantity is this?

6. Using a dropper, measure 15 drops into a medication cup.

    a. By approximation, how many cc do you believe are in the cup?

    b. Is the quantity in the cup more or less than 1 teaspoon?

    c. How many minims are this quantity?

7. Fill an 8 ʒ beaker or other cup with water. Place the cup on a flat surface and observe other measurements equal to this amount of fluid.

    a. By observation, how many cc are in the cup?

    b. By calculation, how many ʒ are in the cup?

    c. By observation, how many pt are in the cup?

CHAPTER REVIEW EXERCISES

For problems 1–6, make the following conversions:

1. 3 cups to fʒ.

2. gr V to mg.

3. 40 ʒ to ml.

4. ʒ iv to tsp.

5. 44 ml to ʒ.

6. 75 kg to lb.

7. You are to give instructions to an adult to take ʒ iii of a liquid over-the-counter preparation. How many tablespoons should you instruct the client to take?

8. An injection of gr 1/300 of a drug is ordered. How many mg of the medication was ordered? If the medication is available as 0.5 mg/ml, how many ml will be injected?

9. A study is being done to consider the side effects of a medication on people who weigh over 100 kg. If a patient weighs 205 lb, will the patient qualify for the study?

10. An over-the-counter (OTC) medication label indicates that adolescents over 12 years of age be given 1 tablespoon. How many cc does this correspond to? How many drams?

11. A medication order reads *gr CLXXX p.o. stat*. How many grams of the medication are ordered?

12. The recommended daily dosage of a medication is listed as 2.5 mg/kg. What would the recommended dosage for a single day be if the patient weighed 165 pounds?

CRITICAL THINKING

1. Suppose your lab partner is converting 2 tsp to milliliters in the following way:

$$\frac{2\ t}{1} \times \frac{1\ ʒ}{1\ t} \times \frac{4\ ml}{1\ ʒ} = 8\ ml$$

and you calculate:

$$\frac{2\ t}{1} \times \frac{5\ ml}{1\ t} = 10\ ml$$

Which answer is the most correct? Why is it more correct? What mistake did the other student make?

2. If you choose to fill a teaspoon with a dropper, approximately how many ♍ would it take to fill the teaspoon?

3. A bottle of diphenhydramine hydrochloride indicates there is 12.5 mg of medication in every 5 ml of solution. If you are to give 1 teaspoon, how much medication is the patient receiving?

4. A 5 ft 6 in tall female patient weighing 154 pounds requires a prescription determined by her size. The medication is ordered as 50 mg/kg. How many grams should she receive?

5. You need to give 7 mg of a drug. The drug comes as 42 mg/ʒ. How many teaspoons will you give?

6. You need to give 6 mg of a drug that is supplied as 30 mg/ʒ. How many ʒ will you give?

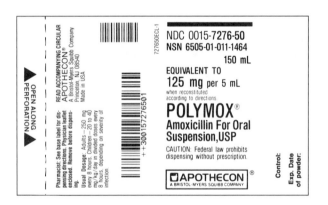

7. Refer to the insert above. Dosage ordered: 250 mg qid po. You instruct the patient to take how many teaspoons at home?

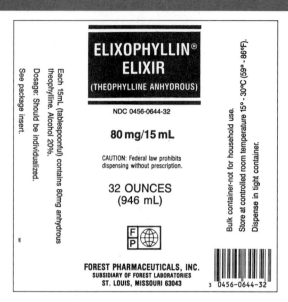

8. The drug Theophylline is available in liquid form. Referring to the label, note that each 15 ml has 80 mg of the drug. The order is for 160 mg. How many tablespoons will you prepare?

9. To revisit calculating oral intake and recording on the sample intake and output record form, the figure below will assist with volume relationships. Enter the equivalent of each picture depicted in cc.

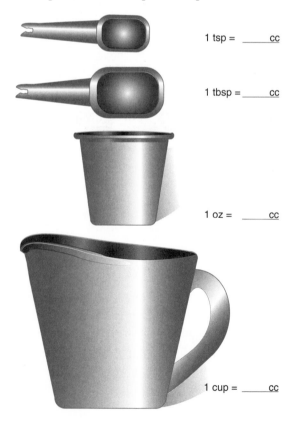

1 tsp = _____ cc

1 tbsp = _____ cc

1 oz = _____ cc

1 cup = _____ cc

For the following example, calculate each quantity and enter the total volume of intake on the intake and output record form. Mr. Jack has just returned to his room following diagnostic tests throughout the morning. He will receive a liquid lunch. Convert the intake and enter for 12:00 on the sample form on the next page:

4 ℨ sherbert

1 glass of water

2 tbsp of orange juice with medication

½ cup of soup

ALBANY MEDICAL CENTER
INTAKE AND OUTPUT

Date: _____

PATIENT IDENTIFICATION PLATE

MR# 321863
SS#: 000 222 5631
Jack, Morton
DOB 12/07/1952 Sex M
ATT: Rogers MD, Lucy

LEFT IN BAG

	0700 SOLUTION/RATE	AMT.	1500 SOLUTION/RATE	AMT.	2300 SOLUTION/RATE	AMT.
#	#1 D5 N5 @85cc/hr 275					

INTAKE

TIME	FEEDINGS	SOL. #	INF.	SOL. #	INF.	SOL. #	INF.	COMMENTS
0810								
0900		#1	250					
1200								
TOTAL								

OUTPUT

							INITIALS
URINE							SB
400							

SIGNATURE _Susan Baker_

INITIALS/STATUS SB /NA

95335 1090

144

Dosage Calculation

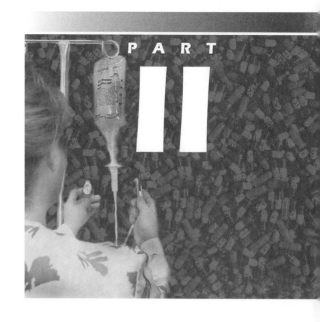

Introduction to Medication Orders

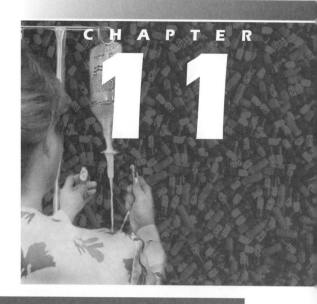

OBJECTIVES

Upon completion of this chapter, you will be able to:

- Describe the parts of a medication order.
- Explain the ability to administer the medication in relation to the volume or quantities supplied.
- Describe the five rights of medication administration.

Introduction

In order to problem solve calculations for medication administration, it is necessary to have an understanding of the common guidelines that govern ordering, transcription, and the delivery of medications. These guidelines are followed by licensed nurses in order to administer medications safely. Knowledge of pharmacology, including the action, therapeutic use and effects, usual dosage, adverse effects, and nursing implications of medications should precede administration of any pharmacologic agent.

Medication

A medication is prescribed by a qualified physician, dentist, or his or her designee. Referring to Figure 11-1, the medication prescribed may be written in generic or trade name terms. Generally speaking, if a trade name medication is prescribed, the hospital pharmacy may dispense a generic form of the medication, but if a generic name of the medication is ordered, it is filled with the generic form. Please refer to the note on the bottom of the physician order sheet in Figure 11-1.

Dosage

The dosage reflects the mass or quantity of medication that has been prescribed. The mass of the drug is ordered in the system of measurement appropriate for the medication. Recall that mass units are quantities such as grains and milligrams.

Medication may be supplied in many forms as well as several strengths or mass quantities including tablets, capsules, solutions for oral use, solutions for injection, solutions for intravenous use, inhalers, and suppositories. The labels in Figure 11-2 show medications in various forms for a variety of routes and

H-90050 (REV. 10/91)

ALBANY MEDICAL CENTER HOSPITAL
Physician's Order Sheet

INSTRUCTIONS:
1. Imprint patient's plate before placing in chart.
2. After each medication order is written, remove first copy and fax to PHARMACY.
3. "X" out remaining unused lines after last copy is used.
4. Imprint new set and place in chart.
5. Each order must be dated, timed and signed by the ordering physician.

MR 76023
SERIAL 303892646

Hood, John
DOB 03/08/1952 Sex M
ATT James MD, Mary 560

PATIENT IDENTIFICATION PLATE

ALLERGIES:

Date Ordered	Time Ordered	USE BLACK BALL POINT PEN ONLY - PRESS FIRMLY
		Present Weight _____ lbs. _____ kg.
3/6		NPH Insulin 15 U SQ qAM @ 0730
		Digoxin 0.125mg po qd @ 0900
		VancOR 500mg q 6h IVMB
		Tagamet 300mg IVMB q 8h
		M James MD

THE PRESCRIBER AUTHORIZES THE USE OF GENERIC EQUIVALENTS AND AUTOMATIC INTERCHANGE OF APPROVED THERAPEUTIC EQUIVALENT DRUGS UNLESS OTHERWISE NOTED.

FIGURE 11-1
Medication Prescriptions

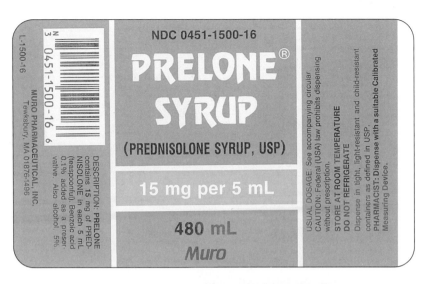
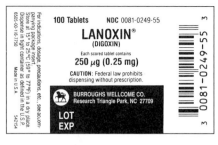
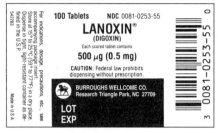
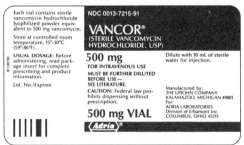
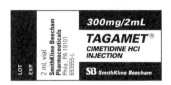

FIGURE 11-2

Medications of Various Quantities

uses. The nurse needs to be knowledgeable of the administration guidelines for each form.

Note the order: *Hycotuss Expectorant™ tsp i pc and HS*. When the medication quantity is ordered, such as an expectorant/antitussive syrup, the order is based on knowledge of the contents of the mass of drug per volume of solution. A solution has two parts: the solute (the drug) and the solvent (the liquid in which the drug is dissolved). Whatever the form of medication, the mass refers to the amount of medication. The volume that follows indicates the amount of solution containing the medication. When preparing to administer the medication, the nurse should have a clear concept of what the volume is that requires preparation. Orders often name the mass of the drug. By interpreting the order and asking yourself, *What will I administer or what is the amount to be prepared,* often it is in terms of the volume that the medication is poured or prepared.

PRACTICE EXERCISE 11.A

In each of the following examples, identify the mass of drug and the quantity or volume in which the mass is supplied.

1. Each tablet contains 50 mg

2. 20 mg per 5 ml

3. gr X per 3 ml

4. 100,000 units per ml

5. 250 mg per ml

7. 100 units per ml

6. Each one capsule contains 500 mg

8. 2 mEq/ml

When the strength or mass of the drug per form supplied by the manufacturer is different from the dose prescribed by the physician, calculation is required. The amount of medication ordered needs to match an available amount per form of medication. Figure 11-2 shows the label for Prelone syrup. Interpret the following example.

EXAMPLE: Ordered: *Prelone syrup 30 mg PT (per tube) q.d.*

On hand: See Figure 11-2 (Prelone syrup)

What will you administer?

$$30 \text{ mg} \times \frac{5 \text{ ml}}{15 \text{ mg}} = 10 \text{ ml}$$

The mass of 30 mg needs to be administered per tube every day. The label indicates that there are 15 mg in every 5 ml. The volume to be administered has been calculated. In order to give 30 mg, you will administer 10 ml.

Route

The route and form for administration requires consideration, as the volume to be administered is calculated. The oral route is abbreviated as po (per oral). For common oral medications, the route may not be included in the order. The assumption is made that the po route is intended. Any questions regarding this interpretation should be resolved before administration. Once a volume is calculated, it needs to be congruent with the form supplied. Other routes of administration are listed in Table 11-1. These routes will be explained in more detail in subsequent chapters. This list reflects the most common routes. (Refer to Appendix 1 for additional terms).

Frequency or Time

The frequency of administration refers to how often the medication should be administered. Medication frequency is based on the therapeutic action of the medication and the desired effect for the individual. Institutional policy often dictates the specific times to be assigned for the common medication frequencies, for example, q.i.d. medications are administered at 9 A.M., 1 P.M., 4 P.M., and 9 P.M. (9-1-4-9). The duration of the administration of a solution may or may not be included in the order depending on the type of order. Drip infusions require hourly rates in the orders. Infusions need to be given in a time frame consistent with the therapeutic action, use, and specific patient needs. Intermittent infusions may or may not have a frequency included in the order. Often their infusion rate is dependent on package information. The specific times for administration are

TABLE 11-1 Medication Administration Routes (Besides Oral)

Intramuscular	IM
Subcutaneous	SC, sc, or SQ
Intravenous	IV
Rectal (per rectal)	PR
Enteral (per feeding tube)	PT

TABLE 11-2 Frequency of Administration

Every day or once per day	QD
Every other day	QOD
Twice per day	BID
Three times per day	TID
Four times per day	QID
As needed	PRN
At hours of sleep or bedtime	HS
Before meals	ac
After meals	pc

set by the nurse transcribing the order. Common abbreviations used are shown in Table 11-2. Nursing implications of administration must be known by the nurse.

PRN (or prn) medications or medications to be administered only as the patient needs them are documented separately from the regular standing medication orders. The total treatment regime of the patient must be assessed prior to the administration of a PRN to determine the appropriateness of the medication.

The time medications are given vary from institution to institution. A typical timetable is shown in Table 11-3.

TABLE 11-3 Institution Frequency Timetable

	0100	0200	0300	0400	0500	0600	0700	0800	0900	1000	1100	1200	1300	1400	1500	1600	1700	1800	1900	2000	2100	2200	2300	2400
QD									♦															
BID									♦												♦			
TID									♦						♦						♦			
QID									♦				♦				♦				♦			
QAM									♦															
QPM																				♦				
AMHS									♦												♦			
QSHIFT							♦									♦								♦
CC							♦					♦				♦								
AC						♦					♦					♦								
PC								♦					♦					♦						
Q2H		♦		♦		♦		♦		♦		♦		♦		♦		♦		♦		♦		♦
Q3H		♦			♦			♦			♦			♦			♦			♦			♦	
Q4H				♦				♦				♦				♦				♦				♦
Q6H						♦						♦						♦						♦
Q8H							♦									♦								♦
Q12H									♦												♦			
Insulin QAM 0730							♦																	
Insulin QPM																	♦							
Insulin (Coverage QID)							0730 ♦				♦					♦					♦			

Physician Prescription

For a medication to be safely administered by nurses, the four parts of the medication order must be provided in the prescription written by the physician. The order must be clearly indicated for the appropriate patient on the order form and dated and signed by the physician. See Figure 11-1 for a sample of a physician order form.

In addition, prescribing guidelines for the specific health care institution or community setting need to be followed. This includes complete and clear written orders on the designated order form. As nurses, we have the responsibility for safe administration; any questions regarding the written order need to be clarified by the physician before the order is acted upon.

Once the order is presented completely and in full, following agency guidelines, it is sent to pharmacy for dispensing.

Transcription

Within health care institutions, the original medication orders are transcribed from the physician order sheet to the medication administration record (MAR) (Figure 11-3). This may be done with the aid of the unit support personnel or it may be a computerized process. When support staff assist with the transcription, nurses must assure the accuracy of the transcribed orders. Medications are most often prepared for administration from the transcribed orders on the MAR. Whenever there is any question regarding the interpretation of the order, the original prescribed order on the physician order sheet is the primary source to consult for clarification. This will be discussed further in Chapter 12.

KEY POINT

A medication order consists of four parts: the medication name, the dosage, the route, and the frequency or time (and duration) of administration. The order must include the signature of the prescribing physician.

The Five Rights of Medication Administration

The goal of medication administration is to administer an *accurate dose* of the *correct medication* by the *ordered route* at the *appropriate time* to the *correct patient*.

KEY POINT

The Five Rights of Medication Administration

1. The right PATIENT

2. The right MEDICATION

3. The right DOSE

4. The right ROUTE

5. The right TIME

H-94268 (Rev. 7/95) ALL ENTRIES MUST BE PRINTED		**ALBANY MEDICAL CENTER HOSPITAL MEDICATION ADMINISTRATION RECORD**													IN PENCIL NUMBER OF FORMS IN USE	
DATE		**MEDICATION - DOSAGE - FREQUENCY RT. OF ADM.**	**HOUR**	3/6	3/7	3/8	3/9	3/10	3/11	3/12	3/13	3/14	3/15	3/16	3/17	3/18	3/19
ORDER	RENEWAL														
3/6		NPH Insulin 15 units SQ q Am	0730 site														
3/6		Digoxin 0.125mg PO qd @ 0900	0900														
3/6		Vancor 500mg q 6h IVMB	0600 1200 1800 2400														
3/6		Tagamet 300mg q 8h IVMB	0800 1600 2400														

SIGNATURE RECORD

SIGNATURE	STATUS	INITIALS	SIGNATURE	STATUS	INITIALS
Mary Stewart	RN	MS			

NAME	ROOM	ALLERGIC TO	DIAGNOSIS	MD
Hood, John	54-1	NONE	Pneumonia	James, M.

FIGURE 11-3

Medication Administration Record

This principle applies to any prescribed therapy whether it be medications, intravenous solutions, parenteral, or enteral therapies. If there is an error, it can be identified that one of the five rights has not been followed.

In addition to the five rights, the patient and/or his or her family should *always be questioned* about any allergies the patient may have. Health care professionals have a responsibility to make sure they assess the allergy status of the individual. Since the number of substances that an individual is allergic to can change with each health care and life experience, this information needs to be updated and documented frequently. Part of the preparation for administration should always include assessing the allergies of the individual.

REMEMBER!

For safe administration always follow the five rights of medication administration. If there is an error, one of the five rights has not been followed for safe administration. Also, check for allergies.

REMEMBER!

As nurses, we have the responsibility for safe administration. Any questions regarding the written order need to be clarified by the physician before the order can be acted upon.

Reading Medication Labels

Medication labels need to be read very carefully. Referring to the medication labels on page 157, note the variety of labels indicating the quantity of medication within the package. Labels will give the name of the medication, mass or quantity of medication with units, lot number and expiration date, manufacturer, and preparation guidelines if they apply. Sometimes this information can be obscure. Medications are administered by determining the volume to be prepared based on the mass of medication. Therefore, reading labels and having the ability to explain the contents of the package are very important.

Selecting Appropriate Strengths

Medications are supplied in many forms. They also are in various concentrations. At times, when choosing between various concentrations it is necessary to consider the convenience and comfort of the patient. If you have a choice, choose volumes or solutions to administer that are smaller and require less effort on the part of the patient. For example, if you can administer the correct dose with one tablet versus two, choose to give the one tablet with the exact amount that has been ordered. Consider what makes sense, what is easier for the patient, and what has less potential for error.

LEARNING ACTIVITIES

The following activities are designed to assist with recognition and calculation of complete medication orders. Answer the questions to prepare for safe administration.

H-90050 (REV. 10/91)

ALBANY MEDICAL CENTER HOSPITAL

Physician's Order Sheet

INSTRUCTIONS:
1. Imprint patient's plate before placing in chart.
2. After each medication order is written, remove first copy and fax to PHARMACY.
3. "X" out remaining unused lines after last copy is used.
4. Imprint new set and place in chart.
5. Each order must be dated, timed and signed by the ordering physician.

MR 65029
SERIAL 202798474
HOLMS, MARY
DOB 02/07/1949 SEX F
ATT BOCK MD, George 640

PATIENT IDENTIFICATION PLATE

ALLERGIES:

Date Ordered	Time Ordered	USE BLACK BALL POINT PEN ONLY - PRESS FIRMLY
		Present Weight ___ lbs. ___ kg.
1/15		Tagamet 800mg po @ HS
		Sinemet 25mg PO TID
		Procan SR 500mg po q 3h
		R. Mach MD

THE PRESCRIBER AUTHORIZES THE USE OF GENERIC EQUIVALENTS AND AUTOMATIC INTERCHANGE OF APPROVED THERAPEUTIC EQUIVALENT DRUGS UNLESS OTHERWISE NOTED.

1. Verify that the four parts of a medication order are present for each prescription written above.

2. Is the patient name and room number clearly identified?

3. What aspects, if any, of the above orders would you potentially have questions about prior to administration and why?

4. Before the orders are transcribed onto the MAR, what will need to be determined?

					DATES ADMINISTERED												IN PENCIL NUMBER OF FORMS IN USE	

H-94268 (Rev. 1/82)

ALBANY MEDICAL CENTER HOSPITAL
MEDICATION ADMINISTRATION RECORD

ALL ENTRIES MUST BE PRINTED

DATE		MEDICATION · DOSAGE · FREQUENCY RT. OF ADM.	HOUR	1/15	1/16	1/17	1/18	1/19	1/20	1/21	1/22	1/23	1/24	1/25	1/26	1/27	1/28
ORDER	RENEWAL																	
1/15		Tagamet 800mg po @ HS	2100	JJ													
1/15		Sinemet 25mg po TID	0900	X	mS												
			1600	JJ													
			2100	JJ													
1/15		Procan SR 500mg po q 3h	0200	X	JN												
			0500	X	JN												
			0800	X	mS												
			1100	X	mS												
			1400	X													
			1700	JJ													
			2000	JJ													
			2300	JJ													

SIGNATURE RECORD

SIGNATURE	STATUS	INITIALS	SIGNATURE	STATUS	INITIALS
Mary Stewart	RN	mS			
Joseu Jones	RN	JJ			
Jill Nap	RN	JN			

NAME Holms, Mary	ROOM 58-1	ALLERGIC TO (RECORD IN RED) NONE	DIAGNOSIS HYPERTENSION	DOCTOR Bock	OP. DATE	DIET RESTRICTIONS BLAND

5. Are all the orders clearly transcribed on the above MAR?

6. What order, if any, would need clarification and how would you accomplish this?

7. You are starting the evening shift at 1500. Is it clear when the last dose of Procan SR was administered?

8. What would you need to ask the nurse previously administering medications before you proceed?

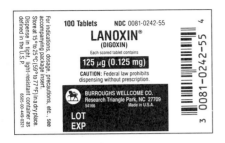
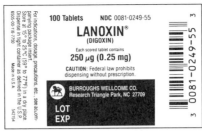
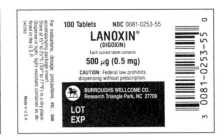

9. What is the mass of the medication in the first figure above?

10. Locate where the expiration date would be recorded during packaging.

11. How many mcg of medication are there in the third label pictured here?

12. Which medication would you choose for the order *Lanoxin 125 mcg po q.d.?*

13. The order reads: Give 2 g po qid. You have available medications in the following concentrations: 125 mg/5 ml and 1 g/10 ml. Which concentration will you choose and why?

14. The order reads: Valium 10 mg po @ HS prn. You have available medications in the following concentrations: Valium 1 mg tabs and Valium 5 mg tabs. Which concentration would you choose and why?

15. The order reads: Meperidine 100 mg IM q4h prn. You have available medications in the following concentrations: Demerol 25 mg/ml and 50 mg/ml. Which concentration would you choose and why?

CHAPTER REVIEW EXERCISES

Interpret the following orders and translate all symbols and abbreviations. Refer to Appendix 1 as needed.

1. Propranolol hydrochloride 40 mg po bid

2. Demerol 50 mg IM q4h prn for pain

3. Acetaminophen 325 mg tabs ii po stat

4. Pilocarpine gtt ii OU q3h

5. Digoxin Elixir 0.25 mg po qd

6. K-lor 30 mEq po bid

7. Heparin 6000 units sc q4h

8. Insulin 15 units sc qd 0730

9. Aspirin gr X po q4h prn for temperature over 101 degrees

10. Prednisone 10 mg po qod

CRITICAL THINKING

1. In each of the following, what is the mass of medication and which is the volume/quantity for administration?

   a. Thorazine 10 mg per 5 ml

   b. Theophylline 200 mg sustained-release tablets

   c. Heparin 1,000 units per ml

   d. Penicillin 1,000,000 units per ml

   e. 1,000 ml 5% dextrose in water

2. Read the following orders. Identify the parts of each order:

   a. Codeine 60 mg po q3h prn

   b. Benadryl Elixir 30 mg po tid

   c. $FeSO_4$ 300 mg po qid

   d. Atropine gr 1/100 IM stat

   e. Vancomycin 1 g IVMB q12h

3. For each of the following labels, determine the mass, volume or how supplied, and generic and trade name:

a.
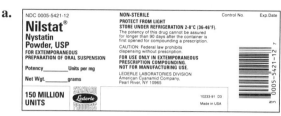

b.
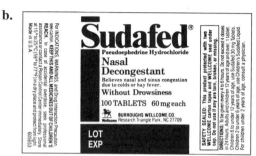

c.
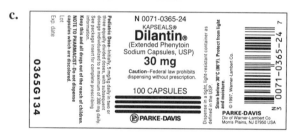

d.
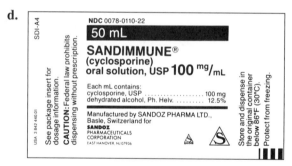

e.
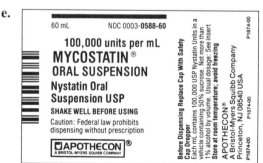

4. Ordered: K-Lor 40 meq po bid

On hand:

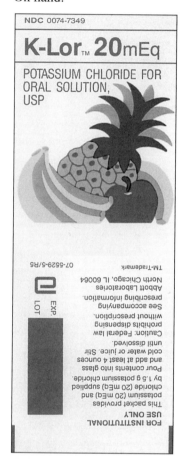

What are the nursing implications of administering this medication?

5. Ordered: Xanax 0.5 mg po HS

On hand: Xanax 0.25 mg tab and Xanax 0.5 mg tab

Which would you choose to administer and why?

6. On hand: Morphine 2 mg/ml; morphine 4 mg/ml; 10 mg/ml; 15 mg/ml

Given the order, Morphine SO$_4$ gr1/4 sc q4h prn, which concentration would you choose? Keep in mind comfort of the patient and ease of administration.

7. You are preparing to administer a medication and find a medication with a similar name, same dose, and preparation for the same route in the drawer for your patient. What do you do?

Medication Administration Records

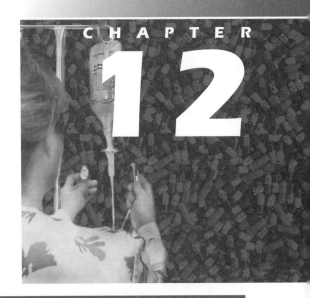

OBJECTIVES

Upon completion of this chapter, you will be able to:

- Describe the purpose of the medication administration record.
- Describe the nursing responsibility for medication administration documentation (computerized and handwritten).
- Explain the principles of medication delivery systems.
- Interpret orders on the medication administration record.
- Explain the three check method utilized to prepare medications for administration.

Introduction

Medication administration records (see Figure 12-1) are part of the patient's health care record. This document provides a permanent record of the prescribed medication treatments the patient received. Whether the patient receives a medication once, receives a single order, or receives regular scheduled medications each day, all medications and prescribed therapies the patient is given must be documented. Parenteral and enteral therapies are often documented on other records such as intake and output records. However, from an aspirin to the additive in an intravenous solution, all prescriptions must be documented.

Reading the Medication Administration Record

The medication record is your guide to the patient's medication regime. This resource provides a record of the medications the patient is receiving, the dose, route, time, and frequency—the five rights—as well as the person who has administered each medication. Because this document reflects the composite of medication therapies that are being given to the patient, an assessment of how well the therapies are working together and their interactions can be made. The record is checked routinely for the last dose administered and the time that the next dose of medications is scheduled to be given.

When preparing to give medications, read the medication administration record (MAR) completely, including the patient name, room number, diagnosis, allergies, and any additional information related to the next dose. A separate section or page of the MAR is used for PRN administration. Read through all the

H-94268 (Rev. 7/95)

ALBANY MEDICAL CENTER HOSPITAL
MEDICATION ADMINISTRATION RECORD

ALL ENTRIES MUST BE PRINTED

IN PENCIL NUMBER OF FORMS IN USE

DATES ADMINISTERED

DATE		MEDICATION - DOSAGE - FREQUENCY RT. OF ADM.	HOUR	3/3	3/4	3/5	3/6	3/7	3/8	3/9							
ORDER	RENEWAL																
3/3		Klor 40 mEg g d	0900	JP	JP												
3/3		Lanoxin 0.125mg po g d (√pulse)	0900	JP	JP												
			Pulse	78	76												
3/3		Elixophyllin 0.49m PO BID	0900	JP	JP												
			2100	MS	JB												
3/3		NPH Insulin 12units SQ g Am	0730	JP	JP												
			site	RA	LA												
3/4		Acetominophen 650mg po g 4h	0900	X	JP												
			1300	X	JP												
			1700	X	JB												
			2100	X	JB												

SIGNATURE RECORD

SIGNATURE	STATUS	INITIALS	SIGNATURE	STATUS	INITIALS
Jane Parter	RN	JP			
Mary Stewart	RN	MS			
John Bogs	RN	JB			

NAME John, Henry ROOM 60-1 ALLERGIC TO Penicillin/ASA DIAGNOSIS CHF PT IS BLIND MD Jackson, M

FIGURE 12-1

Medication Administration Record

orders including the times of administration. Read everything! When first learning to prepare for medication administration, read aloud the entire MAR for clarity, pronunciation of terms, and interpretation of symbols.

Read the MAR each hour of your patient assignment to determine what needs to be administered and how you will plan to achieve this. Changes in orders can occur from one hour to the next. Changes may be communicated to you by other health team members; however, the responsibility for being aware of the change is with the individual assigned to administer medications.

As you read orders for the current hour, read the patient's name and room number, the date, the complete order, and the last recorded time of administration. If any information is unclear, or if the last recorded time of administration is not congruent with the medication schedule, investigate. Clarify any questions that may arise from reading the medication prescription. The physician order sheet remains the primary reference for validating orders.

PRACTICE EXERCISE 12.A

Read the medication administration record in Figure 12-1 aloud and then answer the following questions:

1. What is the patient's last name?
2. What individual patient considerations need to be made when approaching this patient to give him his medication?
3. What are this patient's allergies?
4. When did the patient receive his last dose of K-Lor?
5. Did he get his insulin on time this morning?
6. What medications did the patient receive at 2100 on 3/4? Give the complete order.
7. If you were preparing to administer medications at 1700 on 3/5, what would you administer?

Transcription

The original medication orders are transcribed from the physician order sheet to the MAR. The registered professional nurse is accountable for assuring the accuracy of the transcribed orders. Most medications are prepared for administration from the MAR. The transcription process requires careful consideration of the purpose of the medication and the best timing for the patient based on the rest of the health care regime. Careful attention to spelling and the numbers/quantities used to express the dose are needed. For example, there is a big difference between 0.25 mg and 2.5 mg. Careful placement of decimal points and an extra zero to the left of the decimal can clarify orders greatly. Remember that when MARs are handwritten, the writing needs to be clear and easily read by other health professionals.

Computerized Medication Orders and Transcription

Computerized systems eliminate many concerns related to legibility. These systems provide a mechanism for automatic ordering with the pharmacy at the same time the order is entered in the system by the physician. Access to the system is user dependent. Each health care provider has a user code to enter each time the system is used. The user code dictates the type of access the user has.

Medications may be ordered in these systems in various ways. They may be ordered from a menu of standard prescriptions complete with medication, dose, route, and frequency, or the physician can choose to create his or her own order. Many systems have an alphabetical listing of the hospital formulary from which medications can be chosen. The system will warn against duplication of orders, but does not always safeguard against actual order duplication. Medication orders that are part of ordered protocols are automatically added to the patient's medication regime at the time the protocol is ordered.

The patient's prescribed medication regime can be accessed from more than one display in the computerized information system. The computerized medication record can be accessed as well as a work list of all prescribed nursing interventions to be accomplished over a set period of time on a specific patient. These systems can also provide mechanisms to identify undone work or that which should have been accomplished. For this reason, clinical practice must be in congruence with standard policies entered in the system. For example, if the hospital BID schedule is every 12 hours, 0900 and 2100, but common practice for a specific medication is to give the second dose at 2200, then the system will identify these orders as not given and not in compliance with the system.

One of the best features of these systems is the charting prompt provided to document evaluative notes to administration, for example, charting a response to pain medication after a prn pain medication has been given, or charting the rate, rhythm, and quality of the apical pulse with the administration of digoxin.

When preparing medications, regardless of the system, there must be documentation from which the medication can be prepared. The documentation must provide a mechanism for the nurse to check and double-check the order as it is prepared and administered. Computerized systems provide a printout of the medication administration record and can be double-checked prior to administration at the bedside. These systems can also provide a reference and verification of calculations of complex medication orders.

Medication Delivery Systems

Medications are supplied to the patient care areas within health care institutions according to a variety of delivery systems. Once an order is written, it is most often sent to the pharmacy so that the pharmacist has an accurate record of all the medications and treatments that have an impact on patient outcomes.

The stock supply system is the oldest system. Most medications historically were made available through this system. Today, it is one of the smaller supplies of medications to a patient care area. This decreases the amount of medication available for potential error or overuse. Within each patient care area there is a central supply of medications available. Examples of medications often considered stock are milk of magnesia, acetaminophen, aspirin, and Ducolax.

Narcotics and medications under the controlled substance guidelines are also stock supplied on most hospital units. However, these are under a monitored double-lock system of control. Each dose and all use of this supply is strictly monitored. Computerized systems have improved the monitoring and recording of these potentially harmful medications.

Another system is the individual client supply. With this system, each patient has his or her own labeled section with a medication supply to last several days. The disadvantage of this system is the limited amount of available medication.

The system that is most popular at this time is the unit dose system. Packaging is individualized, by dose, as much as possible (see Figure 12-2). A 24-hour

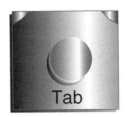

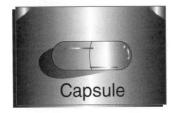

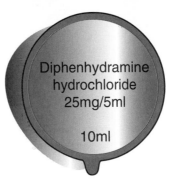

FIGURE 12-2
Unit Dose Packaging

supply is individually prepared. Each patient has their own drawer or compartment, excluding narcotics and refrigerated medications. This system has simplified the amount of calculation and preparation required prior to the administration of medications. More medications come to the patient care unit ready for administration in the dose prescribed and with less required preparation than with previous delivery systems. Many institutions employ a medication cart with individually labeled drawers for each patient that can be wheeled to each patient room. This system has many safety features, for example, singularly packaged medications that can be removed from labeled packages at the bedside prior to administration.

Technological advances continue to redefine systems, reducing the potential for error. Automated dispensing systems, such as the PYXIS system, have revolutionized the dispensing of narcotics. This type of system monitors and controls access and distribution of medications. These systems require personal staff codes to gain access plus patient information to activate opening of the individual drawers of the stacked tool chest–like cart. The controls on the system require answering displayed questions on the view screen, similar to an automated bank teller machine. The medication that is being obtained must be counted and the quantity verified as it is removed from the drawer. This process reduces the time needed to verify the narcotic supply at the end of each shift.

Medication Administration

Read the order. Locate the medication either in the patient's drawer or where it may otherwise be stored, for example, the refrigerator or narcotic cabinet/automated system. Make any necessary calculations. Pour or prepare the medication and read the order again. Compare the complete order to the prepared medication once the medication has been prepared and read the order again.

REMEMBER!

Check the medication order three times with the prepared medication before administration:

1. When removing the medication package from the drawer.
2. Prior to pouring the medication.
3. After preparing the medication.

When administering medications, check the name and room number of the patient on the medication administration record with the name and room number on the room plate. Room numbers should coincide. If the location of the patient has changed, verify changes and modify the MAR appropriately before administration.

After checking the patient room number, greet the patient and explain what you have to give to the patient. Ask the patient his or her name, and check the patient's name band. The patient's name band should be checked prior to each administration. The name band is the best source for assuring the accuracy of delivery to the correct patient.

REMEMBER!

The Five Rights of Medication Administration:

1. The right patient
2. The right medication
3. The right dose
4. The right route
5. The right time

Documentation

Document that the medication has been given by writing your name and/or initialing the appropriate boxes on the MAR immediately after administration. If the MAR is not signed off, there is no way of verifying that medications have been given. If you give a medication at a time different from the time indicated, document the time of administration in the box with your initials. Only sign for what you have given. Never administer what another health care professional has prepared. You are responsible for verifying the medications that you administer, and therefore can only administer and sign for what you give.

Regularly scheduled medications that have not been signed for need to be addressed so that the responsible person can accurately document the administration or give the reason for omitting the dose.

LEARNING ACTIVITIES

1. The patient is asking for pain medication at 2200 on 3/9. What can he have based on the prn medication administration record documentation pictured below?

PRN MEDICATIONS

DATE		NURSE GIVING A PRN MEDICATION ENTERS, NEXT TO THE MEDICATION. VERTICALLY THE DATE-TIME GIVEN AND INITIALS, ROUTE, AND/OR DOSE FOR EACH DOSE ADMINISTERED.
ORDER	RENEWAL	
3/8		Diphenhydramine HCl ⊺–⊺⊺ PO @HS PRN for sleep — 3/03 (2100), 3/9 (2400)
3/8		Acetaminophen 650mg PO q 4h prn
3/8		Meperidine 75mg po q 2h–3 prn for pain — 3/9 0800 JS
3/8		Naproxen 500mg ⊺ q 6-8h pain
3/8		Meperidine HCl 25mg Im q 3-6h PRN for pain — 3/9 0900 JS, 3/9 1300 JS, 3/9 1530 JS, 3/9 1900 JKB
3/8		Hydroxyzine 25mg Im q3-6h PRN — 3/9 0900 JS, 3/9 1300 JS, 3/9 1530 JS, 3/9 1900 JKB

Patient Identification Plate:

MR 95623
SERIAL 624356987
Romano, John
DOB 02/18/25   Sex M
Att. Hackett, Donald   562

SINGLE AND STATS

MEDICATION - DOSE - ROUTE	DATE	TIME	INIT.
MSO4 5mg IV once for pain	3/8	2130	JB

PRE-OPS	DATE	TIME	INIT.

A. NPO FOR SURGERY	E. NON-FORMULARY
B. REFUSED	F. NPO
C. HOLD FOR PHYSICIAN ORDER	G. OTHER CHART IN NURSES NOTES
D. LOA	H. PATIENT TOOK OWN MEDICATION

2. What would your action be if the patient asked for the injection he received the night before in his IV?

3. The patient asks for pain medication but states, "no more shots." What can you offer him?

CHAPTER REVIEW EXERCISES

H-90050 (REV. 10/91)

ALBANY MEDICAL CENTER HOSPITAL

Physician's Order Sheet

INSTRUCTIONS:
1. Imprint patient's plate before placing in chart.
2. After each medication order is written, remove first copy and fax to PHARMACY.
3. "X" out remaining unused lines after last copy is used.
4. Imprint new set and place in chart.
5. Each order must be dated, timed and signed by the ordering physician.

ALLERGIES:

MR 86147
SERIAL 404982658
Lake, Edna
DOB 01/29/26 Sex F
ATT Book MD, Betty 640
PATIENT IDENTIFICATION PLATE

Date Ordered	Time Ordered	USE BLACK BALL POINT PEN ONLY - PRESS FIRMLY
		Present Weight ____ lbs. ____ kg.
3/30		NPH Insulin 12 U q AM
		Digoxin 0.25mg po q AM
		furosemide 40mg po BID
		Tagamet 300mg IV q 6h
		Benadryl 50mg @ HS PRN
		acutaminophen c̄ Codeine 30mg ī - īī q 6h prn
		Docusate Sodium ī PO qd
		Betty Book MD

THE PRESCRIBER AUTHORIZES THE USE OF GENERIC EQUIVALENTS AND AUTOMATIC INTERCHANGE OF APPROVED THERAPEUTIC EQUIVALENT DRUGS UNLESS OTHERWISE NOTED.

1. Using the medication administration record at your institution, transcribe the orders shown on the physician order sheet on the preceding page. Consider the following:

   a. What are the implications of administration that need to be taken into consideration when transcribing these orders?

   b. What times need to be assigned for administration based on hospital policy and the times of other prescribed medications?

   c. If you have access to computerized information systems, print out a medication documentation page. Read the complete page. Study for a complete understanding and clarify any questions related to documented administration.

2. Read the medication administration record on the next page. For each order, interpret the date and time that the next dose is due.

CRITICAL THINKING

1. If you were preparing to administer medications and noted that the last dose was not signed for, what would you do?

2. Why is it important to read and verify the patient's name and room number on all medication documentation?

3. If you were going to prepare the Diphenhydramine HCl 5 ml shown in Figure 12-2, describe when you would perform the three checks.

4. If you had a question about a transcribed medication order, what is the primary source for clarifying the order?

H-94268 (Rev. 7/95)

ALL ENTRIES MUST BE PRINTED

ALBANY MEDICAL CENTER HOSPITAL
MEDICATION ADMINISTRATION RECORD

DATES ADMINISTERED

IN PENCIL
NUMBER
OF FORMS
IN USE

DATE		MEDICATION - DOSAGE - FREQUENCY RT. OF ADM.	HOUR	3/3	3/4	3/5	3/6	3/7	3/8										
ORDER	RENEWAL																		
3/2		KCl 50 meq in	0600	Lg	Lg														
		250 cc D5W over 50min	1800	JM															
3/3		Metronidazole	0900	MT															
		500mg po TID X	1300	MT															
		7 days	2100	JM															
2/28		Procan SR 1.25 g	0200	Lg	Lg														
		q 6 h	0800	MT															
			1400	MT															
			2000	JM															
2/28		Levothyroxine Na	0900	MT															
		0.1 mg po QD																	
2/28		Vitamin A 10,000 units	0900	MT															
		po BID	1700	JM															
2/28		Vitamin C 500 mg po	0900	MT															
		QID	1300	MT															
			1700	JM															
			2100	JM															
3/2		Ofloxacin 200 mg po	0600	Lg	Lg														
		Q 12 h	1800	JM															

SIGNATURE RECORD							
SIGNATURE		STATUS	INITIALS	SIGNATURE		STATUS	INITIALS
Laney Gates		LN	Lg				
Mary Trace		RN	MT				
Jane Mash		RN	JM				

NAME Booker, Margaret	ROOM 59-02	ALLERGIC TO none	DIAGNOSIS Anemia	MD Dr H. Reed

FIGURE 12-3
PRN Medication Administration Record

Oral Medications

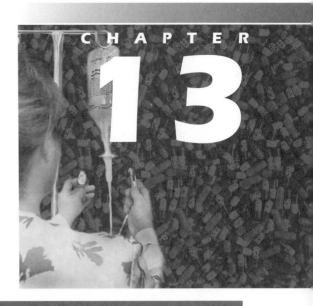

OBJECTIVES

Upon completion of this chapter, you will be able to:

- Explain the various forms of oral medication preparations.
- Apply dimensional analysis to oral medication calculation examples.
- Calculate the amount of oral medication to be administered.
- Assess the appropriateness of calculated answers.

Introduction

Oral medications are supplied in many forms, as well as several strengths or mass quantities. Oral (per oral/po) solid forms of medications include tablets, scored tablets, spansules, capsules, and pills. Liquid forms include solutions, syrups, and elixirs. Whatever the form, calculating and preparing the correct medication in form and dosage is important.

In the following situation, the amount of drug needed versus the amount supplied per tablet requires calculation in order to determine the number of tablets to be administered. The label in Figure 13-1 indicates that these tablets are scored. The tablet can be broken if indicated to prepare the order.

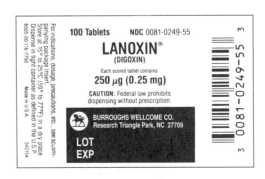

100 Tablets   NDC 0081-0249-55

LANOXIN®
(DIGOXIN)

Each scored tablet contains
250 µg (0.25 mg)

CAUTION: Federal law prohibits
dispensing without prescription.

BURROUGHS WELLCOME CO.
Research Triangle Park, NC 27709

LOT
EXP

For indications, dosage, precautions, etc., see accompanying package insert.
Store at 15° to 25°C (59° to 77°F) in a dry place.
Dispense in tight container as defined in the U.S.P.
Made in U.S.A.
6505-00-116-7750
542154

FIGURE 13-1
Scored Lanoxin Tablet Label

EXAMPLE: The dosage of Lanoxin ordered in Figure 13-2 (order sheet) is 0.125 mg. The medication on hand or supplied in Figure 13-1 is 0.25 mg per scored tablet, which means each tablet contains 0.25 mg of the drug. A calculation needs to be done in order to determine the quantity or number of tablets to be administered accurately for a mass of 0.125 mg.

H-90050 (REV. 10/91)

ALBANY MEDICAL CENTER HOSPITAL
Physician's Order Sheet

INSTRUCTIONS:
1. Imprint patient's plate before placing in chart.
2. After each medication order is written, remove first copy and fax to PHARMACY.
3. "X" out remaining unused lines after last copy is used.
4. Imprint new set and place in chart.
5. Each order must be dated, timed and signed by the ordering physician.

ALLERGIES:

MR 206432
SERIAL 252684564
TOWERS, DONALD
DOB 01/06/1930 Sex M
ATT HUME MD, JANE 530

PATIENT IDENTIFICATION PLATE

Date Ordered	Time Ordered	USE BLACK BALL POINT PEN ONLY - PRESS FIRMLY
		Present Weight ___ lbs. ___ kg.
1/10	0200	Klor 40 meg qd
		Lanoxin 0.125mg po qd
		Elixophyllin 0.4gm po BID
		M. Jackson MD.

THE PRESCRIBER AUTHORIZES THE USE OF GENERIC EQUIVALENTS AND AUTOMATIC INTERCHANGE OF APPROVED THERAPEUTIC EQUIVALENT DRUGS UNLESS OTHERWISE NOTED.

FIGURE 13-2
Physician's Order Sheet

$$\frac{0.125 \text{ mg}}{1} \times \frac{1 \text{ tab}}{0.25 \text{ mg}} = \frac{0.125 \text{ tab}}{0.25} = \frac{1}{2} \text{ tab}$$

Break the tablet for administration.

EXAMPLE: Ordered: Amoxicillin 500 mg po q8h

On hand: Amoxicillin 500 mg/5 ml

What will you administer?

A calculation needs to be done in order to determine the volume to be administered accurately for a mass of 500 mg. This means that each 5 ml contain 500 mg of the drug.

$$\frac{500 \text{ mg}}{1} \times \frac{5 \text{ ml}}{500 \text{ mg}} = \frac{5 \text{ ml}}{1} = 5 \text{ ml}$$

Pour the liquid into a medication cup at eye level.

How many teaspoons is 5 ml? Look on the medicine cup.

$$\frac{5 \text{ ml}}{1} \times \frac{1 \text{ tsp}}{5 \text{ ml}} = 1 \text{ tsp}$$

PRACTICE EXERCISE 13.A

For the following orders, find what is to be administered:

1. Ordered: Aspirin gr X po q4h prn
   On hand: Aspirin 325 mg tablets

2. Ordered: Tagamet 400 mg po hs
   On hand: Tagamet 300 mg per ml

3. Ordered: Codeine gr 1/2 po q3h prn
   On hand: Codeine tablets gr 1/4

Oral Medication Orders

Oral orders will often not include the route of administration. If the route is not indicated in the order, then the assumption is made that the po route is intended. Any question regarding this interpretation should be resolved before preparing the medication for administration.

In general, when calculating oral dosages, question any answer if you calculate more than two tablets, or 1–2 ounces for a solution or syrup. With the variety of manufactured medications and with consideration of the comfort of the patient, most all prescriptions are ordered within this margin. Use this as a safety check when calculating and preparing oral medications for administration.

Preparation of Oral Medications

Once a volume is calculated, it needs to be congruent with the form supplied. If half the tablet is desired and the form of the drug is an enteric-coated pill, prolonged-release tablet, or capsule, which cannot be broken, then another strength of medication needs to be supplied.

Liquid oral medications also require careful preparation. Read accompanying instructions for administration. Some require refrigeration; others are to be shaken well before poured. Liquid medication cups are calibrated to make it easy to prepare and administer this type of medication. When pouring liquid medications, the cup should be placed on a flat surface so that the volume can be verified as it is poured. Bend down at eye level as needed to verify the volume.

There are many forms of medications. Read and know the implications of administration. For example, a sublingual tablet dissolves quickly under the tongue. It is not intended to be swallowed like other tablets.

1. Aluminum hydroxide ℥ i q4h prn is ordered. To what level would you fill the medicine cup? Show the calculation and shade the cup.

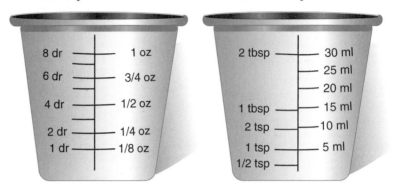

2. Ordered: Diphenhydramine hydrochloride 15 mg po q4h prn

   On hand: Diphenhydramine hydrochloride 12.5 mg/5 ml

   How many teaspoons will you prepare? Is the medicine cup adequate for providing an accurate measure?

3. Review the medication administration record on the next page.

   a. How much prednisone will you give on day 1?

   b. If supplied with 10 mg tablets, what will you give on day 3? Calculate your answer.

   c. What time of day will you administer prednisone on day 5?

REMEMBER!

The Five Rights of Medication Administration
   1. The right patient
   2. The right medication
   3. The right dose
   4. The right route
   5. The right time

REMEMBER!

Check the medication order three times with the prepared medication before administration:
   1. When removing the medication package from the drawer.
   2. Prior to pouring the medication.
   3. After preparing the medication.

H-94268 (Rev. 7/95)

ALBANY MEDICAL CENTER HOSPITAL
MEDICATION ADMINISTRATION RECORD

ALL ENTRIES MUST BE PRINTED

DATES ADMINISTERED

IN PENCIL
NUMBER
OF FORMS
IN USE

DATE ORDER	RENEWAL	MEDICATION - DOSAGE - FREQUENCY RT. OF ADM.	HOUR	3/3	3/4	3/5	3/6	3/7	3/8	3/9	3/10	3/11	3/12				
3/3		Aomoxicillin 250mg	0800	X	MD	1000 SG	MD	MD	MD	SG	SG	SG	SG				
		po Q8h	1600	BY	CC	PD	by	CC	by	PD	PD	PD	PD				
			2400	CC	CC	aw	CC	CC	CC	AW	AW	AW	AW				
3/4		Prednisone 10mg qAM	0900	X	X	SG	MD	X	X	X	X	X	X	X	X		
		X 2days															
		Prednisone 5mg qAM	0900	X	X	X	X	MD	MD	X	X	X	X	X	X		
		X 2days															
		Prednisone 5mg qPm	1600	X	X	PD	by	X	X	X	X	X	X	X	X		
		X 2days															
		Prednisone 5mg po god pm X 2 then D/c	1600	X	X	X	X	X	X	X	by	X	PD	X	X	X	

CHAPTER REVIEW EXERCISES

For problems 1–10, read the questions and use the labels for information if one is supplied. If more than one label is given, describe which you will choose and why. Determine by calculation what you will administer.

1. Ordered: Polymox 0.5 g po TID

   On hand:

   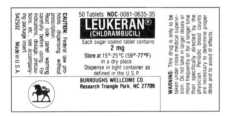

2. Ordered: Leukeran 4 mg po BID

   On hand:

   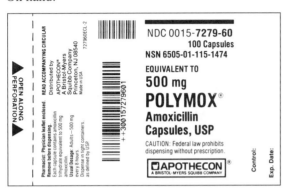

3. Ordered: Lanoxin 0.25 mg po qd

   On hand:

   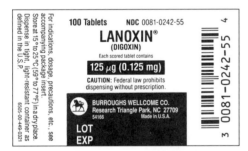

4. Ordered: Tagamet 800 mg po HS

   On hand:

   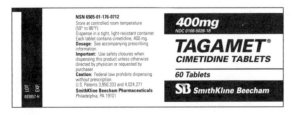

5. Ordered: Mycostatin 1 million units po TID X 48 hours

   On hand:

   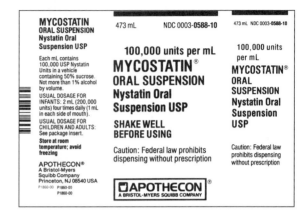

6. Ordered: Dilantin 200 mg BID

   On hand:

   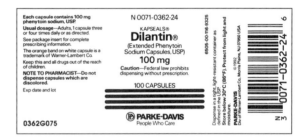

7. Ordered: Theophylline 0.4 g po loading dose

   On hand:

   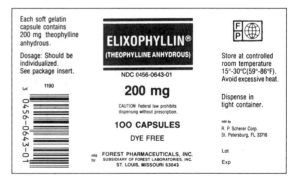

8. Ordered: Prelone syrup 10 mg PO qd

On hand:

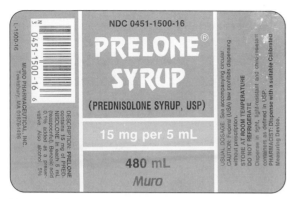

How many teaspoons would you administer?

9. Ordered: Diamox 0.25g q4 hr

On hand:

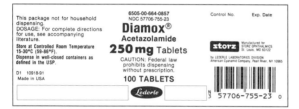

10. Ordered: Procan SR 4,000 mg per day, given in two divided doses

On hand:

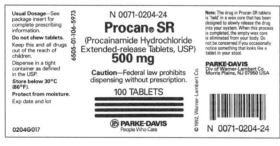

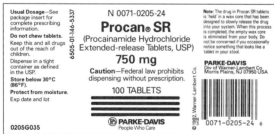

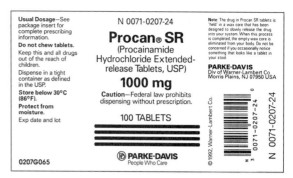

Which strength will you administer?

REMEMBER!

Safety Parameters for Administration

If the amount to be administered is calculated to be:

- More than two tablets po,
- 1–2 ounces po,
- and for parenteral, 2 ml,

question your calculation and/or the order.

The oral medication order is listed for each exercise. Calculate the amount you will give. Show all work. Ask yourself, Does my answer make sense?

11. Ordered: Thorazine 25 mg tid

On hand: Thorazine syrup 10 mg/5 ml

12. Ordered: Lanoxin 0.125 mg po qid

On hand: Lanoxin 0.25 mg scored tablets

13. Ordered: Dilantin 200 mg tid

On hand: Dilantin 100 mg tablets

14. Ordered: Morphine Elixir 15 mg po q4h prn

On hand: Morphine Elixir 20 mg/10 ml

15. Ordered: Levothroid 0.1 mg po qd

On hand: Levothroid 100 mcg/tablet

CRITICAL THINKING

1. You have prepared medications and have three tablets in the medication cup. What actions will you take?

2. When you arrive in a patient's room to administer medications and he does not have a name band, what actions should you take?

3. The patient says to you, "I usually get two diuretic tablets. Where is the other one?" What do you do?

4. You calculate a drug dosage to be one half and the form of the medicine is a sustained-release capsule that is not to be broken. What do you do?

5. You need to prepare 3.3 ml of an oral liquid medicine. How do you accurately measure this volume?

Parenteral Medication Calculations

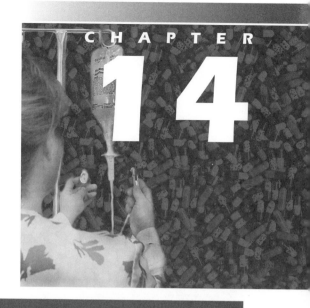

OBJECTIVES

Upon completion of this chapter, you will be able to:

- Describe parenteral routes of administration.
- Utilize concepts of parenteral administration to determine the appropriateness of calculations.
- Apply dimensional analysis to parenteral medication calculation examples.
- Calculate the amount of parenteral medication to be administered.
- Explain the process of reconstitution.
- Assess the appropriateness of calculated answers.

Introduction

Parenteral refers to any medications that are administered via injection. Figure 14-1 illustrates skin layers and muscle, which are common sites for parenteral administration. Table 14-1 identifies the various routes included in the parenteral administration category. Parenteral administration provides the opportunity to deliver medication with a faster rate of absorption than the gastrointestinal (GI) tract. Orally administered medications are affected by food, acidity, and the absorption rate of the GI tract.

Parenteral medications are supplied in many forms: solutions, suspensions, powders, single-dose vials, multiple-dose vials, ampules, prefilled syringes, and

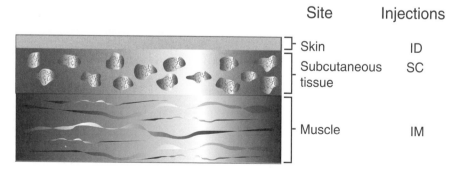

Site	Injections
Skin	ID
Subcutaneous tissue	SC
Muscle	IM

FIGURE 14-1

Skin and Muscle Sites of Parenteral Medication Administration

TABLE 14-1 Parenteral Administration Routes

Intradermal (ID)
Intramuscular (IM)
Intrathecal
Interarticular
Subcutaneous (SC)
Intravenous (IV)
Intracardial

cartridges (Figure 14-2). Preparation for administration includes interpretation of the order in relation to the form of medication supplied.

Common Parenteral Routes

Parenteral medications vary based on the intent of the prescription, size of the client, and specific route of administration.

The intradermal route of injection delivers small quantities, less than 1 ml, into the subcutaneous tissue. This route is desirable for a slow absorption rate.

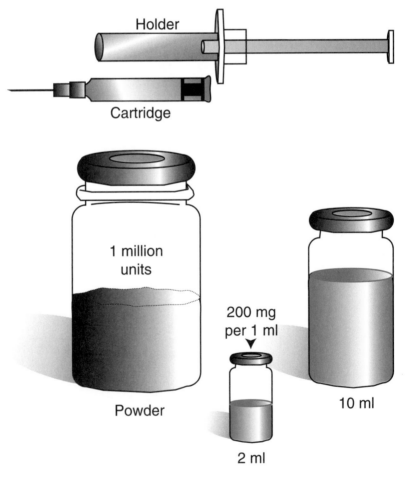

FIGURE 14-2
Parenteral Preparations

For very small volumes—less than 0.5 ml—1 ml syringes with one tenth of 1 cc markings and minim markings assist in preparing an accurate volume. The intradermal route is used for allergy testing and other immunological purposes.

The intramuscular route of injection is for delivering larger quantities for which a greater absorption rate is desired. The larger muscle masses are usually used. The amount of solution per injection should not exceed 2.5 ml. The size of the individual and the development of the major muscles must be taken into consideration. For quantities greater than 2.5 ml, which occur infrequently, the quantity may be split into two syringes and administered in two injection sites.

The intravenous route of administration provides the fastest route for medication absorption. The medication is delivered directly into the venous system and circulated. The amount of medication needed to provide the desired effect is less than for the other routes. It is very important to be aware of the safe ranges for parenteral volumes. The accuracy of the order and the calculated volume to be administered must be double-checked.

In order to deliver volumes of medication into the desired tissues, the correct needle size must be used. Table 14-2 indicates the needle size desired for different routes of administration.

Preparation for Administration

In order to prepare parenteral orders for administration, a relationship should be made between the mass or weight of medication that has been prescribed and the volume to be administered. Orders routinely prescribe a mass of medication; however, syringes are a volumetric measure, and without a conversion to volume, the medication cannot be prepared for administration.

EXAMPLE: Ordered: Meperidine HCl 35 mg IM q4h prn

On hand: Meperidine HCl 50 mg/2 ml in a cartridge

The amount of medication ordered is 35 mg. On hand is a cartridge from which the medication is directly administered. It contains 2 ml of solution in which there is 50 mg of medication. Calculating the volume to be administered:

$$35 \text{ mg} \times \frac{2 \text{ ml}}{50 \text{ mg}} = \frac{14 \text{ ml}}{10} = 1.4 \text{ ml}$$

In order to deliver the amount of medication prescribed, 0.6 ml needs to be discarded from the cartridge.

TABLE 14-2 Needle Sizes for Administration Routes

Route	Volume to Be Administered	Syringe and Needle Size
Intradermal	0.01–0.2 ml	TB syringe 26 g 3/8″
Subcutaneous	0.1–1.0 ml	0.5–3cc 25 1/2″–27 5/8″
Intramuscular	0.5–2.5 ml	3cc 20 1″–22 2″

Reconstitution

Preparation may include reconstitution, which is the addition of a calculated amount of sterile liquid to powders to form a solution prior to preparing the volume to be administered. Reconstitution requires carefully reading the directions included on the box, label, and/or insert of the supplied medication. A diluent, usually sterile water, normal saline, or dextrose 5% water (D5W), is used to transform the solvent into a solution for administration. There are also multi-strength solutions that provide a table or scale of different amounts of diluent to reconstitute based on the desired concentration for the desired amount of administration.

EXAMPLE: Refer to Figure 14-3.

Ordered: Staphcillin 1 g IM

1. How much diluent will you add to prepare Staphcillin 1 g IM for administration? [5.7 ml]

2. What solution will be used as the diluent? [sterile water or sodium chloride]

3. What is the dosage strength of prepared solution? [1 g/2 ml]

4. What volume will you give? [2 ml]

5. How long will the reconstituted solution hold potency? [24 hours at room temperature and 4 days under refrigeration]

6. What information should you indicate on the label? [patient name, room number, time of expiration, and date of expiration]

Units

Some medications are prescribed in units. Units are an expression of the biological action of a drug rather than the actual weight or mass of the drug. Medications expressed in units are heparin, insulin, and some anti-infectives.

Insulin

Unlike other parenteral medications, insulin administration is unique. It is administered in an insulin syringe according to the number of units rather than a calcu-

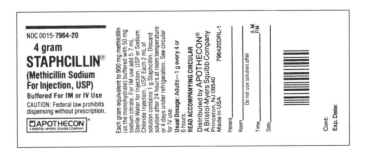

FIGURE 14-3

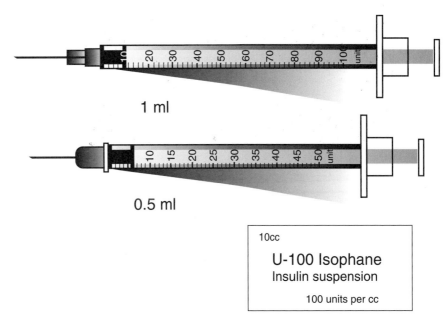

FIGURE 14-4
Insulin Syringes and Label

lated volume (see Figure 14-4). All insulin, no matter what type, is measured and administered in an insulin syringe. Insulin is available in vials in which the concentration is 100 units per 1 cc. Other strengths were once available, but have been phased out. Insulin syringes are utilized for insulin administration in order to accurately prepare the number of units ordered. The calibrations on the 1 ml insulin syringe are in increments of 2 units. The 0.5 ml insulin syringe is in increments of 1 unit. Reading and preparing insulin orders requires special nursing considerations. The client's fasting blood glucose, incremental capillary glucose measures, activity, diet, and types of insulin prescribed need to be monitored. Refer to a pharmacology reference for more information.

KEY POINT

1. Consider the route of administration before preparing the volume to be administered.

2. Consider the patient in relation to the syringe and needle chosen.

3. Ask yourself if your answer makes sense.

REMEMBER!

Question calculated volumes of more than 2–2.5 ml.

PRACTICE EXERCISE 14.A

In each of the following examples, calculate the volume to be administered.

1. Ordered: Hydroxyzine HCl 15 mg IM preop
   On hand: Hydroxyzine 50 mg/1 cc

2. Ordered: Nubain 10 mg sc q4h prn
   On hand: Nubain 10 mg/ml

3. Ordered: Ativan 2 mg IM preop
   On hand: Ativan 2 mg/ml

4. Ordered: Codeine gr 1/2 IM q4h prn
   On hand: 30 mg/ml

5. Ordered: Atropine gr 1/100 sc stat
   On hand: Atropine 1 mg/ml

LEARNING ACTIVITIES

The following activities are designed to assist with developing an awareness of the sizes of syringes and needles in order to determine the appropriateness of calculated answers for the route of administration. With proper supervision and permission, provide syringes and needles in the laboratory setting for review.

1. Determine the volume and incremental markings on syringes supplied.

2. Review various needle sizes.

3. Does the size of the needle get larger or smaller as the gauge of the needle changes?

4. The length of needles is proportional to the site of delivery. Give two examples of needle length and the relationship to the site of delivery.

5. Draw up a volume into a 3 cc syringe. Determine the amount of volume in the syringe to the nearest one tenth of a cc. Most syringes have a plunger with a ring at the top and the bottom. Read the volume at the top ring, which is closest to the volume and reflects the desired measure. The lower ring is part of the barrel.

6. Read the following three examples of prepared syringes below. Determine the prepared volume.

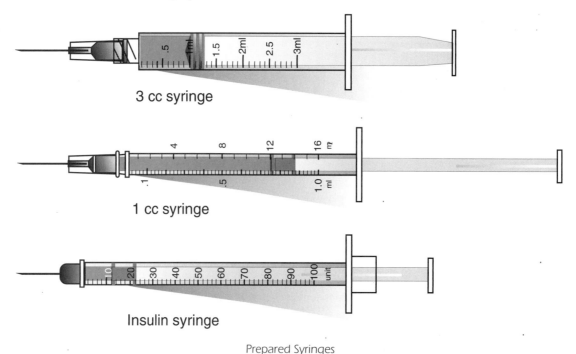

3 cc syringe

1 cc syringe

Insulin syringe

Prepared Syringes

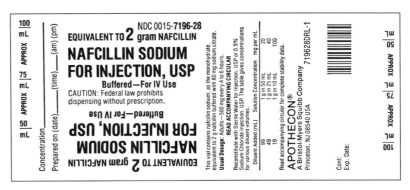

7. Referring to the label above, reconstitute the vial in order to prepare to give the following order of Nafcillin 2 g IV minibag to infuse over 30 minutes.

   a. How many total grams of Nafcillin are in the vial?

   b. What diluent will you add and how much? *Note:* The prepared volume needs to be large enough to be infused over 30 minutes via a programmed IV pump.

   c. What is the dosage per unit after reconstitution?

   d. What is the total amount of solution in the vial after reconstitution?

   e. How much diluent would you add for an order that reads Nafcillin 500 mg IV via 25 ml.

CHAPTER REVIEW EXERCISES

1. Ordered: Morphine sulfate gr 1/5 sc prn

   On hand: Morphine 10 mg/ml

2.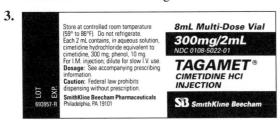

   Ordered: Thorazine 50 mg IM now

3.

   Ordered: Tagamet 300 mg IM q6h

4. Ordered: Ampicillin 250 mg IM q6h

   On hand: Ampicillin 250 mg/ml

   a. What is the route of administration?

   b. What is the volume?

5. Ordered: Penicillin 1.2 million units IM X 1

   On hand: Bicillin L-A 600,000 units per 2 ml tubex

   a. What is the route of administration?

   b. Is the volume to be administered within the safe range for IM injections?

   c. How often is this order to be given?

   d. How is the medication supplied?

CRITICAL THINKING

1. You need to give NPH Insulin 7 units sc. How will you prepare this? What syringe will you use (type and size)?

2. You need to give a volume of 2.0 ml IM to a 70-year-old lady, 5′ and 90 lb. What considerations will you make for the syringe and needle selection?

3. You need to give 1 ml IM. The patient has an excoriated skin condition over both buttocks. The sites commonly used for an IM are the deltoid and gluteus muscles. In this case, what would be the preferred site for administration?

4. Give heparin 5,000 units sc. Prepare from a vial labeled 10,000 units per ml. What will you give? What nursing considerations are specific to heparin administration?

Dosages Based on Body Weight

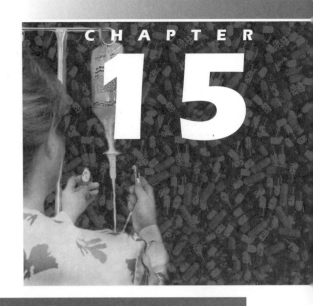

OBJECTIVES

Upon completion of this chapter, you will be able to:

- List situations in which dosages are calculated based on body weight.
- Calculate dosages based on body weight/mass and body surface.
- Discuss age-specific variations for consideration of dosage accuracy.

Introduction

The treatment regime for each individual varies based on age, sex, height, weight, and general health status. For this reason, dosages based on body weight assist in determining a more individualized dose. The distribution and concentration of drugs to all parts of the body are affected by the ratio of the size of the individual to the concentration of the drug (see Figure 15-1). A 5-foot, 90-pound, 65-year-old woman and a 6-foot, 250-pound, 20-year-old man will benefit from very different dosages of the same medication. Within the study of pharmacology, you will learn how medications affect living tissue based on the biochemical and physiological status of the individual.

The prescription is the responsibility of the physician. Typically medication dosing for adults is based on the statistics of the average population. For instance, the average adult dose is determined by the medication effect on 50% of the population who are between 18 and 65. Thus, some prescribing is done with the knowledge of the average dose regime for individuals. Individuals respond differently to therapy. For example, digoxin is a cardiac medication that slows the heart rate and increases the regularity of the heart. The same dose given to the two individuals could have a very different response. The heart rate of the 20-year-old man may be enhanced with no adverse side effects; however, in the 65-year-old woman the same dose may cause the heart rate to slow too much. This individual could exhibit signs of increasing circulatory congestion and problems that would require medical intervention to correct.

Medications are prescribed with consideration of the variation in size and age across the life span. Anyone 12 years old or younger is usually considered to be a child requiring pediatric considerations. Just as adults vary greatly in size, so can children. A 12-month-old child may weigh as little as 16 pounds or as much

185

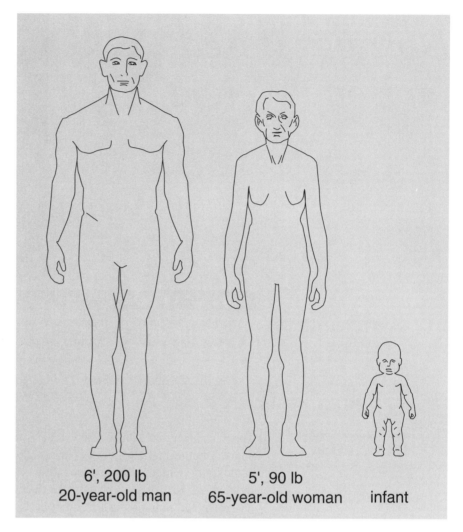

6', 200 lb
20-year-old man

5', 90 lb
65-year-old woman

infant

FIGURE 15-1

as 35 pounds. Children benefit from medications prescribed based on weight. Likewise, a 90-pound adult may benefit from dosages similar to a pediatric dose, avoiding potentially adverse effects from a larger average adult dose. Therefore, many individuals do not fit average parameters. See Chapter 16 for a discussion of pediatric considerations.

Special Therapies

The specialized therapeutic action of some drugs requires dosage determination by body weight. For these therapies, a very exact dose or as minimal a dose as possible should be used due to the severity of adverse effects. Many cardiac medications, antineoplastic medications used in the treatment of cancer, and anti-coagulants used for disorders related to the clotting mechanisms of the blood are examples of medications that are prescribed in this manner. The prescription of these medications will also vary for loading versus maintenance doses.

For this reason, dosages based on body weight assist in determining a more individualized dose. It is the responsibility of the nursing professional to administer medications with the knowledge and accountability for the accurate dose. The nurse must be able to validate dosages according to body weight. Nursing professionals assess, monitor, and evaluate the outcome of administered treatment.

KEY POINT

Purposes of calculating dosage based on body weight:

1. Patient size/type of medication.
2. Validate accurate dosage range.
3. Alter the therapeutic level of the drug.
4. Determine loading or maintenance dosages.

Table 15-1 provides methods for determining body mass.

Total Body Mass

When medication dosages are ordered according to the body mass of the individual, the overall size of the person is taken into account. If the dosage is based on total body weight, then a dosage can be easily computed based on the mass of drug per body mass (see Table 15-1). Milligrams per kilogram (mg/kg) or micrograms per pound (mcg/lb) are the units of measure used for determining the drug mass. Most often you will see kilograms as the body mass unit of measure. If the weight is recorded in pounds and the medication is ordered in relation to kilograms, your equation should include the conversion to kilograms. The nursing implication to be considered is weighing the patient or consulting a current source for the patient's weight. Upon admission to any health care agency or with any health evaluation, the weight is routinely assessed.

Medication calculations, including verification of the dosage in relation to body weight, is often seen in health care today. The height and weight measures are needed with each health care agency visit. Nursing professionals need to validate dosages in relation to the ordered treatment by utilizing their knowledge, reference books, and clinical experts.

TABLE 15-1 Methods for Determining Body Mass Measurements

1. Total body mass—the total mass measurement in units such as pounds, grams, or kilograms.
2. Body surface area—the patient's weight to height ratio is used in conjunction with nomograms to determine a measure in m^2 units.
3. Lean body mass—a formula based on height is used to arrive at a figure in kilograms.

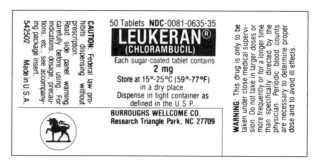

FIGURE 15-2

EXAMPLE: Refer to Figure 15-2.

Ordered: Leukeran 0.03 mg per kg po qd

The client weighs 149½ lb. Referring to the label, the drug is available 2 mg per 1 tab. What will you give? Does your answer make sense?

$$\frac{149½ \text{ lb}}{1} \times \frac{1 \text{ kg}}{2.2 \text{ lb}} \times \frac{0.03 \text{ mg}}{1 \text{ kg}} \times \frac{1 \text{ tab}}{2 \text{ mg}} = 1 \text{ tab}$$

The answer is 1 tab. Note, as indicated throughout this text, the units have been arranged so that the answer will satisfy the question. The question asks, *What will you give?*, not the weight of the individual or the number of milligrams to be administered. Problem solve clinical calculations including body weight carefully and organize the calculation so that the calculated answer is indeed what you are looking for with the one-step method. In examples such as this one, remember that only whole tablets can be administered and only portions of properly scored tablets. Although the arithmetic yielded 1.012, the answer is 1 tab. Remember to ask yourself, *Does my answer make sense?*

PRACTICE EXERCISE 15.A

In each of the following examples, begin by identifying what the units of your answer will be and then proceed with calculating the answer. Remember to use a dimensional analysis equation for each question asked.

1. Ordered: 3 mg/kg po tid, client weight 110 lb

    On hand: 100 mg scored tablets

    a. What will you administer?

    b. What is the dosage (quantity of mg)?

2. Ordered: 50 mcg/lb po qid, client weight 75 lb

    What is the dosage?

3. A patient weighing 132 lb is to receive vinblastine sulfate 0.15 mg/kg IV x 1. How much should you give?

4. Ordered: Heparin 5,800 units IVP (heparin 80 units/kg), client weight 160 lb

    Verify the order by performing the necessary calculations.

5. Ordered: Heparin 6,800 units IVP (heparin 80 units/kg), client weight 85 kg

   Verify the order by performing the necessary calculations.

6. Ordered: 2 mg/kg IM stat, client weight 180 lb

   What will you administer?

7. Ordered: Neomycin sulfate 15 mg/kg, client weight 80 kg

   What is the dosage?

8. Ordered: Nitroprusside sodium 3 mcg/kg, client weight 150 lb

   What is the dosage?

Body Surface Area

Body surface area (BSA) (see Table 15-1) is determined by using a chart or nomogram to interpret the height and weight ratio in terms of the units: square meters (m^2). The chart or nomogram is used to interpret an estimation of body surface area. An example is the chart found on the back of the antineoplastic chemotherapy order sheet (Figure 15-3).

Antineoplastic Chemotherapy

When verifying chemotherapy orders, many factors impact on the dosage determination. It is best to recalculate the BSA from the height and weight. Many references and specialists are available to assist with the verification process. Often institutions require additional education to administer medications from this classification. Antineoplastic agents are administered usually with verification of the dosing by two nurses. The dosage varies depending on regional protocols and the disease process being treated. The rounding off of dosage calculations may be based on the health status of the patient. Dosages are adjusted accordingly with respect to the patient's weight.

EXAMPLE: Cathy weighs 115 kg and is 162 cm tall. She is to receive etoposide 75 mg per square meter BSA.

1. Determine the BSA for Cathy using the chart. The number at the intersection of 115 kg and 162 cm is 1.8 m^2.

2. Calculate the dosage of etoposide that Cathy would receive.

$$\frac{1.8 \ m^2}{1} \times \frac{75 \ mg}{m^2} = 135 \ mg$$

EXAMPLE: The ordered dosage for cisplatin is 86 mg for a 5-foot 11-inch-tall man who weighs 205 lb.

Verify the dosage.

$$5 \ feet \times \frac{12 \ inches}{1 \ foot} = 60 \ inches$$

$$60 \ inches + 11 \ inches = 71 \ inches \ (Total \ height)$$

$$71 \ inches \times \frac{2.54 \ cm}{1 \ inch} = 180.34 \ cm = 180 \ cm$$

$$205 \ lb \times \frac{1 \ kg}{2.2 \ lb} = 93 \ kg$$

ALBANY MEDICAL CENTER HOSPITAL
Antineoplastic Agent Order Sheet
Antineoplastic Agents Must Be Ordered On This Sheet
Include All Information
This Form For One Time Use Only
Use Ball Point Pen

PATIENT IDENTIFICATION PLATE

ALLERGIES:

Date Ordered	Time Ordered	Time Posted	Protocol Name and #

Present Height	in.	cm.	Present Weight	lbs.	kg.	Ideal Weight	kg.	Use lower weight for BSA	BSA	m²

Drug	Dose/m² or kg.	Total Dose	Route of Administration	Schedule

Antiemetic Orders:

None Required: ☐

Laboratory Tests:

None Required: ☐

Expected Adverse Reactions:
(i.e. fever, seizures, hypotension)

Administration and Hydration Orders:

H-95927 (9/85)   M.D. Signature

FIGURE 15-3
Antineoplastic Agent Order Sheet

PATIENT IDENTIFICATION PLATE

Surface area (m²) as a function of height (cm) and weight (kg)　　ECOG

Weight (kg)

Height (cm)	4	6	8	10	12	14	16		18	20	22	24	26	28	30	32	34		36	38	40	44	48	52	56	60
50	0.25	0.31	0.36	0.40	0.44	0.48	0.51		0.54	0.57	0.60	0.63	0.66	0.68	0.71	0.73	0.75		0.78	0.80	0.82	0.86	0.90	0.94	0.97	1.01
55	0.26	0.32	0.37	0.42	0.46	0.50	0.53		0.57	0.60	0.63	0.66	0.68	0.71	0.74	0.76	0.78		0.81	0.83	0.85	0.90	0.94	0.98	1.01	1.05
60	0.27	0.33	0.39	0.43	0.48	0.52	0.55		0.59	0.62	0.65	0.68	0.71	0.74	0.76	0.79	0.81		0.84	0.86	0.88	0.93	0.97	1.01	1.05	1.09
65	0.28	0.34	0.40	0.45	0.49	0.53	0.57		0.61	0.64	0.67	0.70	0.73	0.76	0.79	0.82	0.84		0.87	0.89	0.91	0.96	1.00	1.05	1.09	1.13
70	0.29	0.36	0.41	0.46	0.51	0.55	0.59		0.63	0.66	0.69	0.73	0.76	0.79	0.81	0.84	0.87		0.89	0.92	0.94	0.99	1.04	1.08	1.12	1.16
75	0.30	0.37	0.42	0.48	0.52	0.57	0.61		0.64	0.68	0.71	0.75	0.78	0.81	0.84	0.87	0.89		0.92	0.95	0.97	1.02	1.07	1.11	1.16	1.20
80	0.31	0.38	0.44	0.49	0.54	0.58	0.62		0.66	0.70	0.73	0.77	0.80	0.83	0.86	0.89	0.92		0.95	0.97	1.00	1.05	1.10	1.14	1.19	1.23
85	0.31	0.39	0.45	0.50	0.55	0.60	0.64		0.68	0.72	0.75	0.79	0.82	0.85	0.88	0.91	0.94		0.97	1.00	1.02	1.08	1.13	1.17	1.22	1.26
90	0.32	0.40	0.46	0.51	0.56	0.61	0.65		0.70	0.73	0.77	0.81	0.84	0.87	0.91	0.94	0.97		0.99	1.02	1.05	1.10	1.15	1.20	1.25	1.29
95	0.33	0.40	0.47	0.53	0.58	0.63	0.67		0.71	0.75	0.79	0.83	0.86	0.89	0.93	0.96	0.99		1.02	1.05	1.07	1.13	1.18	1.23	1.28	1.32

Height (cm)	12	14	16	18	20	22	24		26	28	30	32	34	36	38	40	42		44	48	52	56	60	64	68	72
100	0.59	0.64	0.68	0.73	0.77	0.81	0.84		0.88	0.91	0.95	0.98	1.01	1.04	1.07	1.10	1.13		1.15	1.21	1.26	1.30	1.35	1.40	1.44	1.48
105	0.60	0.65	0.70	0.74	0.78	0.82	0.86		0.90	0.93	0.97	1.00	1.03	1.06	1.09	1.12	1.15		1.18	1.23	1.28	1.33	1.38	1.43	1.47	1.52
110	0.61	0.67	0.71	0.76	0.80	0.84	0.88		0.92	0.95	0.99	1.02	1.05	1.08	1.11	1.14	1.17		1.20	1.25	1.31	1.36	1.41	1.45	1.50	1.55
115	0.63	0.68	0.73	0.77	0.81	0.86	0.89		0.93	0.97	1.00	1.04	1.07	1.10	1.13	1.16	1.19		1.22	1.28	1.33	1.38	1.43	1.48	1.53	1.58
120	0.64	0.69	0.74	0.79	0.83	0.87	0.91		0.95	0.99	1.02	1.06	1.09	1.12	1.15	1.19	1.22		1.24	1.30	1.36	1.41	1.46	1.51	1.56	1.60
125	0.65	0.70	0.75	0.80	0.84	0.89	0.93		0.97	1.00	1.04	1.07	1.11	1.14	1.17	1.21	1.24		1.27	1.32	1.38	1.43	1.49	1.54	1.58	1.63
130	0.66	0.71	0.77	0.81	0.86	0.90	0.94		0.98	1.02	1.06	1.09	1.13	1.16	1.19	1.23	1.26		1.29	1.35	1.40	1.46	1.51	1.56	1.61	1.66
135	0.67	0.73	0.78	0.83	0.87	0.92	0.96		1.00	1.04	1.07	1.11	1.15	1.18	1.21	1.25	1.28		1.31	1.37	1.43	1.48	1.53	1.59	1.64	1.69
140	0.68	0.74	0.79	0.84	0.89	0.93	0.97		1.01	1.05	1.09	1.13	1.16	1.20	1.23	1.26	1.30		1.33	1.39	1.45	1.50	1.56	1.61	1.66	1.71
145	0.69	0.75	0.80	0.85	0.90	0.94	0.99		1.03	1.07	1.11	1.14	1.18	1.22	1.25	1.28	1.32		1.35	1.41	1.47	1.53	1.58	1.64	1.69	1.74

Height (cm)	30	34	38	42	46	50	54		58	62	66	70	74	78	82	86	90		94	98	102	106	110	114	118	122
150	1.12	1.20	1.27	1.34	1.40	1.46	1.52		1.58	1.63	1.69	1.74	1.79	1.84	1.88	1.93	1.98		2.02	2.07	2.11	2.15	2.19	2.23	2.27	2.31
155	1.14	1.21	1.29	1.35	1.42	1.48	1.54		1.60	1.65	1.71	1.76	1.81	1.86	1.91	1.96	2.00		2.05	2.09	2.14	2.18	2.22	2.26	2.30	2.34
160	1.15	1.23	1.30	1.37	1.44	1.50	1.56		1.62	1.68	1.73	1.78	1.84	1.89	1.94	1.98	2.03		2.08	2.12	2.17	2.21	2.25	2.29	2.34	2.38
165	1.17	1.25	1.32	1.39	1.46	1.52	1.58		1.64	1.70	1.75	1.81	1.86	1.91	1.96	2.01	2.06		2.10	2.15	2.19	2.24	2.28	2.32	2.37	2.41
170	1.18	1.26	1.34	1.41	1.48	1.54	1.60		1.66	1.72	1.78	1.83	1.88	1.94	1.99	2.04	2.08		2.13	2.18	2.22	2.27	2.31	2.35	2.40	2.44
175	1.20	1.28	1.35	1.43	1.49	1.56	1.62		1.68	1.74	1.80	1.85	1.91	1.96	2.01	2.06	2.11		2.16	2.20	2.25	2.30	2.34	2.38	2.43	2.47
180	1.21	1.29	1.37	1.44	1.51	1.58	1.64		1.70	1.76	1.82	1.88	1.93	1.98	2.04	2.09	2.13		2.18	2.23	2.28	2.32	2.37	2.41	2.45	2.50

Height (cm)	40	44	48	52	56	60	64		68	72	76	80	84	88	92	96	100		104	108	112	116	120	124	128	132
185	1.42	1.49	1.56	1.63	1.69	1.75	1.81		1.87	1.93	1.98	2.03	2.08	2.13	2.18	2.23	2.28		2.33	2.37	2.42	2.46	2.50	2.55	2.59	2.63
190	1.44	1.51	1.58	1.65	1.71	1.77	1.83		1.89	1.95	2.00	2.06	2.11	2.16	2.21	2.26	2.31		2.35	2.40	2.44	2.49	2.53	2.58	2.62	2.66
195	1.45	1.53	1.60	1.67	1.73	1.79	1.85		1.91	1.97	2.02	2.08	2.13	2.18	2.23	2.28	2.33		2.38	2.43	2.47	2.52	2.56	2.60	2.65	2.69
200	1.47	1.54	1.62	1.68	1.75	1.81	1.87		1.93	1.99	2.05	2.10	2.15	2.21	2.26	2.31	2.36		2.40	2.45	2.50	2.54	2.59	2.63	2.68	2.72
205	1.49	1.56	1.63	1.70	1.77	1.83	1.89		1.95	2.01	2.07	2.12	2.18	2.23	2.28	2.33	2.38		2.43	2.48	2.52	2.57	2.62	2.66	2.70	2.75
210	1.50	1.58	1.65	1.72	1.79	1.85	1.91		1.97	2.03	2.09	2.14	2.20	2.25	2.30	2.36	2.41		2.45	2.50	2.55	2.60	2.64	2.69	2.73	2.77
215	1.52	1.59	1.67	1.74	1.80	1.87	1.93		1.99	2.05	2.11	2.17	2.22	2.27	2.33	2.38	2.43		2.48	2.53	2.58	2.62	2.67	2.71	2.76	2.80
220	1.53	1.61	1.68	1.75	1.82	1.89	1.95		2.01	2.07	2.13	2.19	2.24	2.30	2.35	2.40	2.45		2.50	2.55	2.60	2.65	2.69	2.74	2.79	2.83

HEIGHT CALCULATION:

_____cm = 2.54 x _____in.

WEIGHT CALCULATION:

_____kg. = _____lbs ÷ 2.2

IDEAL BODY WEIGHT CALCULATION:

IBW MALE = 50 kg + 2.3 kg x each inch greater than 5 feet

_____kg = 50 kg + 2.3 kg x _____in.

IBW FEMALE = 45.5 kg + 2.3 kg x each inch greater than 5 feet

_____kg = 45.5 kg + 2.3 kg x _____in.

Referring to the table on the Antineoplastic Agent Order Sheet:

$$180 \text{ cm and } 93 \text{ kg} \rightarrow \text{BSA of } 2.16 \text{ m}^2$$

The cisplatin regional dose parameters are cisplatin 40 mg per m²:

$$2.16 \text{ m}^2 \times \frac{40 \text{ mg}}{1 \text{ m}^2} = 86 \text{ mg}$$

The calculation verifies the dosage ordered.

EXAMPLE: The ordered dosage for cisplatin is 40 mg/m². The total dose is 60 mg IVMB Day #1 administered over 1 hour. The patient is a 5-foot 2-inch-tall woman who weighs 110 lb. Is this dose within acceptable administration parameters?

$$5 \text{ feet} \times \frac{12 \text{ inches}}{1 \text{ foot}} = 60 \text{ inches}$$

$$60 \text{ inches} + 2 \text{ inches} = 62 \text{ inches (Total height)}$$

$$62 \text{ inches} \times \frac{2.54 \text{ cm}}{1 \text{ inch}} = 157.48 \text{ cm}$$

$$= 157 \text{ cm}$$

$$110 \text{ lb} \times \frac{1 \text{ kg}}{2.2 \text{ lb}} = 50 \text{ kg}$$

Referring to the table on the Antineoplastic Agent Order Sheet:

$$157 \text{ cm and } 50 \text{ kg} \rightarrow \text{BSA of } 1.48 \text{ m}^2$$

The cisplatin regional dose parameters are cisplatin 40 mg per m²:

$$1.48 \text{ m}^2 \times \frac{40 \text{ mg}}{\text{m}^2} = 60 \text{ mg}$$

The calculation verifies the dosage ordered.

PRACTICE EXERCISE 15.B

In each of the following examples, begin by identifying what the units of your answer will be and then proceed to verify the dosage ordered. When verifying your calculated dose, your value may be approximate to the dose that has been rounded for ease of administration.

1. Patient height: 155 cm, weight: 46 kg

   a. What is the BSA in m², using the chart on the Antineoplastic Agent Order Sheet?

   b. The patient is ordered Taxol 135 mg/m². If the patient is ordered a total dose of 200 mg, does your calculation match?

2. Patient height: 5′5″, weight: 171.5 lb

   a. What is the BSA in m², using the chart on the Antineoplastic Agent Order Sheet?

   b. Verify the following order. Compare your calculation to the ordered total dose:

   Doxorubicin 50 mg/m², total dose ordered: 90 mg

3. Patient height: 68.5 inches, weight: 168 lb, BSA 1.7 m^2

   Ordered: Chemotherapy 3 g/m^2. The total dose ordered is 5.7 g.

   Verify the ordered dose.

4. Patient height: 5′9″, weight 135 lb, BSA 1.7 m^2

   Ordered: Chemotherapy 425 mg/m^2. The total dose ordered is 725 mg.

   Verify the ordered dose.

5. Patient height: 65 inches, weight: 136 lb, BSA 1.7 m^2

   Ordered: Chemotherapy 25 g/m^2. The total dose ordered is 40 mg.

   Verify the ordered dose.

6. BSA 1.7 m^2

   Ordered: Chemotherapy 100 mg/m^2. The total dose ordered is 170 mg.

   Ordered: Chemotherapy 200 mg/m^2. The total dose ordered is 350 mg.

   Verify the ordered dose.

7. BSA 2.08 m^2

   Ordered: Chemotherapy 60 mg/m^2. The total dose ordered is 125 mg.

   Ordered: Chemotherapy 125 mg/m^2. The total dose ordered is 250 mg.

   Verify the ordered dose.

Lean Body Mass

Formulas may be used to convert the body height and weight into a mass amount depending on the type of medication. Lean body mass (LBM) (see Table 15-1) is used to determine dosages for medications poorly distributed and absorbed by adipose tissue. For drugs of this type, LBM measures assure that the amount of drug prescribed matches the amount of lean tissue. This measure is determined by height. Someone who weighs 205 lb and someone who weighs 145 lb of the same sex and height still have the same amount of lean body mass. If the dosage for the 205 lb person was based on the total body weight, then the concentration of the drug would be too high in the nonadipose tissue part of the body. Examples of drugs poorly distributed into the adipose tissue are digoxin, heparin, and many of the aminoglycoside antibiotics.

> **KEY POINT**
>
> Lean Body Mass Formula
>
>   Male: 50 kg + 2.5 kg for each inch over 5 feet
>
>   Female: 45.5 kg + 2.3 kg for each inch over 5 feet

Calculate the dosage based on the lean body mass or ideal body weight of the patient. If the patient is debilitated and underweight, the actual body weight is used to determine dosages for drugs that do not penetrate fat.

EXAMPLE: Calculate the lean body mass of a woman who is 5′2″ and
weighs 180 lb.

$$LBM = 45.5 \text{ kg } (1) + 2.3 (2)$$
$$= 45.5 \text{ kg} + 4.6$$
$$= 50.1 \text{ kg}$$

PRACTICE EXERCISE 15.C

In each of the following examples, begin by identifying what the units of your answer will be and then proceed with calculating the answer.

1. Ordered: 2 mg/kg IM stat, client: female, weight 180 lb, height 5′4″

   On hand: 40 mg/ml

   Based on a lean body mass (LBM) calculation, how much will you administer?

2. Ordered: Heparin 5,200 units IVP, client: male, weight 220 lb, height 5′6″

   a. Find the lean body mass.

   b. The dosage is 80 units/kg. Verify the order for 5,100 units IVP.

3. Ordered: 20 mg/kg, client: male, weight 210 lb, height 5′2″.

   a. Find the lean body mass.

   b. What is the dosage?

4. Ordered: Heparin 6,800 units IVP initial bolus, client: female, weight 187 lb, height 5′6″.

   Verify the order for 6,800 units IVP (80 units/kg)

Administration Considerations

Administration of medications based on body weight is not unlike administering any other medications. Incidentally, medications calculated in this manner are either more toxic or the therapeutic response is more variable. For this reason, dosages and calculations are made under close scrutiny of other resources and often additional checking procedures exist. It is good practice to ask for consultation and verification of another nurse to confirm your calculated dosage.

REMEMBER!

Always evaluate your answer. Stop and ask yourself, *Does the answer make sense?* Always employ the five rights of administration.

Daily Dosages

The following activities are designed to assist with problem-solving dosages involving daily dosages. Daily dosages are the total amount of drug ordered per day (a 24-hour period). To compute daily dosages, consider a 24-hour dosage versus the amount given per one dosage. Your equation needs to reflect this measurement. What would be an example of units of your answer for a daily dose calculation?

EXAMPLE: Ordered: 5 mcg/kg/day in four equal doses, client weight 150 lb

On hand: 0.2 mg scored tablets

1. Find the daily dose. What will be the unit of the answer?

   The unit of the answer is mcg/day.

   $$\frac{150 \text{ lb}}{1 \text{ day}} \times \frac{1 \text{ kg}}{2.2 \text{ lb}} \times \frac{5 \text{ mcg}}{1 \text{ kg}} = 341 \text{ mcg/day}$$

   Interpreting mcg/kg/day as mcg/kg per day, the day unit is placed consistently under the weight unit in order to complete the fractional form. You can loosely identify that on the given day the patient does weigh 150 lb; therefore, 150 lb per day. Note as demonstrated before, units are divided to solve for the desired answer. The answer computed is 340.90 and is rounded to 341 mcg/day. It is important to maintain a focus on the units for which you are solving.

2. Find the individual dose. What will be the unit of the answer?

   The unit of the answer is mcg/dose.

   $$\frac{341 \text{ mcg}}{1 \text{ day}} \times \frac{1 \text{ day}}{4 \text{ doses}} = \frac{85.25 \text{ mcg}}{\text{dose}}$$

3. What will you administer?

   $$\frac{85.25 \text{ mcg}}{\text{dose}} \times \frac{1 \text{ mg}}{1,000 \text{ mcg}} \times \frac{1 \text{ tab}}{0.2 \text{ mg}} = \text{}^1/_2 \text{ tab}$$

PRACTICE EXERCISE 15.D

1. Ordered: 250 mg/m² tid, client weight 61 kg and height 78 inches
   a. Determine the BSA using the chart on the Antineoplastic Agent Order Sheet.
   b. Calculate the amount of drug per dose.
   c. How much will the client receive in 1 day?

2. A 115 lb female patient who is 162 cm tall with a BSA of 1.5 m² has the following order for an antineoplastic agent: 140 mg in 500 cc NS IV over 1h QD x 5.

   On hand: 20 mg/ml
   a. What will you administer?
   b. The recommended IV range is 50–100 mg/m²/day. Is this order within range?

3. Ordered: 300 mg po qid

   On hand: A reference book indicates the recommended dosage is 1 to 2 grams/day.

   Is this medication order in the recommended range?

LEARNING ACTIVITIES

1. What would be the daily dose if a 157½ lb patient were to receive a nitrofurantoin oral suspension 5 mg/kg/day po in four divided doses? On hand is 5 mg per ml. How many ml will be given at each dose?

2. The physician orders an antibiotic to be given IM q6 hours. The drug label reads 1 gram/2.5 ml and the adult dosage is 15 mg/kg/day.

   a. What is the 24-hour dosage?

   b. What is the amount per dose of antibiotic for a 50 kg woman?

   c. What would you administer?

3. The physician orders phenobarbital 4 mg/kg/day IM in three divided doses. The phenobarbital is supplied 65 mg/ml. The man weighs 165 lb.

   a. What is the 24-hour dosage?

   b. What will you administer?

CHAPTER REVIEW EXERCISES

1. A patient is to receive 0.01 mg/kg, and the patient weighs 180 lb. What will you administer?

2. How much do you give if a patient is to receive a medication at a dose of 2.5 mg/kg po qd and the patient weighs 110 lb?

3. A patient weighing 132 lb is to receive vinblastine sulfate 0.15 mg/kg IV x 1. How much will you give?

4. A 155 lb patient has the following order for an initial dose:

   Ordered: Purinethol 2.5 mg/kg/d po x 1 followed by Purinethol 90 mg/m²/d po

On hand:

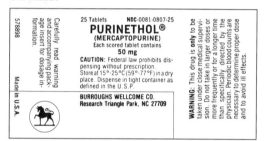

a. What will you administer for the initial dose?

b. If the patient has a BSA of 1.7 m², what will be the dosage for the subsequent dose?

c. What will you administer for the subsequent dose?

CRITICAL THINKING

1. Ordered: 250 mg/m² tid, client weight 61 kg, height 78 inches

   a. Determine the BSA using the chart on the Antineoplastic Agent Order Sheet.

   b. Calculate the amount of drug per dose.

2. Jane weighs 130 lb. She has recently had surgery and has an order for 5 mg morphine IM q4h PRN for pain. The product information indicates that a safe dose is 0.05 to 0.2 mg/kg. Is the dose ordered within the safe range?

3. A physician orders an aminoglycoside antibiotic at a dose of 2 mg/kg IM now, and then a maintenance dose of 1 mg/kg q8 hours. The client is a 70-year-old male who is 6 feet tall and weighs 225 lb.

   a. What is the lean body mass for this individual?

   b. Using the mass determined above, what is the initial dose?

   c. What is the maintenance dose?

   d. What will be the total daily maintenance dose?

4. The dosage ordered is 0.5 mcg IM q2 hours. The patient weighs 220 lb. The medication reference indicates a dosage of 0.04 to 0.05 mcg/kg/day. Is this ordered dosage in the recommended range? In this question two separate equations may need to be calculated. Why?

5. A 185 lb female patient who is 5′8″ tall has the following order for a parenteral antibiotic:

   Ordered: 100 mg IV q8h

   On hand: 40 mg/ml

   a. What is the daily dosage?

   b. The recommended range is 3–5 mg/kg/day. Is this order within the recommended range?

   c. What will you administer?

6. A 115 lb female patient who is 162 cm tall with a BSA of 1.5 m^2 has the following order for an antineoplastic agent:

   140 mg in 500 cc NS IV over 1h QD x 5.

   On hand: 20 mg/ml

   a. What will you administer?

   b. The recommended IV range is 50–100 mg/m^2/day. Is this order within range?

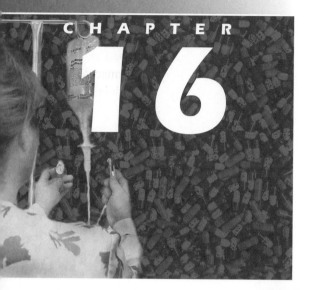

Pediatric Dosages Based on Body Weight

OBJECTIVES

Upon completion of this chapter, you will be able to:

- Calculate pediatric dosages based on body weight.
- Discuss age-specific variations for consideration of dosage accuracy.

Introduction

The administration of medication to the pediatric population is best met by following the concept presented in Chapter 15: basing calculations on body weight. The height and weight of children must be assessed with each health care agency visit due to their growing patterns. The nursing/health science considerations for administration go beyond the scope of this book. Professionals need to validate dosages by utilizing their knowledge, reference books, and clinical experts as needed. Drug dosages are adjusted in proportion to body mass in order to maintain a desired drug concentration in individuals of various sizes. An average (6–12 years) pediatric dose is, relatively speaking, one half of the average adult dose. However, the dose should *never* be determined on this basis. Infants and children of the same age may vary greatly in their size. A 12-month-old child may weigh as little as 16 pounds or as much as 35 pounds. Infants and children benefit from medications prescribed based on weight.

> **KEY POINT**
>
> Very lean patients, very obese patients, and children require special consideration. Drug dosages for these individuals are frequently determined on the basis of the *amount of drug per kilogram of body weight or body surface area.*

As we have contended throughout this text, our one method for calculating eliminates the need to memorize additional formulas. Clark's, Young's, and Fried's Rules can be used to check the safety of dosages, but not to calculate dosages.

Administration

Pediatric medications, when administered orally, are given via the most appropriate volumetric container (Figure 16-1). Many products are on the market to assist with easier administration, for example, the elongated hollowed spoon, droppers, and syringe-like cylinders. Please refer to a pediatric or pharmacology text for more specific information on safety rules, administration techniques, and the nursing implications of administration to the pediatric population.

REMEMBER!
Always evaluate your answer. Stop and ask yourself, *Does the answer make sense?*

A drug dosage is adjusted in proportion to body mass in order to maintain a desired drug concentration in individuals of various sizes.

PRACTICE EXERCISE 16.A

1. Ordered: 50 mcg/lb po qid, client weight: 75 lb

   a. What is the dosage?

   b. How many mg is this?

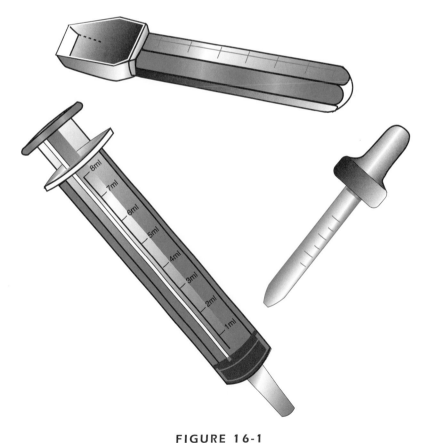

FIGURE 16-1
Pediatric Medication Administration Devices

2. Ordered: 3 mg/kg po tid, client weight: 110 lb

On hand: 100 mg scored tablets

a. What will you administer?

b. What is the dosage?

3. The physician orders an antibiotic to be given IM q6 hours. The drug label reads 1 gram/2.5 ml and the normal pediatric dosage is 100 mg/kg/day.

a. What is the child's 24-hour dosage?

b. What is the amount per dosage of antibiotic for a child weighing 20 kg?

c. What would you administer?

Body Surface Area

Body surface area (BSA) is determined by using a chart to interpret the height and weight ratio in terms of the units: square meters (m^2). A nomogram is used to interpret an estimation of BSA.

West's nomogram (see Figure 16-2) is frequently used for pediatric conversions. The boxed column is used when the weight of the child is known and the child is of normal height. The quantity intersecting the surface area column on a straight line drawn corresponding to the height and weight of the individual represents the measurement for the individual in m^2. There are other nomograms for both children and adults.

EXAMPLE: Cathy weighs 50 pounds and is 46 inches tall. She is to receive daunorubicin 25 mg IV per square meter BSA and vincristine 1.5 mg IV per square meter BSA today.

1. Determine the BSA for Cathy using the nomogram.
Using a straight edge, the number representing the intersection of 50 pounds and 46 inches is 0.86 m^2.

2. Calculate the dosage of daunorubicin that Cathy would receive:

$$\frac{0.86 \text{ m}^2}{1} \times \frac{25 \text{ mg}}{\text{m}^2} = 21.5 \text{ mg}$$

3. Calculate the dosage of vincristine for Cathy:

$$\frac{0.86 \text{ m}^2}{1} \times \frac{1.5 \text{ mg}}{1 \text{ m}^2} = 1.2 \text{ mg}$$

LEARNING ACTIVITIES

In each of the following examples, begin by identifying what the units of your answer will be and then proceed with calculating the answer.

1. Ordered: 250 mg/m^2 tid, client weight 32 kg and height 134 cm

Using Figure 16-2, determine the BSA from the nomogram.

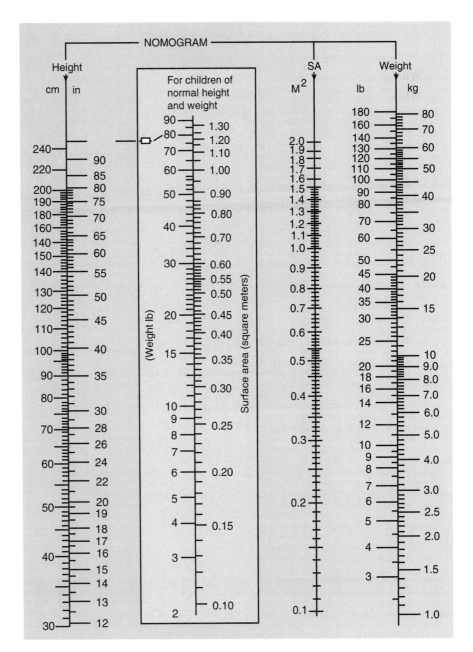

FIGURE 16-2

West's Nomogram for Estimation of Body Surface Area. Reprinted with permission from Behrman, R. E., Kliegman, R. M., and Ervin, A. M. *Nelson Textbook of Pediatrics,* 15th ed., W. B. Saunders Company, Philadelphia, PA 19105.

2. Ordered 150 mg/m^2 tid, client weight 40 lb and height 32 inches

   a. Determine the BSA from the nomogram.

   b. Calculate the amount of drug per dose.

   c. How much will the child receive in 1 day?

CHAPTER REVIEW EXERCISES

1. A 5½-month-old child weighing 40 pounds has been receiving acetaminophen 2 tabs every 6 hours for the past 48 hours. The child's mother tells you that the medication label reads to give 120 mg every 4 to 6 hours and not to exceed 2.6 g/day. Each tablet contains 80 mg.

   a. Is she giving the child an amount that falls within the recommended range?

   b. In another reference you find the dosage for a 5-year-old to be 10 mg/kg/day. What recommendations can you make regarding the mother's current dosing?

2. The physician orders phenobarbital 4 mg/kg/day IM. The phenobarbital is supplied 65 mg/ml. The child weighs 30 lb.

   a. What is the 24-hour dosage?

   b. What will you administer?

3. A 12-year-old patient weighing 70 pounds has the following order for hormone therapy:

   Ordered: 0.06 mg/kg IM q3d

   On hand: 1 mg/ml in a 5 ml vial (when reconstituted)

   What will you administer?

4. Theophylline is ordered for a 10-year-old child who weighs 72 lb. The loading dose is 6 mg/kg and the maintenance dose is 3 mg/kg every 6 hours. The medication is available in 100 mg and 200 mg capsules.

   a. What will you administer for a loading dose?

   b. What will you administer for a maintenance dose?

5. A 25 lb child has an order for an antibiotic 100 mg/kg/day qid.

   On hand: 1 g/25 ml

   a. What is the daily dosage?

   b. What is the amount per dose?

6. Ordered: 10 mg/kg/day IV in 4 divided doses

   Patient weight: 20 kg

   a. What is the daily dosage?

   b. What is the individual dose?

7. Ordered: Ibuprofen 5 mg/kg PO every 4–6 hours

   Patient weight: 60 lb

   a. What is the individual dose?

   b. If the maximum daily dose is 40 mg/kg and the patient has already had three doses today, can she have another dose today?

8. An 1,100 g neonate has an order for erythromycin 50 mg/kg/day in four divided doses.

   a. What is the daily dosage?

   b. What is the individual dose?

CRITICAL THINKING

1. A 60 lb male patient has the following order:

   Ordered: Ativan 2 mg IM preop

   The recommended dosage is 0.05 mg/kg up to 4 mg. Is the dosage ordered closer to the minimum or the maximum dosage?

2. Jane weighs 36 lb. She has recently had surgery and has an order for 2 mg morphine q4h PRN for pain. The product information indicates that a safe dose is 0.05 to 0.2 mg/kg. Is the dose ordered within the safe range?

3. A 4-year-old weighs 36 lb.

   Ordered: Morphine 0.1 mg/kg sc

   On hand: Morphine individual vials 2 mg/1 ml and 4 mg/1 ml

   a. What is the dosage?

   b. What will you choose to administer and how much?

4. a. What would be the daily dose if a 57½ lb patient were to receive a nitrofurantoin oral suspension 5 mg/kg/day po in four divided doses? On hand is 5 mg per ml.

   b. How many ml will be given at each dose?

Intravenous and Other Solution Calculations

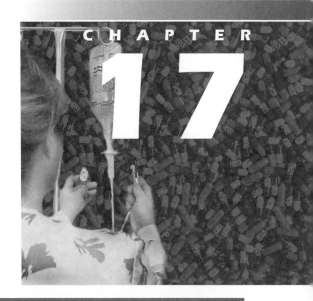

CHAPTER 17

OBJECTIVES

Upon completion of this chapter, you will be able to:

- Calculate infusion set rates for administration.
- Calculate hourly infusion rates.
- Calculate rate settings for infusion pumps.
- Calculate the duration of infusions.
- Recognize the different types of infusions.
- Assess the appropriateness of calculated answers.

Introduction

Infusions are continuous volumes of solution entering the body according to a prescribed rate of flow by way of a catheter, which is a soft plastic tube inserted into the venous system (Figure 17-1). These infusion devices may be placed into the peripheral or central vasculature depending on the needs of the patient and the types of solutions or medications prescribed. Infusions are delivered by rate and are used to treat a variety of conditions. Eighty percent of hospital patients receive some sort of infusion therapy and many infusions are also delivered in the home setting. Rate as previously discussed is an amount, mass or volume, per time—for example, gtt/min, ml/hr, mg/min. Regardless of the type of infusion, the problem-solving process for calculating rates of infusion remains the same.

Infusion Set Administration

When interpreting the prescription for administration, the infusion rate is calculated in relation to the equipment for delivery. Infusion sets are manufactured with a variety of drip chamber sizes. The size of the drip chamber and therefore the size of the drops delivered by the infusion set depend on the features of the tubing specific to the manufacturer. The product information needs to be consulted for the drop factor, which is based on the size of the drops created by the configuration of the drip chamber (Figure 17-2). The drop factor is the number of drops that are equal to 1 cubic centimeter. The unit of measure for the drop factor is gtt/cc. Macrodrip tubing delivers larger drops, either 10, 12, 15, or 20 drops per 1 cubic centimeter. Microdrip or minidrip infusion sets are calibrated to deliver 60 drops per 1 cubic centimeter. This type of tubing is used when smaller

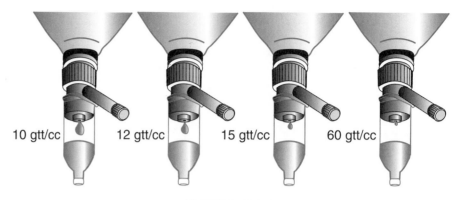

FIGURE 17-2
Variety of Drop Factors

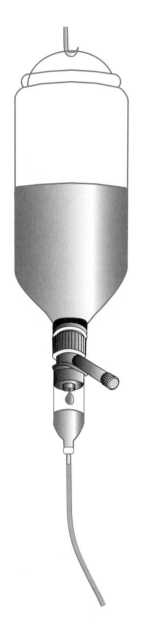

FIGURE 17-1
Intravenous Fluid and Tubing

volumes and slower rates of more toxic medications have been ordered. Micro-drips are also used with the pediatric population.

In order to administer the prescribed volume via the infusion set, the drop rate must be calculated. Most infusion therapy is ordered by volume per time. The prescriber does not usually consider the specific administration techniques or equipment. The order is based on a need for the fluid or medication according to the needs of the client, for example, 1,000 cc normal saline over 8 hours. It is the health care provider's responsibility to calculate the drip rate for monitoring the infusion. The following example illustrates solving for gtt/min. Start with the order and calculate according to the principles you have learned thus far.

EXAMPLE: Ordered: 1,000 cc normal saline over 8 hours

    a. How much volume is ordered to be infused in 8 hours?

        1,000 cc of normal saline

    b. If the infusion is delivered via an infusion set with a drop factor of 15 gtt/cc, what would be the drip rate?

$$\frac{1,000 \text{ cc}}{8 \text{ hr}} \times \frac{15 \text{ gtt}}{1 \text{ cc}} \times \frac{1 \text{ hr}}{60 \text{ min}} = 31.2 \approx \frac{31 \text{ gtt}}{\text{min}}$$

    Does your answer make sense?

    c. How much volume is ordered to be infused each hour?

$$\frac{1,000 \text{ cc}}{8 \text{ hr}} = \frac{125 \text{ cc}}{\text{hr}}$$

Via an infusion set, the IV is monitored by observing the number of drops that fall into the drip chamber. The computation needs to be rounded to a whole number because a partial drop cannot be counted. For the infusion to remain on time, 31 drops need to fall into the drip chamber over 1 minute. Health professionals, maximizing use of time, often monitor the drops for a 15-second time period and then multiply the amount by 4 to arrive at a quantity for 1 minute. For this time period, approximately 7 drops would be expected to drop in the drip chamber. Until the accurate rate is achieved, often the rate will need to be counted repeatedly. Infusions require vigilant monitoring and evaluation to ensure that the solution is delivered according to the prescription via the calculated rate.

> **KEY POINT**
>
> **1.** What is the *total amount of solution* to be infused?
>
> **2.** What is the *type of solution* or medication?
>
> **3.** What is the *time period* over which the volume needs to be infused?
>
> **4.** What is the *method of delivery* or type of equipment to be used?
>
> **5.** What is the *calculated rate of the infusion?*

PRACTICE EXERCISE 17.A

In each of the following examples, calculate the drop rate:

  1. Ordered: 1,000 cc of D5W over 8 hours, drop factor 15 gtt/ml

  2. Ordered: 500 ml 0.9% NS over 8 hours, drop factor 15 gtt/ml

  3. Ordered: D5W 100 ml/hr, drop factor 10 gtt/ml

  4. Ordered: D5 1/2 NS 150 ml/hr for 4 hours, then decrease to 125 ml/hr, drop factor 12 gtt/ml

  5. Ordered: 1,000 cc NS @ 75 cc/hr, drop factor 20 gtt/ml

  6. Ordered: 1,000 cc D5 1/4NS @ 20 ml/hr via microdrip infusion set

  7. Ordered: D5 NS @ 60 cc/hr via microdrip infusion set

  8. Ordered: D5 1/2 NSc̄ 20 mEq KCl @ 125 cc/hr, drop factor 10 gtt/ml

  9. Ordered: 1,000 cc D5 1/2 NS increase to 200 cc/hr × 4 hours, then 125 cc/hr, drop factor 15 gtt/ml

10. Ordered: D2 1/2 + 1/2 NS @ 80 cc/hr × 3 liters, may d/c when taking po, drop factor 20 gtt/cc

---

Infusion Pumps

Many infusions, regardless of the type, are delivered via an infusion pump. Depending on the solution and the acuity of the patient, the decision as to how an infusion is delivered is often a nursing judgment. There are many types of pumps produced by many manufacturers; however, most of them deliver the volume based on cubic centimeters per hour (cc/hr). Pumps are also programmed to monitor the amount to be infused. This setting is dialed to indicate the total volume in the infusion bag to be administered. This assists the nurse in monitoring and reporting the infused volume. For the same example previously discussed, determine the cc/hr in order to set the pump.

EXAMPLE: If the order in the previous example, 1,000 cc normal saline over 8 hours, was delivered via an infusion pump that monitors in units of cc/hr, what would be the rate setting in cc/hr on the machine? 125 cc/hr

$$\frac{1,000 \text{ cc}}{8 \text{ hr}} = \frac{125 \text{ cc}}{\text{hr}}$$

As you work with infusions and the variety of rates that can be prescribed, remember to stop and ask yourself, *What will be the units of my answer? Does my answer makes sense?* Determine what will be the units of your answer before proceeding.

PRACTICE EXERCISE 17.B

In each of the following examples, calculate the hourly rate for infusion pump administration. Also determine the amount to be infused to be indicated on the pump setting.

1. Ordered: 500 cc D5W to run 12 hours

2. Ordered: 1,000 cc D5/0.45 NS q8 hours continuously

3. Ordered: 500 ml NS to run over 8 hours

4. Ordered: 100 ml D5W to infuse over 2 hours

5. Ordered: 1,000 ml NS to run 7 hours

6. Ordered: 200 ml 0.9% NS over 60 minutes

7. Ordered: 1,000 cc D5 1/2NS c 20 mEq KCl to run over 12 hours

8. Ordered: 1000 cc D5 1/2NS over 10 hours

9. Ordered: 50 ml over 30 minutes

10. Ordered: 150 ml over 30 minutes

REMEMBER!

An infusion is calculated based on various quantities per amount of time:

cc/hr—infusion pumps provide monitoring of the hourly rates and information regarding infused volumes or volumes to be infused based on programming of the pump settings.

gtt/min—the drop factor must be known in order to calculate the drop rate.

Flow Meters

Flow meters or time tapes may be used to monitor an infusion (Figure 17-3). Flow meters are paper strips applied to the length of the infusion bag that indicate where the level of the solution should be at hourly intervals. They provide a quick reference for verifying if the infusion is on time. A flow meter can be made with tape or obtained from infusion companies. Commercially prepared flow meters often have color-coded columns or striping to discriminate one hourly rate from another. Regardless of the administration equipment chosen, the infusion requires monitoring, assessment, and evaluation.

Monitoring Infusions

Infusions need to be evaluated and monitored closely to verify that an accurate volume is being delivered at the prescribed rate. Although drop rates, hourly rates, and containers are assessed, the client needs to be evaluated to be sure that the intended response of the therapy is occurring. Assessment of the infusion for accurate delivery is a nursing responsibility. Factors such as the position of the patient, the activity of the patient, and the height of the infusion can affect the rate of the infusion. If the intravenous infusion started at 0900, vigilant nursing would assess the infusion periodically to verify that the infusion remained on time. If the

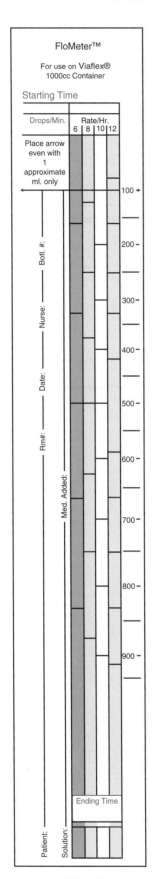

FIGURE 17-3
Commercially Prepared Flow Meter

infusion remained on time, at 1400, one half of the 1,000 cc of D5%W or 500 cc would have infused. If the infusion was not on time, other nursing interventions would need to take place to keep the prescribed order on time.

The following infusion examples require utilization of problem-solving skills. These questions are designed for you to consider at what point the solution will be during various points of delivery, and when the infusion will finish.

EXAMPLE: Calculate the drip rate of 1,000 cc of D5W to infuse over 10 hours, using an infusion set that delivers 15 gtt/ml:

$$\frac{1,000 \text{ cc}}{10 \text{ hr}} \times \frac{15 \text{ gtt}}{1 \text{ cc}} \times \frac{1 \text{ hr}}{60 \text{ min}} = \frac{25 \text{ gtt}}{\text{min}}$$

This IV was started at 4 A.M. At 10 A.M. 600 ml remain in the bottle. Is the IV on time?

First calculate the hourly rate:

$$\frac{1,000 \text{ cc}}{10 \text{ hr}} = \frac{100 \text{ cc}}{\text{hr}}$$

Consider that from 4 A.M. to 10 A.M. is 6 hours, so the amount that is expected to be infused is:

$$\frac{6 \text{ hr}}{1} \times \frac{100 \text{ cc}}{1 \text{ hr}} = 600 \text{ cc infused}$$

The actual amount infused is:

$$1000 \text{ cc} - 600 \text{ cc} = 400 \text{ cc infused}$$

So, the IV is infusing too slowly.

Recalculating the drip rate will assist in infusing the volume in the time prescribed. However, the patient may not tolerate a faster rate. Consider the patient's condition before adjusting the infusion rate. To recalculate, solve for the remaining volume to be infused in the remaining time:

$$\frac{600 \text{ cc}}{4 \text{ hr}} \times \frac{15 \text{ gtt}}{1 \text{ cc}} \times \frac{1 \text{ hr}}{60 \text{ min}} = \frac{38 \text{ gtt}}{\text{min}}$$

a. Administer 500 ml of D5 NS over 8 hours. What is the hourly rate? How much should be infused in 3 hours?

b. Administer 1,000 ml D5W over 8 hours via a drop factor of 20 gtt/ml. If the IV is started at 1400, when should the volume be infused? At 1800, 400 ml is left in the IV bag. Is the IV on time? If the IV is not on time, recalculate the drip rate.

c. Administer 1,000 cc D5 1/2NS via a 20 gtt/ml infusion set at 150 cc/hr for 4 hours, then decrease to 125 cc/hr. What is the initial drip rate? After 4 hours, how much is left in the bag? At the new rate, how long will it take the bag to finish? What is the new drip rate?

Primary and Secondary Infusions

Primary infusions are prescribed for replacing body fluids and maintaining body fluids in a balanced solution. Usually these volumes are ordered in larger quantities and are delivered over a long period of time, for example, NS 1,000 cc/8 hours continuously, such as the examples discussed in this chapter thus far.

Secondary infusions are an intermittent therapy usually prescribed for another purpose than replacement of fluid or electrolytes. Various conditions require medications and solutions that can best help the patient if delivered via the parenteral route. Prescriptions for this purpose are ordered with the same requirements as any other medication. Usually the volumes are much smaller and the time period over which they are administered is much shorter. The primary line is the point of access for the secondary infusion. For these reasons, this type of infusion is referred to as a minibag or piggyback infusion, for example, Cefazolin 1 g IVMB q 8 hours (see Figure 17-4). The rate of the secondary line infusion depends on the administration implications of the medication. The rate is calculated and the secondary infusion is administered according to the required rate.

This system of administration for the secondary line, by utilizing gravity and height, allows the secondary infusion to run rather than the primary line even though the primary line is not shut off. When the secondary line finishes and the level of the solution in the secondary line is at the level of the primary line drip chamber, the primary line starts to flow again. The implication here is to take note of when the secondary line is due to finish so that adjustments can be made in the rate of flow. The roller clamp on the primary line is the regulator for the infusion of both lines. If the rate of the secondary line is different than the primary infusion, which is often the case, the rate needs to then be adjusted back to the rate of the primary line. If these infusions are on an infusion pump, the indicators can be set for the primary and secondary infusions. The indicator for the amount to be infused for the secondary infusion assists in monitoring the completion of the minibag so that the rate of the primary line can be reestablished as soon as the minibag is completed.

Other Infusions

In addition to common intravenous solutions, hyperalimentation or total parenteral nutrition (TPN) is an infusion administered via a central port. This solution provides a balanced nutrition of carbohydrates, amino acids, vitamins, and minerals. Note the prescribed infusion in Figure 17-5.

Enteral feedings are delivered via the gastrointestinal tract. They are not a parenteral infusion. However, the rate of flow is calculated and monitored the same. These feedings may be delivered via the nasogastric route to various junctures along the gastrointestinal system. Gastrostomy tubes and jejunostomy tubes deliver feedings directly into these parts of the gastrointestinal tract. The prescriptions for these types of infusions are calculated similarly so that the rate may be administered via the intended route, to the right patient at the prescribed frequency. These therapies must also be delivered according to the five rights. Note the prescribed infusion in Figure 17-6.

Some orders for infusions of medication are prescribed in the mass unit of the drug per minute, for example, 50 mg nitroglycerine in 500 ml @ 50 mcg/min, or mass units of the drug per body weight, per time, for example, dopamine HCl IV @ 5 mcg/kg/min. These prescriptions need to be interpreted and calculated to be administered via an infusion pump. Chapter 18 will address these calculations.

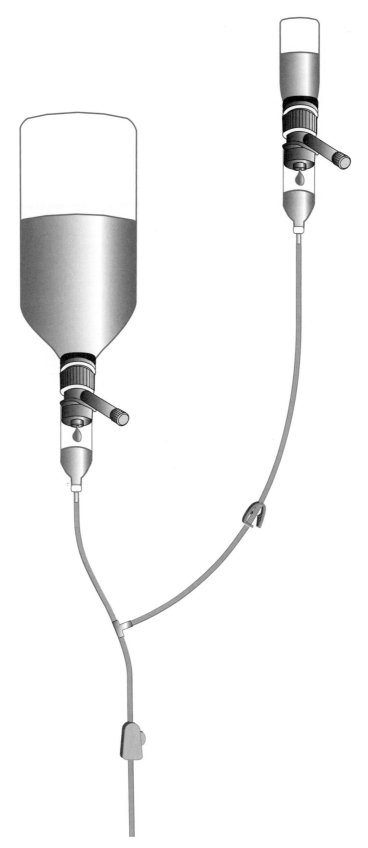

FIGURE 17-4
Secondary Line Piggybacked to Primary Line

11-29-95

ALBANY MEDICAL CENTER HOSPITAL
ADULT
PARENTERAL NUTRITION ORDER SHEET
Each order has 24-hr. automatic stop
unless specified here x ___**3**___ days.
Standard start time for ordered solution is 1700
Standard multivitamins and trace elements added daily
Infusion rate will vary with volume, infuse at rate on label

ALLERGIES: ___*None*___

Start 11/30/95

D4E 454
MR 9765498
Bird, Clara
DOB 02/19/67   Sex F
Att. Rogers, B

Patient Identification Plate

A.   STANDARD DEXTROSE-AMINO ACID SOLUTIONS (Amount supplied per day)
Circle mode of delivery and check box for desired solution

TOTAL PROTEIN/DEX KCAL	PROTEIN G	DEX G	MINIMUM VOLUME(L)	RATE GIVEN OVER 24 HR	Na mEq	K mEq	Cl mEq	Ac mEq	Mg mEq	P mM	Ca mEq
PERIPHERAL / CENTRAL / PICC SOLUTION											
☐ 500	50	90	1.5	63ml/hr	60	55	60	95	9	25	10
CENTRAL / PICC SOLUTIONS											
☐ 1000	65	220	1.5	63ml/hr	55	45	55	110	8	23	10
☐ 1250	75	280	1.5	63ml/hr	60	55	60	125	9	25	10
☐ 1500	75	350	1.5	63ml/hr	60	55	60	125	9	25	10
☐ 1750	75	430	2.0	84ml/hr	60	55	60	125	9	25	10
☒ 2000	75	470	2.0	84ml/hr	60	55	60	125	9	25	10

Standard electrolytes added unless options chosen below.

B.   NON-STANDARD DEXTROSE-AMINO ACID SOLUTIONS
☐ Central   ☐ Peripheral - (check desired concentration of dextrose) ☐ 50 g/liter   ☐ 75 g/liter .
(a) Dextrose ___*400*___ g/day (maximum dextrose concentration = 350g/L)
(b) Protein ___*100*___ g/day
(c) Standard electrolytes added, unless specified below (Section C)
(d) Volume & rate options - order below (Section D)
(e) Fat (optional) - order below (Section E)

C.   ELECTROLYTE OPTIONS AND OTHER ADDITIVES (Check one):
Optional additives will be added to above electrolytes unless checked below:
☐ Give only additives listed below.

OPTIONAL ADDITIVES (designate amount to be added per day)

Sodium chloride ___*30*___ mEq	Sodium phosphate* _____ mEq	Sodium acetate _____ mEq	
Potassium chloride _____ mEq	Potassium phosphate* ___*10*___ mEq	Potassium acetate _____ mEq	
Magnesium (sulfate) ___*5*___ mEq	Calcium (gluconate) _____ mEq	Vitamin K _____ mg	
Human insulin _____ units	Other: *B12 1mg Zn 10mg Pepcid 40mg 5/300mcg*		

*(1mEqNaPO4 = 23mgP = 0.75mMP and 1mEq KPO4 = 21mg P = 0.68mMP)

D.   VOLUME AND RATE OPTIONS
Dextrose/Amino Acid solution dispensed in minimum volume or volume specified below whichever is greater.
For specific volume needs, please check options desired/day:
☐ 1 L (42ml/hr)   ☐ 1.5 L (63ml/hr)   ☒ 2 L (84ml/hr)   ☐ 3 L (125 ml/hr)   ☐ _____ L
Dextrose/Amino Acid solution infused over 24 hours unless otherwise specified:
Cycle _____ Liters over ___*24*___ hours

E.   FAT EMULSION (check desired g/day of fat to be given)   **INFUSE FAT OVER *20* HOURS**
(No fat dispensed unless dose specified below)   (recommended infusion time ≥ 12hr)
☐ 20g   ☐ 50g   ☐ 70g   ☒ 100g   Other _____
(100ml, 200kcal)   (250ml, 500kcal)   (350ml, 700kcal)   (500ml, 1000kcal)

F.   OTHER INSTRUCTIONS _____

Date Ordered	Time Ordered	Time Posted	Order must be received in pharmacy by 1200
11/29/95	*10 am*		**Physician Signature** *B. Rogers MD*

FIGURE 17-5
Example of Parenteral Nutrition Order

11-17-95

D4E 451

MR 8762345

Burns, Cora

DOB 5/7/64   Sex F

Att. Rogers, B

Patient Identification Plate

ALBANY MEDICAL CENTER HOSPITAL

ADULT TUBE FEEDING ORDERING FORM
ORDERS MUST BE RECEIVED IN FOOD AND NUTRITION SERVICES BY 1200

Attention Nursing: For new Orders after 1200, refer to the
Materials Management Quick Reference Guide

A.   TYPE OF TUBE FOR INSERTION:
[X] Small-bore weighted feeding tube OR_____

B.   SELECT TYPE OF PRODUCT NEEDED: *See Reverse for indications
[X] STANDARD FORMULA (1.0 Kcal/ml)

[ ] Low Protein	[ ] Fluid Restricted (2.0 Kcal/ml)
[ ] High Protein	[ ] Partially Hydrolyzed
[ ] Fiber Enriched	[ ] Other _____

C.   ADMINISTRATION AND RATE OF INFUSION:

    ** A New Order Form must be completed daily until final volume is reached.
    ** Please Check Mode of Tube Feeding Desired AND Select One Rate/ Volume Per Day

[X] CONTINUOUS FEEDING

    [ ] **DAY ONE:** Start feeding at 25 ml/hr full strength. Increase 20 ml/hr q 8 hrs (1080 ml/day 1)
              OR until reach *65* ml/hr.   **Order discontinued after 24 hours**

    [ ] **OTHER** _____
    [ ] **DAY TWO:** Advance feeding by 20 ml/hr q 8 hrs (2520ml/day 2)
              OR until reach _____ml/hr.   **Order discontinued after 24 hours**
    [ ] **FINAL RATE/VOLUME:** Continue feeding at _____ml/hr., over _____hrs., and _____ml/day.
    [ ] Flush tube with 30 ml sterile water q 4 hours OR _____q shift.

[ ] **BOLUS FEEDING:** NG/G tube Only. Bolus rate not to exceed 100 ml over 5 minutes.
    [ ] **FIRST DAY:** Start feeding 120 ml/feeding at full strength q 3 hours between 0600 to
            2200 OR _____. Advance by 120 ml/feeding to maximum of
            360 ml/feeding OR _____.Order discontinued after 24 hours.
    [ ] **OTHER RATE/VOLUME:** _____
    [ ] **FINAL RATE/VOLUME:** _____ml/feeding, _____ ml/day, and _____ feedings/day.
    [ ] Flush tube with 50 ml sterile water or _____before and after each feeding.

D.   [ ] DISCONTINUE TUBE FEEDING.

E.   MONITORING AND PLACEMENT STANDARD ORDERS:
    ** Check Box Only if Non Standard Options Desired

    Chest X-ray after insertion to verify placement of small bore weighted feeding tube (MD must complete requisition).
    Dietitian consult.
    Check residuals per Nursing protocol. Notify MD for persistent residuals > 200 ml, cramping, distention, nausea, vomiting, diarrhea, OR [ ] Other_____
    Record weight on Monday, Wednesday, and Friday.
    Monitor Input/ Output for 7 days.
    Daily Profile I and PO4 X 3 days. Fingerstick glucose q shift X 2 days, continue if glucose > 240 mg/dl.

    [ ] Baseline CBC with differential, Profile II, and Mg + + (if not documented within past 72 hours).
    [ ] Other Labs _____

B. Rogers, MD	*11/17/95*	*1810*
PHYSICIAN SIGNATURE	**DATE**	**TIME**

FIGURE 17-6
Example of an Adult Tube Feeding Order Form

LEARNING ACTIVITIES

1. Utilizing the supplied equipment, adjust the infusions to the drip rates calculated in Practice Exercise 17.A. Equipment needed includes wristwatch with second hand, IV bags, infusion sets (micro and macro), and sink or waste receptacle in which to allow the solution to run.

2. Infusions require careful monitoring. Flow meters provide a means of monitoring the start, duration, and stop time of an infusion. Some institutions utilize flow meters or time tapes to provide a mechanism to assess the level of solution in the container in relation to time. Commercially prepared flow meters (Figure 17-3) are available from some companies with their infusion products. However, one can easily be made by following these steps:

Making a Time Tape
A physician orders an IV of 1,000 cc of D5W started on your patient to infuse over 8 hours. The IV is started at 0900. The drop factor is 10 gtt/cc. Prepare a flow meter. Perform the calculations required to complete the flow meter.

   a. Cut a piece of tape lengthwise the size of the infusion container.

   b. Place the tape on the container lengthwise to include the level of solution when the container is full. The tape should also be long enough to include the level of solution at the lowest point.

   c. Indicate the date, rate of the infusion, start time, and completion time.

   d. Draw a vertical line on the tape at the level indicating a full 1,000 cc in the bag at the start time. (If a tape is initiated at another time besides when the bag is hung, indicate the level of the solution when you begin the time tape monitoring.) This technique is usually used for primary infusions.

   e. Calculate the hourly rate. Draw successive lines to indicate the level of the solution at each hourly interval based on the hourly rate.

   f. Indicate the completion time.

CHAPTER REVIEW EXERCISES

For the following orders, answer these questions:

   a. What is the total amount of solution to be infused?

   b. What is the type of solution or medication?

   c. What is the time period over which the volume needs to be infused?

   d. What is the method of delivery or type of equipment to be used?

   e. What is the hourly rate of the infusion and the rate via the infusion set if indicated?

1. 1,000 cc Dextrose 5% normal saline with 20 mEq KCl over 8 hours via 15 gtt/cc infusion set.

2. 1,000 cc Dextrose 5% normal saline @ 75 cc/hr via 10 gtt/cc infusion set.

3. 1,000 cc Dextrose 5% 1/2 normal saline @ 80 cc/hr via 10 gtt/cc infusion set.

4. 1000 cc Dextrose 5% normal saline with 40 mEq KCl @ 100 cc/hr × 2 via microdrip infusion set, then call for orders.

5. 1,000 cc Dextrose 5% 1/2 normal saline with 40 mEq KCl @ 75 cc/hr via an infusion pump.

6. 50 cc Dextrose 5% Water with 50 mEq KCl over 5 hours via an infusion pump.

7. 700 cc Ensure 3/4 strength enteral feeding via J-tube @ 110 cc/hr via feeding pump.

8. Tagamet 300 mg in 50 cc NS q 6 hour IVMB over 20 minutes via an infusion pump.

9. 500 cc Osmolyte 1/2 strength enteral G-tube continuous feeding @ 35 cc/hr via feeding pump.

10. Hyperalimentation order: 1,000 cc TPN @ 94 cc/hr and 500 cc lipids @ 31 cc/hr via central line.

11. Mrs. Jones is to receive 1,000 cc of D5 1/2NS q 8 hours continuously. A new bottle is due to be hung at 1300. The drop factor is 10 gtt/cc. At what time will the bottle be finished? At what time will half of the bottle be infused? Prepare a flow meter. Regulate the IV to the prescribed rate.

12. Mrs. Mope's IV order is for 500 ml NS to run over 10 hours. You choose a microdrip infusion. The infusion is started at 0200. When will the bottle finish? At what time will half the bottle be infused?

CRITICAL THINKING

1. You are monitoring an intravenous infusion, and assess it to be infusing at 28 gtt/min. The ordered rate is 31 gtt/min. What do you do?

2. You are asked to check an IV infusion on a patient on your team. Before going to the patient's room, what information do you need?

3. At the change of shift, it was reported to you that there were 600 cc remaining in an infusion on one of your patients. The ordered infusion rate is 100 cc/hr. Now, 2 hours into the shift, there are 400 cc remaining. Is the IV on time? Show your calculations.

4. Primary Line Infusion Order: 1,000 cc D5%W @ 100 cc/hr. Secondary Line Infusion Ordered: Zantac 50 mg q 8 hours IVMB. Zantac 50 mg/100 ml mini-bag is to be infused over 30 minutes via 20 gtt/ml infusion set. What is the primary line drip infusion rate? What is the secondary line drip infusion rate? The Zantac was administered as scheduled to be given at 0800. When will the minibag finish? Perform all calculations.

5. Primary Line Infusion Order: 1,000 cc D5% 1/2NS over 10 hours via infusion pump. Secondary Line Infusion Ordered: 250 mg in 250 cc dextrose 5% water at 20 mg/30 min via infusion pump. What is the primary line infusion rate? What is the secondary line infusion rate? What is the total infusion time of the minibag?

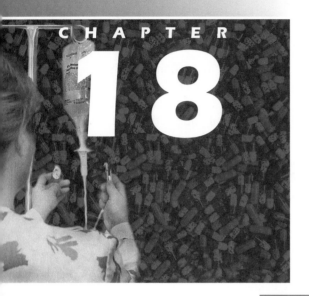

18

Advanced Intravenous and Other Solution Calculations

OBJECTIVES

Upon completion of this chapter, you will be able to:

- Problem solve complex infusion calculations.
- Recognize the benefit of one consistent calculation method for a variety of prescribed therapies.
- Calculate the duration of infusions.

Introduction

In Chapter 17, the process of solving for rates of infusion for common intravenous therapy and nutritional therapy was presented. It was demonstrated that volumes of solutions ordered for a period of time can be calculated, assessed, monitored, and evaluated. Remembering to identify the units you are solving for and if your answer makes sense are very important.

Due to the efficacy of the parenteral route and the increased accessibility of this route of administration, more and more medications are administered this way. Advanced or complex intravenous therapy can be simplified by consistently using the dimensional analysis method of solving. When solving, keep in mind where you are headed and the units of your answer. In most cases, you will solve for the rate to be administered via an infusion pump, so cc/hr are the units of choice. The nature of these orders and the complexity require very close monitoring of the infusion via the pumps.

Reading Complex Orders

Complex orders can seem confusing because of the amount of information that needs to be included in the prescription; however, they really are not very different from other orders.

KEY POINT

1. What is the *total amount of solution* to be infused?

2. What is the *type of solution* or medication?

3. What is the *time period* over which the volume needs to be infused?

4. What is the *method of delivery* or type of equipment to be used ?

5. What is the *calculated rate of the infusion?*

EXAMPLE: Ordered: Morphine drip 8 mg/hr. Infusion prepared as 50 mg/250 cc D5W. To interpret such an order, start by visualizing what is represented: A 250 cc bag of D5W has 50 mg of morphine. This information provides us with the amount of medication, which is the focus of the order, not the intravenous volume, which is important for determining the length of the infusion. The morphine is to be administered via the prescribed time frame of 8 mg within a 1-hour period. Both pieces of information are needed to arrive at the units that are being solved for, which is cc/hr.

1. What is the total amount of solution to be infused?

250 cc D5W with 50 mg of morphine

2. What is the type of solution or medication?

Morphine 8 mg

3. What is the time period over which the volume needs to be infused?

1 hour

4. What is the method of delivery or type of equipment to be used?

IV pump

5. What is the calculated rate of the infusion?

Start with what you have, 50 mg/250 cc. Set up the equation to foster arriving at the units you need. Remember that proportions/ratios/conversion factors can be expressed in an inverted form and can still express the same relationship. After successfully setting up the equation, the rest falls into place very easily. The units intended for the answer dictate the process:

$$\frac{250 \text{ cc}}{50 \text{ mg}} \times \frac{8 \text{ mg}}{\text{hr}}$$

By starting with cc in the numerator, the desired units of the answer are halfway completed. Next, choose a relationship that will link mg in the denominator to the intended units of the denominator in the answer. Solve the equation.

$$\frac{250 \text{ cc}}{50 \text{ mg}} \times \frac{8 \text{ mg}}{1 \text{ hr}} = 40 \text{ cc/hr}$$

PRACTICE EXERCISE 18.A

In each of the following examples, calculate the hourly rate for infusion pump administration.

1. Ordered: $MgSO_4$ 20 mg/min. The medication is supplied as 2 g in 50 cc.
2. Ordered: Pronestyl 1/mg/min supplied as 1 g/1,000 ml D5W.
3. Ordered: Tagamet 300 mg in 50 ml IVMB over 30 min.
4. Ordered: Aminophylline 1 g/1,000 cc to infuse at 35 mg/hr.
5. Ordered: Nitroglycerine 10 mcg/min. Supplied as 100 mg/500 cc D5W.
6. Ordered: Isuprel 1 mg/250 cc D5W. Start at 2 mcg/min and increase to 5 mcg/min.
7. Ordered: Nitroglycerin 50 mcg/min. Supplied as 100 mg in 500 ml D5W.
8. Ordered: Dopamine HCl 200 mcg/min. Supplied as 200 mg/50 ml.
9. Ordered: Procanimide HCl 1,500 mcg/min. Supplied as 500 mg/500 ml.

Medication Infusions Based on Body Weight

Just as PO or IM prescriptions are most therapeutic when ordered by body weight, the same is true for infusions. Many infusions of medications are ordered by the mass of the medication in relation to body weight per unit of time. This type of calculation is one of the most complex that will be encountered.

EXAMPLE: A patient weighing 150 lb is ordered to receive dopamine IV @ 5 mcg/kg/min. A 250 ml solution with 400 mg of dopamine has been prepared to be delivered via an infusion pump. What is the hourly rate?

$$\frac{150 \text{ lb}}{\text{min}} \times \frac{1 \text{ kg}}{2.2 \text{ lb}} \times \frac{5 \text{ mcg}}{1 \text{ kg}} \times \frac{1 \text{ mg}}{1,000 \text{ mcg}} \times \frac{250 \text{ ml}}{400 \text{ mg}} \times \frac{60 \text{ min}}{1 \text{ hr}} =$$
$$12.8 \text{ cc/hr} = 13 \text{ cc/hr}$$

Remember that when solving a calculation that includes body weight, start with the body weight. By thinking through the problem and approaching the units one at a time, relationships can be made easily. Notice how the units of each numerator are divided successively by the following denominator.

Infusion of Units

Biological units ordered for infusion are usually delivered via an infusion pump because these medications are administered for patients with acute medical problems. Whether it be heparin, insulin, or antibiotics, the implications of administration must be known.

EXAMPLE: Regular U-100 insulin 2 units per hour. Available 25 units per 250 ml of NS. What is the hourly rate via the infusion pump?

$$\frac{2 \text{ units}}{1 \text{ hr}} \times \frac{250 \text{ ml}}{25 \text{ units}} = \frac{20 \text{ ml}}{\text{hr}}$$

LEARNING ACTIVITIES

Read the information as it corresponds to the circled numbers on the Heparin Anticoagulation Protocol in Figure 18-1 on the next page. Complete the examples.

1. Follow the corresponding circled numbers in the figure.

   a. Prior to initiating the Heparin Anticoagulation Protocol, the protocol should be imprinted with the patient's name plate. The order must be dated, timed, and signed by the ordering physician. If an order is written in addition to the protocol, then stop the protocol.

   b. The protocol must also have the box checked indicating the desired therapeutic range.

2. Fill in the patient's height and weight. The patient's weight should be recorded on the protocol. The patient's mass in kilograms is needed for the calculation. If the patient is severely obese, consult with the pharmacy. Since heparin is poorly absorbed into adipose tissue, the patient's adjusted body weight should be calculated by the pharmacy.

   a. Prior to initiation, verify with the physician doses of heparin greater than 12,000 units IVP and/or greater than 2,000 units/hour for infusions.

   b. Baseline CBC (complete blood count) and APTT (activated partial thromboplastin time) should be done prior to heparin therapy.

3. Check the calculation of the order for the initial bolus.

   Ordered: Heparin 5,800 units IVP (recommended dose 80 units/kg, round to the nearest 100 units). The patient weighs 160 lb.

   $$\frac{160 \text{ lb}}{1} \times \frac{1 \text{ kg}}{2.2 \text{ lb}} \times \frac{80 \text{ units}}{1 \text{ kg}} = 5{,}816 \text{ units} \approx 5{,}800 \text{ units}$$

   Keep track of units. Make sure they divide and that the calculation is labeled with the correct units. When the answer is rounded to the nearest 100 units, the 5,816 becomes 5,800 units, so the order checks. Administer 5,800 units IVP.

   a. Number 2 on the Heparin Anticoagulation Protocol further indicates to repeat the APTT 8 hr after the bolus.

   b. Check the order for the infusion rate:

   (same example continued): Ordered: Heparin drip 20,000 units 500 cc D5W. Initiate drip at 1,320 units/hr (recommended dosage 18 units/kg/hr).

   When performing this type of calculation, always start with the weight of the patient, kg or lb, so that you will be more likely to convert to the units you are solving.

   $$\frac{160 \text{ lb}}{1} \times \frac{1 \text{ kg}}{2.2 \text{ lb}} \times \frac{18 \text{ units}}{1 \text{ hr}} = 1{,}308.6 \text{ units/hr}$$

4. The Heparin Anticoagulation Protocol states to round the IV infusion rate to nearest 40 units/hr.

   $$1{,}308.6 \text{ units/hr} \approx 1{,}308 \text{ units/hr}$$

Albany
Medical
Center

PHYSICIAN'S ORDER SHEET - DEPENDENT PROTOCOL

> ① Must be completed!
> " Mr. Jones "
> 11/4

Instructions:

① {
1. Imprint patient's plate before placing in chart.
2. The order must be dated, timed, and signed by the ordering physician.
3. Check appropriate boxes.
4. Fill in height and weight, prior to faxing to pharmacy
}

Allergies:

HEPARIN ANTICOAGULATION PROTOCOL

② Supportive Data: The recommended dosage guidelines outlined below and in the tables are based on the patient's actual body weight except when the patient is severely obese. For severely obese patients, contact pharmacy (extension 3258) for determination of proper dosing weight for calculations (also known as, adjusted body weight). Doses of heparin > 12,000 units IVP and/or > 2000 units/h infusion should be verified with MD prior to initiation.

② 1. Patient's height:_____ ; actual body weight: _160 lb_
for the severely obese patient, adjusted body weight (determined by pharmacy and used for calculations):_____

③ {
2. Baseline CBC, APTT prior to heparin therapy
Heparin _5800_ units IVP (recommended dose 80 units/kg, round to the nearest 100 units). Repeat APTT in 8 h.
4. Heparin drip 20,000 units/500 cc D5W. Initiate drip at _1320_ units/h (recommended dosage 18 units/kg/hr).
}

④ 5. Adjust maintenance dose based on the therapeutic range checked below and APTT results (round IV infusion rate to the nearest 40 units/hr and IV bolus dose to the nearest 100 units):

⑤ ☒ a. APTT 1.5-2.0: low therapeutic range
⑥

APTT RATIO	REBOLUS	HOLD INFUSION	CHANGE INFUSION	Next APTT
<1.2	80 units/kg	no	increase 4 units/kg/h	8h
1.2-1.4	40 units/kg	no	increase 2 units/kg/h	8h
1.5-1.6	none	no	increase 2 units/kg/h	6h
1.7-2.3	none	no	none	6h
2.4-3.0	none	1/2 hour	decrease 2 units/kg/h	6h
> 3.0	none	1 hour	decrease 4 units/kg/h	6h

⑥

OR

⑤ ☐ b. APTT 2.0-2.5: high therapeutic range

APTT RATIO	REBOLUS	HOLD INFUSION	CHANGE INFUSION	Next APTT
<1.2	80 units/kg	no	increase 4 units/kg/h	8h
1.2-1.4	40 units/kg	no	increase 4 units/kg/h	8h
1.5-2.0	none	no	increase 2 units/kg/h	6h
2.1-2.5	none	no	none	6h
2.6-3.0	none	no	decrease 2 units/kg/h	6h
> 3.0	none	1 hour	decrease 4 units/kg/h	6h

⑦ 6. Repeat APTT as outlined in the column above until 3 consecutive APTT's fall into therapeutic range and repeat this sequence with any change in therapy. Once 3 consecutive APTT's obtained, repeat APTT q am until heparin discontinued. Repeat hgb, hct, plt in 24h then q3d if stable.

① Physician Signature/Date/Time _Dr. Mary albany 11/4 0700_

FIGURE 18-1

The infusion is based on a heparin concentration of 20,000 units/500 cc D5W. This can be reduced mathematically to 40 units per 1 cc in order to calculate the cc/hr for the infusion pump.

$$\frac{1,308 \text{ units}}{1 \text{ hr}} \times \frac{1 \text{ cc}}{40 \text{ units}} = 32.7 \text{ cc/hr} \approx \text{cc/hr}$$

5. The protocol continues by following the therapeutic range indicated. The physician, upon initiating the protocol, must indicate by checking the box either APTT 1.5–2.0: low therapeutic range, or APTT 2.0–2.5: high therapeutic range. The adjustment of the maintenance dose is based on the therapeutic range checked and the APTT results.

6. In this example, the APTT 1.5–2.0: low therapeutic range, is checked.
   The APTT ratio is reported as 1.3. What will you do? Follow the columns of the box across on the protocol to see what your actions will be.
   Do you rebolus? Yes, at 40 units/kg.

$$\frac{160 \text{ lb}}{1} \times \frac{1 \text{ kg}}{2.2 \text{ lb}} \times \frac{40 \text{ units}}{1 \text{ hr}} = 2,909 \text{ units/hr}$$

When rounded to the nearest 100 units, ≈ 2,900 units. So, rebolus with 2,900 units IVP.
   Do you hold the infusion? No.
   Do you change the infusion rate? Yes, increase 2 units/kg/hr.

$$\frac{160 \text{ lb}}{1 \text{ hr}} \times \frac{1 \text{ kg}}{2.2 \text{ lb}} \times \frac{2 \text{ units}}{1 \text{ kg}} = 145.4 \text{ units/hr}$$

$$1,308.6 \text{ units/hr} + 145.4 \text{ units/hr} = 1,454 \text{ units/hr}$$

$$\frac{1,454 \text{ units}}{1 \text{ hr}} \times \frac{1 \text{ cc}}{40 \text{ units}} = \frac{36.3 \text{ cc}}{\text{hr}} \approx 36 \text{ cc/hr}$$

When is your next APTT? 8 hr. The next APTT is 8 hours from when you make the change in rate.

7. Once three consecutive APTTs fall in range, then repeat the APTT q AM until heparin is discontinued.
   Document on the Heparin Protocol Flow Sheet (see next page).

8. Mr. Mop's actual body weight is 75 kg. He is ordered to receive heparin via the Heparin Anticoagulation Protocol.
   The initial bolus is 6,000 units IVP and initial infusion is 1,760 units/hr.

   a. Mr. Mop's first APTT is 1.2. Follow the table on the protocol. Do you rebolus?

   b. Do you hold the infusion?

   c. Do you change the infusion?

9. Mrs. Berry weighs 85 kg. She is ordered to receive heparin via the Heparin Anticoagulation Protocol. The initial bolus is 6,800 units IVP and the initial infusion ordered is 1,530 units/hr.

10. Mr. Shack is 5 feet 6 inches tall and weighs 220 lb. He is ordered to receive heparin via the Heparin Anticoagulation Protocol. The initial bolus is 5,100 units IVP and the initial infusion ordered is 2,550 units/hr.

Albany
Medical
Center

Heparin Protocol Flowsheet

"Mr. Jones"

Instructions:

1.   Imprint patient's plate before placing in chart.

Weight: ___72.7___ kg. for the severely obese patient, adjusted body weight
(determined by pharmacy and used for calculatons: _____
Therapeutic Range: (circle one) 1.5-2 or 2.0-2.5

Heparin Protocol Flowsheet

Date	Time	Current Heparin Dose (Units/hour)	PTT		Dosage Adjustment				Next PTT	RN Initials
			Time	Result	Time	Rebolus	Drip rate	Held x_h	TIme Posted	
11/4	0900	5800 units IVP	1700	1.3	1900	2900 IVP	36 cc/hr	NA	0800	KCXB
		1320 units /hr								

CHAPTER REVIEW EXERCISES

1. A 115 lb female patient who is 162 cm tall with a BSA of 1.5 m² has the following order for an antineoplastic agent: 140 mg in 500 cc NS IV over 1 h QD x 5.

On hand: 20 mg/ml

a. What is the dosage?

b. What is the hourly rate?

2. Ordered: 200 mg in 500 cc D5W over 24 hours. What is the hourly rate?

3. Ordered: 90 mg in 500 cc NS to be given over 1 hour. What is the hourly rate?

4. Ordered: 40 mg in 250 cc NS to be given over 30 minutes. What is the hourly rate?

5. Ordered: 1 liter NS @ 500 cc/hr x 2 pre-chemotherapy. What is the hourly rate?

6. Ordered: 20 mEq KCl in NS @ 250 cc/hr x 2 post-chemotherapy. What is the hourly rate?

CRITICAL THINKING

For the following orders, answer these questions:

a. What is the total amount of solution to be infused?

b. What is the type of solution or medication?

c. What is the time period over which the volume needs to be infused?

d. What is the calculated rate of infusion?

1. Ordered: Amphotericin B 0.5 mg/kg/day via central line. Pharmacy prepares medication in 500 cc NS. Patient weighs 134 lb.

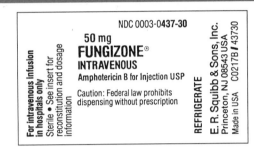

2. Ordered: 500 cc NS with heparin drip 1,200 units q hr continuously. Heparin solution is supplied as 20,000 units per 500 ml NS. What is the hourly rate?

3. Ordered: Heparin 900 units/hr. Heparin solution is supplied as 20,000 units per 500 ml NS. What is the hourly rate?

Advanced Mathematics

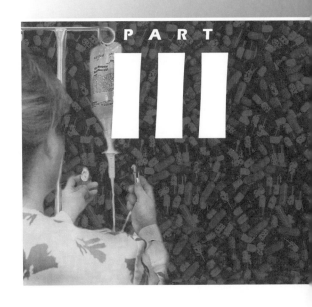

Significant Digits

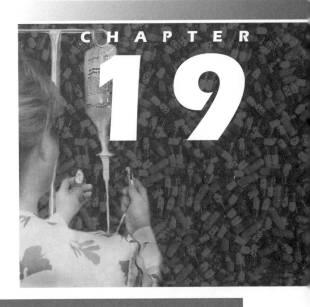

CHAPTER 19

OBJECTIVES

Upon completion of this chapter, you will be able to:

- Identify significant numbers in measured numbers.
- Round measured numbers to appropriate precision.
- Perform operations on measured numbers.

Introduction

When measuring quantities, especially within a scientific context, there are two related concepts: quantity and precision. Measurement accuracy is dependent on the precision of the measuring instrument (meter stick, graduated cylinder, etc.) as well as consideration of the individual situation. When discussing the amount of IV fluid that is remaining, we might say there are 400 cc left. The implication is that there are approximately 400 cc left in the bag, but this is not a very precise measurement. That is okay because there is no reason for it to be more precise. It is not likely given the indications on an IV bag that we could say there was 397.1 cc left. Since we cannot, our measurement is less precise and therefore has fewer significant digits. Suppose we wished to measure 25 milligrams of a drug in a laboratory. There is a difference between measuring 25 mg, 25.0 mg, and 25.00 mg. While numerically they represent the same number, the second and third amounts are more precise and therefore have more significant digits.

KEY POINT

Significant digits are the result of measurement and reflect the precision of the result.

Rules for Significant Digits

There are several rules for determining the number of significant digits in a measurement. It will be necessary for us to make sense of these rules by thinking about precision.

> ### REMEMBER!
> Rule 1: In a whole number all digits are significant except zeros on the right (also known as trailing zeros).

EXAMPLE: How many significant digits in 4,280 kg?

There are three significant digits in 4,280, as the zero on the right is not significant.

EXAMPLE: How many significant digits in 4,300 kg?

There are two significant digits in 4,300, as the zeros on the right are not significant.

EXAMPLE: How many significant digits in 4,000 kg?

There is one significant digit in 4,000, as the zeros on the right are not significant.

With the previous examples we can see that all of these measurements could have been taken of the same mass. (The second and third measurements were less precise than the first one most likely due to the inability of the instrument to provide the accuracy or precision.) The third measurement was probably measured to the nearest thousand kilograms for the purpose of giving a rough estimate.

> ### REMEMBER!
> Rule 2: In a decimal number all digits are significant except zeros on the left (also known as leading zeros).

EXAMPLE: How many significant digits in 0.00003 kg?

There is only one significant digit in this measurement. Only the numeral 3 is a result of measurement.

EXAMPLE: How many significant digits in 0.050 g?

There are two significant digits in 0.050. The two zeros on the right are leading zeros and the last zero on the left, since this is a decimal number, is the result of measurement and therefore is significant.

EXAMPLE: How many significant digits in 2.5700 L?

All of the digits in this number are significant. It is a decimal number with no leading zeros, so there are five significant digits, indicating quite a bit of precision. This amount is measured to the nearest ten thousandth of a liter (nearest tenth of a milliliter).

> ### REMEMBER!
>
> Rule 3: A nonsignificant digit, according to the previous rules, may be made significant by placing a bar over the top.

EXAMPLE: How many significant digits in 45,0$\overline{0}$0 mi?

The bar over the next to last zero indicates that the first four digits are significant. The last zero remains as a trailing zero and is not significant.

PRACTICE EXERCISE 19.A

How many significant digits in each of the following quantities?

1. 3,400 mi _____

2. 3,400.1 mi _____

3. 0.00200 kg _____

4. 10.00200 kg _____

5. 6,001 kg _____

6. 0.0120 mg _____

7. 93,000,000 mi _____

8. 93,000,$\overline{0}$00 mi _____

Rounding Numbers in Significant Digits

Because of some of the operations we will perform on numbers with significant digits, we need to consider the process of rounding a number to one that has fewer significant digits. We certainly can never round and gain precision!

The rules for rounding are the same general principles we have encountered previously, plus the idea that if a number ends in exactly a 5 or a 5 followed only by zeros, we round the value to the nearest even number.

EXAMPLE: Round 4,287.0 mi to three significant digits.

The number currently has five significant digits. We consider the first three and move to the fourth, which is a 7. Since the number is more than 5, we round the previous digit up (to a 9). We must remember to place a zero in the fourth position (it will be a trailing zero as a whole number) to keep the approximate value of the number—otherwise, we would have 429, which is not a less precise version of 4,287.0; it is a different number completely. Our result is 4,290 mi.

EXAMPLE: Round 0.013489 g to two significant digits.

We are asked to take this fairly precise measurement (five significant digits) and make it less precise with only two significant digits. Since we are looking for two significant digits, we find the third (the 4). Since this number is less than 5, we simply drop it and everything to the right. We do not need to put zeros in as place holders here, as we are in a decimal and zeros to the right would increase the precision and the number of significant digits. Therefore, 0.013 g is our result.

EXAMPLE: Round 92,495,000 mi to four significant digits.

There are currently five significant digits in this measurement—the rest are trailing zeros. We count the first four and consider the fifth. Since the fifth is a 5 followed only by zeros, we round to the nearest even number, which is a 10 (which increases the 4 by one), and then we fill with trailing zeros. The problem we encounter at first is that the number is 92,500,000, which has only three significant digits instead of four. To remedy this, we use Rule 3 and place a bar over the first zero: 92,5$\bar{0}$0,000 mi is our result. This quantity has four significant digits.

PRACTICE EXERCISE 19.B

Round each of the following measurements to three significant digits:

1. 34,789 mi _____ **2.** 5,445 g _____ **3.** 0.002308 kg _____

4. 4,570,001 mi _____ **5.** 0.01234 kg _____ **6.** 4950 g _____

7. 0.099999 L _____ **8.** 0.003769 g _____

Operations

The key concept in working with significant digits and performing operations on them is to recognize that by adding, subtracting, multiplying, or dividing we cannot increase the precision of the numbers we began with and therefore our result may not contain more precision than the original measurements. As in many arithmetic operations that we have studied, the rules for addition and subtraction are very different than those for multiplication and division. However, they are similar in the idea of not increasing precision.

Addition and Subtraction

> **KEY POINT**
>
> When adding or subtracting measurements, the least precise place value common to all will determine the precision of the result.

EXAMPLE: Add the following measured quantities: 1.70 g, 3.578 g, 4.2 g, 1.003 g.

We would add the quantities first simply as decimals:

$$4\frac{3}{6} = 4\frac{1 \times 3}{2 \times 3} = 4\frac{1}{2} \times \frac{3}{3}:$$

Since the least precise measurement was to the tenth's place, our result is rounded to the tenth's place as well:

$10.481 \rightarrow 10.5$ g

We have obtained a sum that indicates it is precise to the nearest tenth, which was the minimal precision in the list of values we considered.

Multiplication and Division

Multiplication and division are a bit more complicated in terms of significant digits. Recall that when we multiply decimal numbers, the number of places following the decimal point is the sum of all the number places in the numbers being multiplied. So, if we multiply a three-digit decimal by a two-digit decimal, we obtain a result that has a five-digit decimal. The problem with significant digits becomes clearer. Suppose you are multiplying those numbers again now as measurements. In your result you have an answer that is far more precise than either of the original values.

> **KEY POINT**
>
> When multiplying or dividing measured quantities, the number of significant digits in the result will be the least number of significant digits from either of the measured quantities.

EXAMPLE: Multiply the following quantities: 3.20 cm × 4.1 cm.

We would multiply the quantities first as decimals and obtain 13.12. Since the first measurement has three significant digits and the second has only two, our result must have only two significant digits. Therefore, our result is 13 cm^2. (Recall that cm times cm yields cm^2).

Occasionally we need to multiply or divide measured numbers that are in scientific notation. That does not create any new problems once we recognize that the number of significant digits of a number in scientific notation is not affected by the power of 10—it only creates trailing or leading zeros. The precision of the number is completely held with the quantity preceding the power of 10.

EXAMPLE: Divide 6.02×10^{23} by 16.0.

From our previous work we divide 6.02 by 16.0 and obtain 0.37625. Appending the power of 10, we have:

0.37625×10^{23}

The result is too precise and is not in scientific notation. First, converting to scientific notation, we obtain:

3.7625×10^{22}

Since each of our measured numbers has three significant digits, our result must have three. Rounding to three, we have:

3.76×10^{22}

PRACTICE EXERCISE 19.C

Add the following measured numbers:

1. 2.30 g, 3.478 g, 5.723 g, 1.2 g

2. 0.0050 kg, 0.234 kg, 1.00 kg

3. Suppose you and your lab partner are trying to determine the mass of a beaker and its contents. Suppose you measure the beaker to be 54.0 g, the first liquid has a mass of 23.45 g, and the second liquid weighs 2.75 g. What would you claim to be the total weight of the two liquids and the beaker?

Multiply the following measured numbers:

4. 2.3 m by 4.1 m

5. 2.0 cm by 3.1 cm

6. 3.5×10^{12} mm by 3×10^2 mm

7. Find the volume of a box that is measured to have dimensions 20.3 cm by 10.50 cm by 5.1 cm.

8. If there are 1.00×10^7 U in a container, how many measured doses of 2.5×10^6 U are there available?

Ratio Proportion and Formula Method

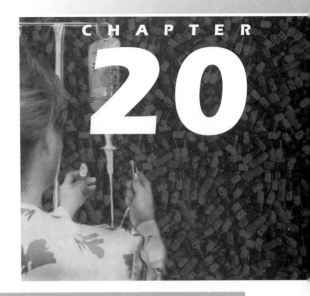

OBJECTIVES

Upon completion of this chapter, you will be able to:

- Recognize alternative calculation methods to the dimensional analysis approach.
- Identify the process of the ratio proportion method.
- Identify the process of the formula method.

Introduction

Throughout this text, the method of problem solving that we have used is the dimensional analysis (or factor label) method. We have included other methods of solving, however, so that the reader can make a comparison of this method to other methods.

The Ratio Proportion Method

A popular method, although more symbolic and often confusing to beginning students, is the ratio proportion method. We have encountered proportions in a number of settings including within dimensional analysis. A conversion factor of 1,000 mg = 1 g can be thought of as a proportion and written either of two ways:

$$\frac{1000 \text{ mg}}{1 \text{ g}} \text{ or in ratio notation 1,000 mg: 1 g}$$

We also encounter ratios within solutions, for example. A 25% W/V solution is often denoted as a 1:4 solution—that is, one part solid dissolved within four parts of solution.

The actual ratio proportion method has long been used within nursing/health care education. We will illustrate the method using examples.

EXAMPLE:

Convert 12 yards to feet using the ratio proportion method.

This problem is fairly straightforward using any method because there is a direct connection between measurement in yards and one in feet. The solution to this problem hinges on the relationship that 3 ft = 1 yd. Any conversion from yards to feet (or feet to yards) must stay in this proportion. This method also requires that we name the unknown. By convention, the unknown is most often identified by an unknown variable such as the letter x. We begin by setting up the proportions:

$$\frac{3 \text{ ft}}{1 \text{ yd}} = \frac{x \text{ ft}}{12 \text{ yd}}$$

We are saying that 3 feet must be to 1 yard as the unknown number of feet must be to 12 yards. Usually at this point we remove the labels and consider the values of the quantities:

$$\frac{3}{1} = \frac{x}{12}$$

Through properties of fractions, we can multiply both sides of this equation by 12×1. This is usually stated more conveniently as the product of the means equaling the product of the extremes. In this problem the 1 and the x are in the means positions and the 3 and the 12 are in the extreme positions. In other words, we multiply $1 \times x = 3 \times 12$ and obtain that $1x = 36$ or that $x = 36$.

One of the inherent problems with ratio proportion is that it is incumbent on us to now remember the label of the answer—that is, in this case, the 36 represents 36 ft.

The ratio proportion method becomes a bit more tedious if there is not a direct link between what you are given and what you are looking for as an answer.

EXAMPLE: Convert 2 cups to tablespoons.

Since there is not a direct link between cups and tablespoons, we will make a connection between cups and ounces and then ounces and tablespoons. Each new connection with ratio proportion requires a new equation. To begin with:

$$\frac{8 \text{ ʒ}}{1 \text{ C}} = \frac{x \text{ ʒ}}{2 \text{ C}} \rightarrow \frac{8}{1} = \frac{x}{2}$$
$$1 \times x = 8 \times 2$$

or $x = 16$. This x represents the number of ounces in 2 cups. We can then use this equivalent to finish the problem:

$$\frac{1 \text{ ʒ}}{2 \text{ T}} = \frac{16 \text{ ʒ}}{x \text{ T}} \rightarrow \frac{1}{2} = \frac{16}{x}$$
$$2 \times 16 = 1 \times x \text{ or } x = 32$$

Recall this is not the same x as the last equation. This 32 is 32 tablespoons. Therefore, there are 32 tablespoons in 2 cups.

EXAMPLE: Ordered: Diphenhydramine 25 mg tid. po

On hand: Diphenhydramine 12.5 mg/5 ml

How many teaspoons should the patient take?

$$\frac{12.5 \text{ mg}}{5 \text{ ml}} = \frac{25 \text{ mg}}{x \text{ ml}} \rightarrow \frac{12.5}{5} = \frac{25}{x}$$

or $5 \times 25 = 12.5 \times x$

$$125 = 12.5x$$

and dividing both sides by 12.5, we obtain:

$x = 10$ (which represents the number of ml to be taken).
To continue,

$$\frac{1 \text{ t}}{5 \text{ ml}} = \frac{x \text{ t}}{10 \text{ ml}} \rightarrow \frac{1}{5} = \frac{x}{10}$$

or $5x = 10$, and therefore, $x = 2$. The patient should take
2 teaspoons 3 times a day.

PRACTICE EXERCISE 20.A

Convert the following using the ratio proportion method:

1. 3 cups to f ʒ .
2. gr V to mg.
3. 40 ʒ to ml.
4. ʒ iv to tsp.
5. 45 ml to ʒ .
6. 75 kg to lb.
7. You are to give instructions to an adult to take ʒ iii of a liquid over-the-counter (OTC) preparation. How many tablespoons should you instruct the client to take?
8. An injection is ordered for a patient. The amount of the drug is gr 1/300. How many mg of the medication was ordered? If the medication is available 0.5 mg/ml, how many ml will be injected?
9. An OTC medication label indicates that children over 12 years of age should be given 1 tablespoon. How many cc does this correspond to? How many drams?
10. The recommended daily dosage of a medication is listed as 2.5 mg/kg. What would be the recommended dosage for a single day if the patient weighed 165 pounds?

The Formula Method

The formula method is less conceptual than the ratio proportion method, so we caution that there are fewer built-in checks and greater chances for error. We must carefully think about what is an appropriate amount and dose for a given situation.

KEY POINT

The Formula Method:

$$\frac{\text{Desired}}{\text{Have}} \times \text{Quantity} = \frac{D}{H} \cdot Q$$

When using the formula method, The D stands for the desired amount (the amount that is ordered), the H for "have" represents how the medication supplied is measured, and the Q for "quantity" is the form in which the medication is supplied. Because this method does not concern itself with the units of the drug, whether milligrams or micrograms, etc., we must be very careful to be sure that the amounts used for D and H are the same. This may require a separate conversion. In addition, there will be times in which the quantity will have to be converted if it is not the same as the form in which the medication is supplied. We will use several problems solved earlier to examine this method.

EXAMPLE:

Ordered: Diphenhydramine 25 mg tid. po

On hand: Diphenhydramine 12.5 mg/5 ml

How many teaspoons should the patient take?

Using the formula method, the desired amount is 25 mg, the have amount is 12.5 mg, and the quantity is 1 teaspoon. This requires a conversion from milliliters to teaspoons using the convenient 1 t = 5 ml. Therefore,

$$\frac{D}{H} \times Q = \frac{25 \text{ mg}}{12.5 \text{ mg}} \times 1 \text{ teaspoon} = 2 \text{ teaspoons}$$

The patient should receive 2 teaspoons.

EXAMPLE:

Ordered: Lanoxin 0.125 mg

On hand: Lanoxin 0.25 mg scored tablets

What should the patient receive?

In this case, D = 0.125 mg, H = 0.25 mg, and Q = 1 tablet. Therefore,

$$\frac{D}{H} \times Q = \frac{0.125 \text{ mg}}{0.25 \text{ mg}} \times 1 \text{ tablet} = \frac{1}{2} \text{ tablet}$$

A half tablet is allowable here, because the tablets were scored. This example is useful in that we can easily see we must carefully identify the desired and the have values; if they were interchanged by accident, we could potentially administer the wrong amount.

EXAMPLE:

Ordered: Meperidine HCl 35 mg IM q4h prn

On hand: Meperidine 50 mg/2 ml in a cartridge

What will be administered?

For this example, the desired amount is 35 mg, the have value is 50 mg, and the quantity is 2 ml. Therefore,

$$\frac{D}{H} \times Q = \frac{35 \text{ ml}}{50 \text{ ml}} \times 2 \text{ ml} = 1.4 \text{ ml}$$

EXAMPLE:

Ordered: Atropine gr 1/100 sc stat

On hand: Atropine 1 mg/ml

What will be administered?

For this example, initially D = 1/100 gr, H = 1 mg, and Q = 1 ml. However, in this case the values for D and H are not in the same units, so they must be converted using another method (either dimensional analysis or ratio and proportion). If we recall that 1 gr = 60 mg, we can make the conversion so that gr 1/100 = 0.6 mg. Therefore,

$$\frac{D}{H} \times Q = \frac{0.6 \text{ mg}}{1 \text{ mg}} \times 1 \text{ ml} = 0.6 \text{ ml}$$

It becomes clear from this last example that if the units of the desired and have quantities are not the same, it may be more efficient to use one of the other methods entirely, since we will have to use another conversion method anyway.

REMEMBER!

When using the formula method, be sure to check that the desired and have quantities are in the same units!

Be sure to always check the reasonableness of your result.

PRACTICE EXERCISE 20.B

Find what will be administered for each of the following orders:

1. Ordered: Polymox 0.5 gm po tid
   On hand: Polymox 500 mg capsules

2. Ordered: Aspirin gr X po q4h prn
   On hand: Aspirin 325 mg tablets

3. Ordered: Leukeran 4 mg po bid
   On hand: Leukeran 2 mg tablets

4. Ordered: Lanoxin 0.25 mg po qd
   On hand: Lanoxin 250 mcg tablets

5. Ordered: Tagamet 800 mg po HS
   On hand: Tagamet 0.4 g tablets

6. Ordered: Ampicillin 250 mg IM q 6h
   On hand: Ampicillin 250 mg/ml

7. Ordered: Morphine sulfate gr 1/5 sc prn
   On hand: Morphine 10 mg/ml

8. Ordered: Thorazine 50 mg IM now
   On hand: Thorazine 25 mg/ml

9. Ordered: Tagamet 300 mg IM q6h
   On hand: Tagamet 0.3 g/2 ml

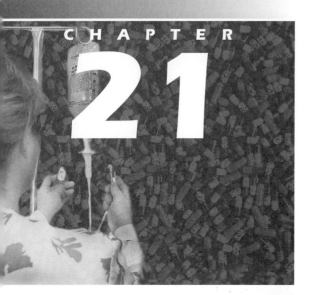

CHAPTER 21

Temperature Conversion

OBJECTIVES

Upon completion of this chapter, you will be able to:

- Explain the relationship between the Fahrenheit and Celsius scales.
- Convert temperatures between the Fahrenheit, Celsius, and Kelvin scales.

Introduction

There are two popular scales for measuring temperature: the Fahrenheit and Celsius scales. These two scales are similar in that they are both relative temperature scales—they measure change in temperature. They do not measure the amount of heat present as an absolute scale would. Both scales are used commonly in nursing/health care situations, and the use of a specific scale is often dependent on the individual institution or setting.

Fahrenheit and Celsius

The Fahrenheit scale is generally referenced from 32° to 212°, the freezing and boiling point, respectively, of water (Figure 21-1).

The Celsius scale is generally referenced from 0° to 100°, the freezing and boiling point, respectively, of water (Figure 21-2).

These scales measure the same temperatures, however, assign them different labels, thus allowing for comparisons (Table 21-1).

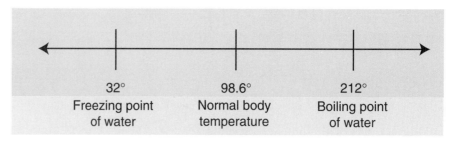

| 32° | 98.6° | 212° |
| Freezing point of water | Normal body temperature | Boiling point of water |

FIGURE 21-1
The Fahrenheit Scale

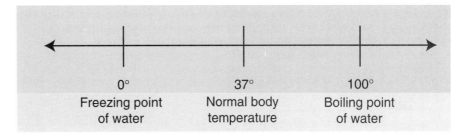

FIGURE 21-2
The Celsius Scale

TABLE 21-1 **Temperature Equivalents**

Fahrenheit Temperature	Celsius Temperature
32°	0°
98.6°	37°
212°	100°

In order to convert between the scales, we first need to recognize that the Fahrenheit temperature scale covers 180° and the Celsius scale covers 100°. That fact leads us to a conversion factor that in a reduced form says for every 9° Fahrenheit, there are 5° Celsius.

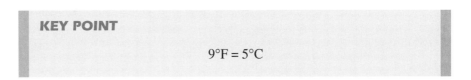

KEY POINT

$$9°F = 5°C$$

This key point becomes a conversion factor that we will use in converting between these two scales. The conversion is basically a series of arithmetic steps that connects the two scales. We will notice in the strategy to follow that the value 40 plays a prominent role. Actually, −40° is the place where both scales are exactly the same—that is, −40°C is equal to −40°F. The negative forty then acts as starting place to begin converting with our conversion scale. Our strategy will be as follows:

REMEMBER!

1. Take the degrees given and add 40.
2. Place the original label following this value.
3. Place the conversion factor 9°F = 5°C using dimensional analysis so that the label we are converting from disappears.
4. Perform the necessary arithmetic.
5. Subtract 40 from the result.
6. Carry along the label of the new scale.

EXAMPLE: Convert 32°F to Celsius.

(32 + 40)°F We add 40 and place the original label:

$$(32+40)°F \ \frac{5C}{9F} = (72)°F \ \frac{5C}{9F} = 40°C - 40 = 0°C$$

We added 32 and 40, yielding 72. We then placed the conversion factor in such a way that the label F dropped out. Performing the arithmetic (72)(9)/5 gave us 40, and then subtracting 40 brought us to 0°C as we expected.

As we can see, there are some inherent problems with this conversion. It is very easy to forget to subtract the final 40 from the result. It is very important for us to estimate what we expect the answer to be as a check to test the reasonableness of our obtained answer. If our answer does not seem reasonable, we might first check to see if we remembered to subtract the final 40.

EXAMPLE: Convert 100°C to Fahrenheit.

Our equation becomes:

$$(100 + 40)°C \ \frac{9F}{5C} - 40 =$$

$$140°C \ \frac{9F}{5C} - 40 = 252°C - 40 = 212°C$$

EXAMPLE: Convert 37.5°C to Fahrenheit.

Our equation becomes:

$$(37.5 + 40)°C \ \frac{9F}{5C} - 40 =$$

$$77.5°C \ \frac{9F}{5C} - 40 = 139.5°C - 40 = 99.5°C$$

We can see in this last example that starting with a Celsius temperature that is slightly higher than normal body temperature should certainly yield a temperature slightly higher than 98.6 on the Fahrenheit scale. By realizing this, we can see that had we forgotten to subtract the 40 in the equation, 139.5° would have been an unreasonable value.

EXAMPLE: Ordered: Tylenol gr V for temp over 101 q4h po.

On hand: Celsius thermometer.

At what temperature should the Tylenol be administered?

$$(101 + 40)°F \ \frac{5C}{9F} - 40 =$$

$$(141)°F \ \frac{5C}{9F} - 40 = 78.3°C - 40 = 38.3°C$$

Therefore, at any temperature of 38.3°C or above the medication should be administered.

Kelvin

As we mentioned earlier, there is a temperature scale that is absolute—it measures the amount of heat present. It is commonly referred to as the Kelvin scale. Because there is either heat present or not, the Kelvin scale has no negative temperatures. The scale begins at 0 K, which indicates the total absence of heat—this is referred to as absolute zero (it corresponds to –273°C). The Kelvin scale is a companion scale to the Celsius scale and conversions from Celsius to Kelvin can be made using K = °C + 273.

KEY POINT

$$K = °C + 273$$

EXAMPLE: Mercury freezes at –39°C. Convert this to Kelvin.

$$K = –39°C + 273 = 234 \text{ K}$$

Therefore –39°C converts to 234 K.

We should note that if the original temperature is measured using the Fahrenheit scale and we wish to convert to Kelvin, first we must convert the temperature to Celsius and then use our rule to obtain the corresponding Kelvin temperature.

PRACTICE EXERCISE 21.A

Make the following temperature conversions:

1. 72°F = _____ °C

2. 40.6°C = _____ °F

3. 0°F = _____ °C

4. 5°C = _____ °F

5. 100°F = _____ °C

6. 39°C = _____ °F

7. 32°C = _____ K

8. 100°F = _____ K

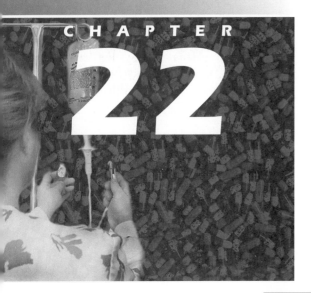

Logarithms and pH

OBJECTIVES

Upon completion of this chapter, you will be able to:

- Interpret the logarithmic notation of a number.
- Express the connection between pH and logarithms.
- Recall the pH scale in relation to acids and bases.

Introduction

Within the nursing/health care setting, we occasionally run into the need to discuss the meaning of pH. pH is a scale that can be used to determine the acidity of a certain solution. We are often interested, for example, in the current pH of a patient's blood.

In order to have some sense of what pH is, we need to first consider a mathematical idea called logarithms.

Basics of Logarithms

Logarithms are a mathematical creation used to solve exponential equations—that is, equations in which the unknown quantity is in the exponent. These types of equations cannot be solved with ordinary arithmetic. Mathematicians created logarithms as a notation for a quantity that is an exponent.

REMEMBER!

Logarithms are exponents.

Since logarithms are simply exponents, there is a direct connection between logarithms and the exponential notation that we studied earlier. We can consider an equation such as:

$$10^2 = 100$$

In its logarithmic form it is written:

$$\log_{10} 100 = 2$$

This is read that the log base 10 of 100 is 2. We notice that the base in either form is the same and that the log, 2, is the exponent on a base of 10 that yields 100.

Logarithms can be considered to a variety of bases. However, for practical purposes logarithms are often used with a base of 10. When we have a logarithm to the base 10, we call it a common logarithm. When we are dealing with a common logarithm, the subscript of 10 is omitted. Therefore,

$$10^2 = 100 \rightarrow \log_{10}100 = 2 \rightarrow \log 100 = 2$$

REMEMBER!

The common logarithm of a given number is the power (exponent) to which you raise 10 to in order to obtain the given number.

EXAMPLE: Find the common log of 1,000.

Since 1,000 can be represented as 10^3, we can say $\log 1,000 = 3$.

EXAMPLE: Find the common log of 0.1.

Since 0.1 can be represented as 10^{-1}, we can say $\log 0.1 = -1$.

What if the given number is not a perfect power of 10 such as our other examples? Suppose that we wish to calculate the log 20. We can estimate our answer to be between 1 and 2 (much closer to 1 than 2) since 20 lies between 10 and 100. However, if we want a more precise answer, we will have to depend on a logarithmic table of values, or more likely a scientific calculator. On a scientific calculator we input 20 and press the key labeled "log" and our result is approximately 1.301. This says that $10^{1.301} \approx 20$.

PRACTICE EXERCISE 22.A

Find the common logarithms of each of the following numbers:

1. log 10,000   **2.** log 10   **3.** log 0.01

4. log 10,000,000   **5.** log 10^7 **6.** log 0.001

Applications of Logarithms: pH

Earlier in our text, we considered solutions. It is important to recall that solute + solvent = solution.

REMEMBER!

Solute + Solvent = Solution

Most solutions encountered in the laboratory setting are dissolved in water. Whether the solution under consideration is pure water or a water-based solution, some water molecules (H_2O) will break apart, forming hydrogen ions (H^+) and hydroxide ions (OH^-).

$$H_2O \quad \rightarrow \quad H^+ \quad + \quad OH^-$$

(water molecule)	(hydrogen ion)	(hydroxide ion)

An acid is a substance that releases H^+ in solution. A base is any substance that releases OH^- in solution.

For every 1 liter of water (at 25°C) there are 1×10^{-7} moles of H^+ and 1×10^{-7} moles of OH^- present. The hydrogen ion concentration, denoted $[H^+]$, may be expressed as pH. pH is defined to be the opposite of the logarithm of the hydrogen ion concentration (in moles/liter).

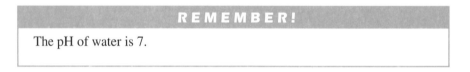

REMEMBER!

$$pH = -\log [H^+]$$

Therefore, if we know the hydrogen ion concentration, we can find the pH. For water (at 25°C), $[H^+] = 10^{-7}$. So, $\log [H^+] = \log 10^{-7} = -7$. Since $pH = -\log [H^+] = -(-7) = 7$, the pH of water (neutral) is 7.

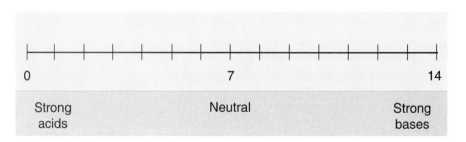

REMEMBER!

The pH of water is 7.

The pH scale ranges from 0 for very acidic solutions to 14 for very basic solutions (Figures 22-1 and 22-2).

The pH of arterial blood has a normal range of 7.35 from 7.45. The body has regulatory mechanisms for keeping the acid base balance.

![pH scale from 0 (Strong acids) to 7 (Neutral) to 14 (Strong bases)]

FIGURE 22-1
The pH Scale

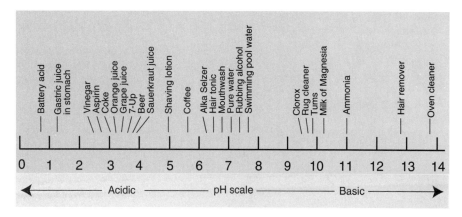

FIGURE 22-1

pH of Common Solutions

PRACTICE EXERCISE 22.B

1. Based on the pH of each solution found below, what would you say would be the effect of each drink on the acid content of the stomach?

   Beer: 4.3

   Tomato juice: 4.1

   Milk: 6.6

2. After a patient has been vomiting, you would expect the pH of the patient's blood to be _____.

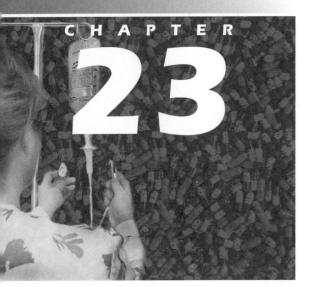

Molarity

Upon completion of this chapter, you will be able to:

- Recognize the application of significant digits and exponents to elements and chemical compounds.
- Calculate moles, grams, and atoms using principles of dimensional analysis.

Introduction

In the lab setting, we encounter solution concentrations in a unit called molarity. Molarity is a ratio that is defined to be:

$$\text{Molarity} = \frac{\text{Moles of solute}}{\text{Liters of solution}}$$

As an introduction, we need to recall what a mole is.

REMEMBER!

$$1 \text{ mole} = 6.02 \times 10^{23} \text{ particles}$$

While we cannot see (with just our eye) a mole of an element, it is a standard amount that is often considered. It is important for us to think about a mole as the amount of a substance. We commonly think of the word *dozen* without a reference as to whether it is a dozen eggs or a dozen donuts—it is simply 12 of something. The same thing holds true for a mole. Whether it is a mole of a substance or a mole of a compound, it is simply 6.02×10^{23} of something.

Mole of an Element

The mole of an element is the amount of a substance equal to the atomic weight expressed in grams (also known as gram atomic weight). Specifically, if we consider the element oxygen (symbol O), it has an atomic weight of 16.0 amu (atomic mass units). If we consider a mole of oxygen, it has a mass of 16.0 grams. In other words, the mass of 6.02×10^{23} atoms of oxygen is 16.0 grams.

PRACTICE EXERCISE 23.A

Complete the individual values in Table 23-1 using Table 23-2. Find the atomic weight (to the nearest tenth) and the weight of 1 mole of each of the following elements. Be sure to include the label.

TABLE 23-1 Examples of Atomic Measures

		Atomic Weight	*(Mass of One Mole) Gram Atomic Weight*
Calcium	Ca	40.1 amu	40.1 g
Sodium	Na		
Potassium	K		
Sulfur	S		
Fluoride	F		
Iron	Fe		
Zinc	Zn		
Iodine	I		

TABLE 23-2 Table of Atomic Weights Based on Carbon-12

Element	*Symbol*	*Atomic Number*	*Atomic Weight*	*Element*	*Symbol*	*Atomic Number*	*Atomic Weight*
Actinium	Ac	89	[227]*	Chlorine	Cl	17	35.453
Aluminum	Al	13	26.9815	Chromium	Cr	24	51.996
Americium	Am	95	[243]	Cobalt	Co	27	58.9332
Antimony	Sb	51	121.75	Copper	Cu	29	63.546
Argon	Ar	18	39.948	Curium	Cm	96	[247]
Arsenic	As	33	74.9216	Dysprosium	Dy	66	162.50
Astatine	At	85	[210]	Einsteinium	Es	99	254
Barium	Ba	56	137.34	Erbium	Er	68	167.26
Berkelium	Bk	97	[247]	Europium	Eu	63	151.96
Beryllium	Be	4	9.0122	Fermium	Fm	100	[253]
Bismuth	Bi	83	208.980	Fluorine	F	9	18.9984
Boron	B	5	10.811	Francium	Fr	87	[223]
Bromine	Br	35	79.909	Gadolinium	Gd	64	157.25
Cadmium	Cd	48	112.40	Gallium	Ga	31	69.72
Calcium	Ca	20	40.08	Germanium	Ge	32	72.59
Californium	Cf	98	[249]	Gold	Au	79	196.967
Carbon	C	6	12.01115	Hafnium	Hf	72	178.49
Cerium	Ce	58	140.12	Helium	He	2	4.0026
Cesium	Cs	55	132.905	Holmium	Ho	67	164.930

continues

TABLE 23-2 Continued

Element	Symbol	Atomic Number	Atomic Weight	Element	Symbol	Atomic Number	Atomic Weight
Hydrogen	H	1	1.00797	Protactinium	Pa	91	[231]
Indium	In	49	114.82	Radium	Ra	88	[226]
Iodine	I	53	126.9044	Radon	Rn	86	[222]
Iridium	Ir	77	192.2	Rhenium	Re	75	186.2
Iron	Fe	26	55.847	Rhodium	Rh	45	102.905
Krypton	Kr	36	83.80	Rubidium	Rb	37	85.47
Lanthanum	La	57	138.91	Ruthenium	Ru	44	101.07
Lawrencium	Lw	103	[257]	Samarium	Sm	62	150.35
Lead	Pb	82	207.19	Scandium	Sc	21	44.956
Lithium	Li	3	6.939	Selenium	Se	34	78.96
Lutetium	Lu	71	174.97	Silicon	Si	14	28.086
Magnesium	Mg	12	24.312	Silver	Ag	47	107.870
Manganese	Mn	25	54.9380	Sodium	Na	11	22.9898
Mendelevium	Md	101	[256]	Strontium	Sr	38	87.62
Mercury	Hg	80	200.59	Sulfur	S	16	32.064
Molybdenum	Mo	42	95.94	Tantalum	Ta	73	180.948
Neodymium	Nd	60	144.24	Technetium	Tc	43	[99]
Neon	Ne	10	20.183	Tellurium	Te	52	127.60
Neptunium	Np	93	[237]	Terbium	Tb	65	158.924
Nickel	Ni	28	58.71	Thallium	Tl	81	204.37
Niobium	Nb	41	92.906	Thorium	Th	90	232.038
Nitrogen	N	7	14.0067	Thulium	Tm	69	168.934
Nobelium	No	102	[253]	Tin	Sn	50	118.69
Osmium	Os	76	190.2	Titanium	Ti	22	47.90
Oxygen	O	8	15.9994	Tungsten	W	74	183.85
Palladium	Pd	46	106.4	Uranium	U	92	238.03
Phosphorus	P	15	30.9738	Vanadium	V	23	50.942
Platinum	Pt	78	195.09	Xenon	Xe	54	131.30
Plutonium	Pu	94	[212]	Ytterbium	Yb	70	173.04
Polonium	Po	81	[210]	Yttrium	Y	39	88.905
Potassium	K	19	39.102	Zinc	Zn	30	65.37
Praseodymium	Pr	59	140.907	Zirconium	Zr	40	91.22
Promethium	Pm	61	[145]				

*A value given in brackets denotes the mass number of the longest-lived or best-known isotope. (From Nelson, J. H., Kemp, K. C. *Laboratory Experiments for Brown and LeMay Chemistry,* Englewood Cliffs, N.J.: Prentice-Hall, 1977.)

Mole of a Compound

We can also consider a mole of a compound. The mole of a compound is the amount of a substance equal to the formula weight of the substance expressed in grams (also known as the gram formula weight). A mole of a compound contains 6.02×10^{23} molecules of that compound. Suppose we consider a mole of water (H_2O). If we check Table 23-2 and round to the nearest tenth, we can find the weight of hydrogen and the weight of oxygen. Each atom of hydrogen has a mass of 1.0 amu and each atom of oxygen has a mass of 16.0 amu. We need to find the formula weight for water, which contains 2 hydrogen atoms and 1 oxygen atom.

$$2 \times \ 1.0 = \ 2.0$$
$$1 \times 16.0 = \underline{16.0}$$
$$18.0 \text{ amu}$$

Therefore, we can say that 1 water molecule has a mass of 18.0 atomic mass units. One mole of water must therefore have a mass of 18.0 grams.

PRACTICE EXERCISE 23.B

Find the mass of a mole of the following compounds:

1. Salt (NaCl)

2. Sodium nitrate ($NaNO_3$)

3. How many molecules of sodium nitrate are contained in a mole of the compound?

In a practical setting, there are essentially three types of questions we encounter:

How many grams?

How many moles?

How many atoms?

We will consider each of these questions, and explore them with individual examples.

How Many Grams?

EXAMPLE: What does 1 mole of potassium nitrate (KNO_3) weigh?

First, we can find the formula weight for 1 molecule of potassium nitrate.

K	39.1
N	14.0
O_3 $3 \times 16.0 =$	$\underline{48.0}$
	101.1 amu

Therefore, 1 molecule of potassium nitrate has a mass of 101.1 amu. We can conclude that 1 mole of KNO_3 has a mass of 101.1 grams.

EXAMPLE: Find the weight of 2.50 moles of potassium nitrate.

Using our result from the previous example, we can set up our dimensional analysis equation:

$$\frac{2.50 \text{ moles}}{1} \times \frac{101.1 \text{ g}}{1 \text{ mole}} = 252.75 \text{ g}$$

However, we must be careful of significant digits because these are measured quantities. Since 2.50 only has three significant digits, our result can have no more precision. Therefore, 2.50 moles of potassium nitrate has a mass of 253 g.

How Many Moles?

EXAMPLE: How many moles are there if you have 659 g of KNO_3?

Since 1 mole contains 101.1 g of potassium nitrate, we can set up our dimensional analysis equation:

$$\frac{659 \text{ g}}{1} \times \frac{1 \text{ mole}}{101.1 \text{ g}} = 6.518 \text{ moles} \approx 6.52 \text{ moles}$$

Again, since our measured quantity, 659 g, was measured to a precision of three significant digits, our result must have three significant digits as well. Therefore, 659 g of potassium nitrate constitutes 6.52 moles.

EXAMPLE: How many moles are there in 1.25×10^{25} molecules of KNO_3?

We recognize that we can set up our dimensional analysis equation and that our answer will have three significant digits:

$$\frac{1.25 \times 10^{25} \text{ molecules}}{1} \times \frac{1 \text{ mole}}{6.02 \times 10^{23} \text{ molecules}} =$$

$$20.764 \text{ moles} \approx 20.8 \text{ moles}$$

How Many Atoms?

EXAMPLE: How many atoms are there in 2.500 moles of potassium?

Since there are 6.02×10^{23} atoms in a mole of any substance, we can set up our dimensional analysis equation (our result should have four significant digits):

$$\frac{2.500 \text{ moles}}{1} \times \frac{6.02 \times 10^{23} \text{ atoms}}{1 \text{ mole}} =$$

$$15.05 \times 10^{23} \text{ atoms} = 1.505 \times 10^{24} \text{ atoms}$$

PRACTICE EXERCISE 23.C

1. A beaker of water contains 40.0 g of water. How many moles of water are present?
2. Find the weight of a mole of carbon dioxide (CO_2).
3. Find the weight of 1 mole of milk of magnesia (MgOH).
4. Determine the number of moles in 162.04 g of sodium nitrate ($NaNO_3$).
5. How many grams are there in 5.25 moles of iron?
6. We have 450 g of zinc (Zn). How many moles are there?
7. How many atoms are there in 3.50 moles of zinc?
8. How many moles are there in 1.204×10^{26} atoms of zinc?

Post-test

1. Which is heavier: a pound or a kilogram?

2. Write Arabic numerals for the following roman numerals:

$$\overline{\text{xxixss}}$$

3. Perform the following arithmetic operations:

   a. $(-2) + (-3)$

   b. $(-5) - (-6)$

   c. $(-5) \times (-2)$

   d. $(12) \div (-2)$

   e. $1.95 + 7.0701 + 5.2$

   f. $5 - 0.327$

   g. $(1.001) \times (1.1)$

   h. $1.1 \div 0.05$

   i. $\frac{2}{3} + \frac{1}{4} + \frac{1}{6}$

   j. $\left(3\frac{2}{5}\right) \times \left(\frac{1}{5}\right)$

   k. $\left(3\frac{2}{5}\right) \div \left(\frac{1}{5}\right)$

4. Convert the following percentages to decimals:

   a. 2.1%

   b. 0.45%

5. Convert the following ratio to a percentage: $1:20$.

6. Place the following numbers in scientific notation:

   a. $6,392$

   b. 0.0006392

249

7. Perform the multiplication and division on the following measured numbers. Place your answer in scientific notation:

$$\frac{(3.20 \times 10^4)\ (4.2 \times 10^3)}{2 \times 10^{-2}}$$

8. Convert 37.8°C to Fahrenheit. (Recall 5°C = 9°F.)

9. Make the following conversions. Show your conversion equations:

   a. 8 ℨ = _____ ml

   b. 2 g = _____ mcg

   c. 15 kg = _____ lb

   d. 1 C = _____ T

   e. gr $\overline{\text{iss}}$ = _____ mg

   f. 1 fℨ = _____ ♏

**Part II:
Applications**

1. Ordered: 250 mg q5h

   On hand: 100 mg/5 ml

   What would you administer?

2. Ordered: Thorazine 50 mg IM stat

   On hand:

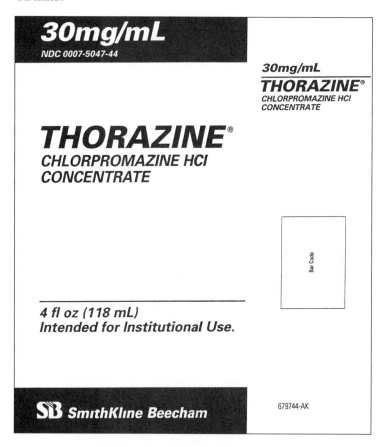

a. What would you administer?

b. Shade in the volume you would administer on the appropriate syringe.

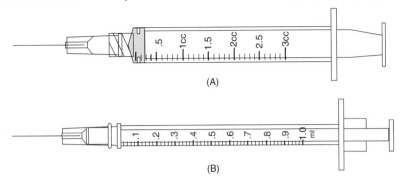

(A)

(B)

3. Ordered: Ampicillin N 350 mg IM stat

On hand:

Ampicillin sodium	For IM use, add 3.5 ml diluent (read accompanying circular). Resulting solution contains 250 mg ampicillin per ml.
for IM or IV use	**Use solution within 1 hour.** This vial contains ampicillin sodium equivalent to 1 gram ampicillin.
Equivalent to 1 gram ampicillin	Usual dosage: Adults—250 to 500 mg IM q6h
Caution: Federal law prohibits dispensing without prescription.	**Read accompanying circular** for detailed indications, IM, or IV dosage and precautions.

a. How many ml should be added to the vial?

b. How many ml should the patient receive?

4. Dosage ordered: Furadantin oral suspension 5 mg/kg/day po given in four equal doses. Client weight is 57½ lb. The drug is available in 25 mg/ml.

a. What is the daily dosage of Furadantin?

b. How much will be administered per dose?

5. Dosage ordered: 500 mg q4h po using lean body mass. The client is a 6′2″ male weighing 210 lb. Recommended dosage range: 20–50 mg/kg/day. (Recall formula for lean body mass: Male: 50 kg + 2.5 kg for each inch over 5 feet; Female: 45.4 kg + 2.3 kg for each inch over 5 feet.)

a. What is the client's lean body mass?

b. Is the dosage within the dosage range? Explain.

6. A box has a top that measures 67 cm by 54 cm and is 200 cm tall.

a. Find the area of the top of the box.

b. Find the volume of the box.

c. Convert the height of the box to meters.

7. Ordered: Mycostatin 200,000 U qid po.

On hand:

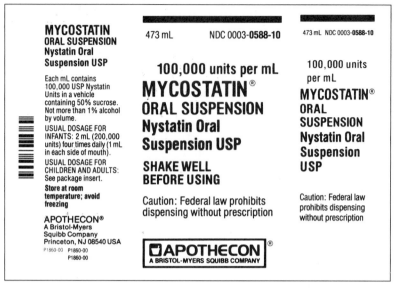

a. Is the on-hand medication a unit dose? Explain your answer.

b. What would you administer?

8. Suppose we wish to prepare 500 ml of 0.50% solution of sodium chloride.

a. How much sodium chloride will we use?

b. How much diluent will we use?

9. Prepare 800 ml of a 5.0% solution from a 25.0% stock solution.

a. How much solute will you need?

b. How much solvent will you need?

10. An IV of 1,000 ml of D5W was started at 12 noon using a microdrip infusion set (60 gtt/ml). The IV is to run 8 hours.

a. What is the drip rate?

b. At 5 P.M., 500 ml is in the bag. Is the IV on time, too fast, or too slow?

11. Ordered: Heparin 8,000 U q8h sc.

On hand: Heparin sodium injection USP 10,000 U/ml

What would you administer?

12. A patient weighing 175 lb has orders for Zovirax 5 mg/kg to be administered in 100 ml D5W over 1 hr. The drop rate is 20 gtt/ml.

a. What dosage should the patient receive?

b. Calculate the hourly rate.

c. Calculate the correct drop rate.

13. a. Determine the molar mass of CaO (Calcium oxide).

b. Determine the number of moles in 500 g of CaO.

c. How many molecules are there in 2.5 moles of CaO?

The following are common abbreviations used in the nursing/health care situation:

ABG	arterial blood gas	kg	kilogram
a.c.	before meals	KVO	keep vein open
ad	to, up to	L, l	liter
A.M.	morning	M², m²	square meter
aq	water	m, ℳ	minim
a.d.	right ear	max	maximum
a.l.	left ear	mcg, μg	microgram
ASAP	as soon as possible	mEq	milliequivalent
a.u.	each ear, both ears	mg	milligram
b.i.d.	two times a day	min	minute
BP	blood pressure	ml	milliter
C	Centigrade/Celsius, or Cup	NaCl	sodium chloride
c̄	with	n&v	nausea and vomiting
caps	capsules	NG	nasogastric
CBC	complete blood count	ng	nanogram
cc	cubic centimeters	noct	at night, during the night
cm	centimeter	NPO	nothing by mouth
d.	day	NR	do not refill
dc, d/c	discontinue	NS	normal saline (0.9% salt)
dil.	dilute	½NS	half-strength normal saline (0.45% salt)
dl	deciliter	¼NS	quarter-strength normal saline (0.2% salt)
dr, ʒ	dram	O.D.	right eye
D5W	5% dextrose in water	O.S.	left eye
elix	elixir	os	mouth
emuls.	emulsion	OTC	over the counter
ext.	extract	O.U.	each eye, both eyes
F	Fahrenheit, fluoride	oz, ʒ	ounce
g	gram	per	by, through
gal	gallon	pH	hydrogen ion concentration
GI	gastrointestinal	PMH	past medical history
gr	grain	PO, po	by mouth
gtt	drop, drops	PR	by rectum
h, hr	hour	PRN, prn	when needed or necessary
h.s.	at bedtime	PT	enteral (by feeding tube)
I&O	intake and output	pt	pint
IM	intramuscular	q	every
IV	intravenous	q.d.	every day
IVMB	IV mini-bag	q.h.	every hour
IVPB	IV piggyback, a secondary IV line	qhs	every night

q2h	every 2 hours	s.o.s.	if necessary, once only
q4h	every 4 hours	$\overline{ss}$	one half
q6h	every 6 hours	stat	immediately, first dose
q8h	every 8 hours	syr	syrup
q.i.d.	four times a day	tab	tablet
q.o.d.	every other day	tbsp (T)	tablespoon
q.s.	as much as is needed or required	t.i.d.	three times a day
qt	quart	T.O.	telephone order
RBC	red blood count	TPN	total parenteral nutrition
Rx	take, symbol for prescription	tsp (t)	teaspoon
$\overline{s}$	without	μg, mcg	microgram
SC, sc, SQ	subcutaneous	U	unit
SL	sublingual (beneath the tongue)	WBC	white blood count
sol	solution		

APPENDIX 2 *Answers to Exercises*

ARITHMETIC PRETEST

1. a. 5; **b.** –5; **c.** –5; **d.** –7; **e.** 2; **f.** –10; **g.** 15; **h.** 3; **i.** –6; **j.** 2; **k.** 0; **l.** 0

2. a. $\frac{13}{12}$; **b.** $\frac{3}{2}$; **c.** $\frac{17}{25}$; **d.** 17

3. a. 14.5453; **b.** 4.613; **c.** 2.20242; **d.** 22

4. a. 0.021; **b.** 0.0045

5. a. 0.9%; **b.** 37.5%

CHAPTER 1

PRACTICE EXERCISE 1A
1. 2 < 5; **2.** 7 > –4; **3.** –5 < 5; **4.** –3 < 0; **5.** –3 < –2; **6.** –2 > –4

PRACTICE EXERCISE 1B
1. 4; **2.** 5; **3.** –5; **4.** –4; **5.** 2; **6.** –5; **7.** –4; **8.** 6; **9.** –5; **10.** 5

PRACTICE EXERCISE 1C
1. –10; **2.** 12; **3.** 12; **4.** 0; **5.** –3; **6.** 5; **7.** 4; **8.** 0

LEARNING ACTIVITIES
1. a. –2°C; 97.8°F; **c.** –12°F
2. a. 650 cc; **b.** 1000cc – 650 cc = 350 cc
3. a. 550 cc; **b.** 1000cc – 550 cc = 450 cc

CHAPTER REVIEW EXERCISES
1. 10; **2.** –7; **3.** 4; **4.** –4; **5.** –8; **6.** –2; **7.** –15; **8.** –5; **9.** 1; **10.** 11; **11.** 1; **12.** 1; **13.** 4; **14.** 14; **15.** 6; **16.** –6; **17.** 0; **18.** 10; **19.** 4; **20.** –16; **21.** 4; **22.** –11; **23.** –21; **24.** 4; **25.** –5; **26.** 7; **27.** 0; **28.** 5; **29.** 0; **30.** –18; **31.** 12; **32.** –13; **33.** –8; **34.** 6; **35.** –24; **36.** –3; **37.** 21; **38.** 5; **39.** 1; **40.** –3; **41.** –3 < 3; **42.** 2 > 0; **43.** –2 < 0; **44.** –5 > –6; **46.** –100 > –101

CRITICAL THINKING
1. grains; **2.** Fahrenheit; **3.** drops; **4.** blood pressure; **5.** minim; **6.** ounce;
7. If the systolic pressure is more than 180 and the diastolic pressure is more than 90, the medicine will be administered.
8. Give acetaminophen for temp > 101°.
9. a. 800cc – 600 cc = 200 cc;
 b. 1000cc – 1300cc = –300cc;
 c. 200cc + (–300cc) = –100cc;
 d. 1600cc – 1400cc = 200cc, 200cc + (–100cc) = 100cc
10. 4867 ft – (–200 ft) = 4867 ft + 200 ft = 5067 ft
11. $289 – $137 = $152

CHAPTER 2

PRACTICE EXERCISE 2A
1. a. improper; **b.** proper; **c.** proper; **d.** mixed; **e.** improper; **f.** mixed.
2. a. 1 1/12; **b.** 3 1/2; **c.** 1 1/6; **d.** 10 1/3

PRACTICE EXERCISE 2B
1. 2/3; **2.** 1 2/5; **3.** 1 1/2; **4.** 1 1/3; **5.** 2/3; **6.** 3 1/3

PRACTICE EXERCISE 2C
1. 5/2; **2.** 41/7; **3.** 11/3; **4.** 7/4

PRACTICE EXERCISE 2D
1. 3/10; **2.** 5/9; **3.** 6/11; **4.** 10; **5.** 6

PRACTICE EXERCISE 2E
1. 5/6; **2.** 6/25; **3.** 3/5; **4.** 2 2/5; **5.** 12/25; **6.** 1/2

PRACTICE EXERCISE 2F
1. 6; **2.** 12; **3.** 24; **4.** 30; **5.** 120

PRACTICE EXERCISE 2G
1. 3/6, 5/6; **2.** 6/12, 8/12, 9/12; **3.** 18/24, 15/24, 16/24; **4.** 15/30, 10/30, 12/30; **5.** 45/120, 80/120, 96/120

PRACTICE EXERCISE 2H
1. 1 1/3; **2.** 1/4; **3.** 1 11/12; **4.** 5/6; **5.** 17/24; **6.** 13/30

PRACTICE EXERCISE 2I
1. <; **2.** =; **3.** >; **4.** >

LEARNING ACTIVITIES
Answers will vary.

CHAPTER REVIEW EXERCISES
1. a. 7/2; **b.** 5/3; **c.** 37/7
2. a. 2/3; **b.** 1 1/3; **c.** 1 2/5; **d.** 2/3; **e.** 1 1/2; **f.** 3 1/3
3. a. 10; **b.** 24; **c.** 30; **d.** 20
4. a. LCD = 24   **b.** LCD = 20

$$\frac{1\times 6}{4\times 6}=\frac{6}{24} \qquad \frac{1\times 10}{2\times 10}=\frac{10}{20}$$

$$\frac{3\times 3}{8\times 3}=\frac{9}{24} \qquad \frac{3\times 5}{4\times 5}=\frac{15}{20}$$

$$\frac{5\times 8}{3\times 8}=\frac{40}{24} \qquad \frac{2\times 4}{5\times 4}=\frac{8}{20}$$

5. a. >; **b.** <; **c.** =; **d.** >; **e.** <; **f.** <

6. a. $\frac{1}{2}+\frac{1}{4}=\frac{2}{4}+\frac{1}{4}=\frac{3}{4}$

 b. $\frac{4}{5}+\frac{8}{15}=\frac{12}{15}+\frac{1}{15}=\frac{13}{15}=1\frac{5}{15}=1\frac{1}{3}$

c. $1\frac{1}{8} + \frac{7}{12} = \frac{9}{8} + \frac{7}{12} = \frac{27}{24} + \frac{14}{24} = \frac{41}{24} = 1\frac{17}{24}$

d. $1\frac{3}{4} + 2\frac{1}{2} + 3\frac{1}{6} = \frac{7}{4} + \frac{5}{2} + \frac{19}{6} =$

$\qquad \frac{21}{12} + \frac{30}{12} + \frac{38}{12} = \frac{89}{12} = 7\frac{5}{12}$

e. $\frac{12}{5} - \frac{2}{5} = \frac{10}{5} = 2$

f. $\frac{13}{18} - \frac{4}{9} = \frac{13}{18} - \frac{8}{18} = \frac{5}{18}$

g. $1\frac{1}{2} - \frac{3}{4} = \frac{3}{2} - \frac{3}{4} = \frac{6}{4} - \frac{3}{4} = \frac{3}{4}$

h. $3\frac{1}{4} - 2\frac{5}{6} = \frac{13}{4} - \frac{17}{6} = \frac{39}{12} - \frac{34}{12} = \frac{5}{12}$

i. $\frac{1}{2} \times \frac{1}{4} = \frac{1}{8}$

j. $\frac{3}{5} \times \frac{2}{4} = \frac{6}{25}$

k. $\frac{11}{10} \times \frac{8}{5} = \frac{88}{50} = \frac{44}{25} = 1\frac{19}{25}$

l. $8\frac{1}{2} \times \frac{3}{4} = \frac{17}{2} \times \frac{3}{4} = \frac{51}{8} = 6\frac{3}{8}$

m. $\frac{2}{3} \times 3\frac{1}{2} \times \frac{5}{8} \times 12 = \frac{2}{3} \times \frac{7}{2} \times \frac{5}{8} \times \frac{12}{1} = \frac{35}{2} = 17\frac{1}{2}$

n. $\frac{7}{6} \div \frac{3}{5} = \frac{7}{6} \times \frac{5}{3} = \frac{35}{18} = 1\frac{17}{18}$

o. $\frac{5}{6} \div 15 = \frac{5}{6} \times \frac{1}{15} = \frac{5}{80} = \frac{1}{18}$

p. $3\frac{3}{4} \div 2\frac{1}{3} = \frac{15}{4} \div \frac{7}{3} = \frac{15}{4} \times \frac{3}{7} = \frac{45}{28} = 1\frac{17}{28}$

CRITICAL THINKING

1. one half; **2.** tablet; **3.** cubic centimeter;
4. subcutaneous; **5.** sodium chloride; **6.** normal saline;
7. ½ normal saline; **8.** ¼ normal saline; **9.** ½ cup;
10. ¾ teaspoon; **11.** ½ teaspoon; **12.** ½ gallon;
13. ½ ounce; **14.** 2 tablespoons; **15.** ½ quart;
16. ½ pint; **17.** ¼ cup;
18. 4/3 cups butter; 3 C sugar; 8 eggs; 3 C milk; 8 C flour;
2 tsp soda; 2 tsp baking powder; 2 tsp salt;
2 C chopped nuts

CHAPTER 3

PRACTICE EXERCISE 3A
1. thousands; **2.** tenths; **3.** hundred thousandths;
4. hundredths; **5.** thousandths

PRACTICE EXERCISE 3B
1. 2.1939; **2.** 30.915; **3.** 2.247; **4.** 4.625; **5.** 0.097

PRACTICE EXERCISE 3C
1. 28.782; **2.** 0.0136; **3.** 165; **4.** 80; **5.** 2.35

PRACTICE EXERCISE 3D
1. a. 0.75; **b.** 0.1$\overline{6}$; **c.** 0.375; **d.** 0.$\overline{2}$; **e.** 1.$\overline{6}$
2. a. 33/100; **b.** 7/8

LEARNING ACTIVITIES
1. 0.375; **2.** 1.53 cc; **3.** 0.6 g; **4.** 0.25 g; **5.** ½ g

CHAPTER REVIEW EXERCISES

1. a.
102.3400
5.7304
0.7890
108.8594

b.
3.575
−0.884
2.691

c.
2.5
3.45
125
100
75
8.625

d.
$\begin{array}{r} 85 \\ 22\overline{)1870} \\ \underline{176} \\ 110 \\ \underline{110} \end{array}$

e.
100.00
32.56
82.00
214.56

f.
2.000
−0.875
1.125

g.
1.0001
3.0
00000
30003
3.00030 = 3.0003

h.
$\begin{array}{r} 135.2 \\ 23\overline{)3109.6} \\ \underline{23} \\ 80 \\ \underline{69} \\ 119 \\ \underline{115} \\ 46 \\ \underline{46} \end{array}$

i.
0.0075
0.7500
0.0750
7.5000
8.3325

j.
32.500
− 0.079
32.421

k.
55.2
2.2
1104
1104
121.44

l.
$\begin{array}{r} 32.\overline{2} \\ 09\overline{)290.0} \\ \underline{27} \\ 20 \\ \underline{18} \\ 20 \\ \underline{18} \\ 2 \end{array}$

m.
$\begin{array}{r} 110.8108 \ldots \\ 111\overline{)12300.0000} \quad = 110.8\overline{10} \\ \underline{111} \\ 120 \\ \underline{111} \\ 900 \\ \underline{888} \\ 120 \\ \underline{111} \\ 900 \\ \underline{888} \\ 12 \end{array}$

n.
12.500
+ 0.725
13.225
− 3.560
9.665

2. a. 1.$\overline{6}$; **b.** 2.25; **c.** 0.00625; **d.** 0.$\overline{285714}$; **e.** 1.8; **f.** 0.$\overline{5}$

3. a. $0.125 = \frac{125}{1000} = \frac{1}{8}$; **b.** $0.11 = \frac{11}{100}$

CRITICAL THINKING
1. 2.0907, 2.9007, 2.907, 2.97
2. 0.5 strength normal saline
3. The patient weighs 65.3 kilograms.
4. To clearly understand how the given quantity is
measured. 2 grams and 2 milligrams are significantly
different.
5. 0.01 mg

6. The zero is for emphasis to help focus attention on the decimal point. It is very important in written medication orders.

7. $0.75 = \dfrac{75}{100} = \dfrac{3}{4}$ cc

8. 0.125 mg $= \dfrac{125}{1000} = \dfrac{1}{8}$ mg,

0.25 mg $= \dfrac{25}{100} = \dfrac{1}{4}$ mg $= \dfrac{2}{8}$ mg,

0.25 is larger, 2 tablets

9.

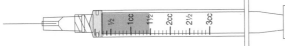

10. 96.43 g	**11.** 3.4 km
$\underline{-30.02\text{ g}}$	$\underline{10.5\text{ km}}$
66.41 g	13.9 km

12. No., probably the decimal point was placed incorrectly. It was most likely 303.0 miles.

CHAPTER 4

PRACTICE EXERCISE 4A
1. a. $3 \times 3 \times 3 \times 3$; **b.** $4 \times 4 \times 4$; **c.** 10×10; **d.** $1/(10 \times 10)$
2. a. 81; **b.** 64; **c.** 100; **d.** 0.01; **e.** 1

PRACTICE EXERCISE 4B
1. 9.178×10^3; **2.** 9.178×10^8; **3.** 9.178×10^{-2};
4. 9.178×10^2 **5.** 9.178×10^{-7}; **6.** 9.178×10^{21}
7. They all have the same 9.178. They all differ in the exponent on 10.

PRACTICE EXERCISE 4C
1. 4^5; **2.** 10^{11}; **3.** 2^1; **4.** 10^{-7}; **5.** 10^{-5}; **6.** 10^0

PRACTICE EXERCISE 4D
1. 4.08×10^6; **2.** 1.2×10^{10}; **3.** 7.056×10^{-3};
4. 1.806×10^2

PRACTICE EXERCISE 4E
1. 4^1; **2.** 10^{-3}; **3.** 2^{-7}; **4.** 10^{-3}; **5.** 10^7; **6.** 10^6

PRACTICE EXERCISE 4F
1. 2.31×10^4; **2.** 1.9×10^{-8}; **3.** 6.88×10^{-3};
4. 2.67×10^9

LEARNING ACTIVITIES
1. $13.5 \times 10^3 = 13,500$ WBC; not in the normal range
2. $3.2 \times 10^6 = 3,200,000$ RBC; not in the normal range
3. 21.6 cm $\times$ 27.9 cm $= 602.64$ cm^2 (approx. 603 cm^2)
4. 21.6 cm $\times$ 27.9 cm $\times$ 5.00 cm $= 3013.2$ cm^3 (approx. 3010 cm^3)
5. 8.0 ft $\times$ 6.5 ft $= 52$ ft^2
6. 24 in $\times$ 12 in $\times$ 3 in $= 864$ in^3 (approx. 860 in^3)

CHAPTER REVIEW EXERCISES
1. a. 2^4; **b.** 5^2; **c.** 10^1; **d.** 10^{-3}
2. a. $3^2 = 3 \times 3 = 9$; **b.** $5^4 = 5 \times 5 \times 5 \times 5 = 625$;
c. $10^8 = 10 \times 10 \times 10 \times 10 \times 10 \times 10 \times 10 \times 10 = 100,000,000$;
d. $10^{-3} = 1/(10 \times 10 \times 10) = 1/1000 = 0.001$; **e.** $3^0 = 1$

3. a. $10^2 \times 10^3 = 10^{2+3} = 10^5$; **b.** $5^2 \times 5^{-3} = 5^{2+(-3)} = 5^{-1}$;
c. $4^{-3} \times 4^{-2} = 4^{-3+(-2)} = 4^{-5}$; **d.** $10^6 \times 10^0 = 10^{6+0} = 10^6$
4. a. $10^2/10^5 = 10^{2-5} = 10^{-3}$; **b.** $5^2/5^{-3} = 5^{2-(-3)} = 5^5$;
c. $4^{-3}/4^{-2} = 4^{-3-(-2)} = 4^{-1}$; **d.** $10^6/10^0 = 10^{6-0} = 10^6$
5. a. 8.1×10^6; **b.** 4.75×10^4; **c.** 9.2×10^{-5}; **d.** 7.6×10^{-1}
e. 8×10^3; **f.** 6.1×10^{-9}
6. 0.001550003;   **7.** 2589988
8. a. $(2.0 \times 10^{-3}) \times (2.2 \times 10^2) = 4.4 \times 10^{-1}$
b. $(3.0 \times 10^2) \times (4.00 \times 10^3) =$
   $12 \times 10^5 = 1.2 \times 10^1 \times 10^5 = 1.2 \times 10^6$
c. $(2.1 \times 10^5) \times (16.0 \times 10^{-3}) = 12.6 \times 10^2 =$
   $1.26 \times 10^1 \times 10^2 = 1.26 \times 10^3$
d. $\dfrac{2.0 \times 10^5}{4.0 \times 10^2} = 0.5 \times 10^3 = 5.0 \times 10^{-1} \times 10^3 = 5.0 \times 10^2$

e. $\dfrac{6.02 \times 10^{23}}{2.00 \times 10^{-10}} = 3.01 \times 10^{33}$

f. $20(1.2 \times 10^{-5}) = 24 \times 10^{-5} = 2.4 \times 10^1 \times 10^{-5} = 2.4 \times 10^{-4}$

g. $(6.02 \times 10^{23}) \times (5.0 \times 10^{-2}) = 30.1 \times 10^{21} = 3.01 \times 10^1 \times 10^{21} = 3.01 \times 10^{22}$

h. $\dfrac{6.02 \times 10^{23}}{1.4 \times 10^{25}} = 4.3 \times 10^{-2}$

i. $(3.0 \times 10^4) \times (4.5 \times 10^{-3}) = 13.5 \times 10^1 = 1.35 \times 10^1 \times 10^1 = 1.35 \times 10^2$

j. $\dfrac{5.0 \times 10^{12}}{8 \times 10^{-2}} = 0.625 \times 10^{14} = 6.25 \times 10^{-1} \times 10^{14} = 6.25 \times 10^{13}$

9. a. $\dfrac{(3.0 \times 10^2) \times (1.0 \times 10^{-6})}{6 \times 10^3} = \dfrac{3.0 \times 10^{-4}}{6 \times 10^3} = 0.5 \times 10^{-7} = 5.0 \times 10^{-1} \times 10^{-7} = 5.0 \times 10^{-8}$

b. $\dfrac{(1.2 \times 10^6) \times (8.5 \times 10^{-2})}{2.4 \times 10^{-3}} = \dfrac{10.2 \times 10^4}{2.4 \times 10^{-3}} = 4.25 \times 10^7$

c. $\dfrac{(3.25 \times 10^2) \times (4.1 \times 10^{-1})}{4.52 \times 10^{-3}} = \dfrac{13.325 \times 10^1}{4.52 \times 10^{-3}} = 2.948 \times 10^4$

d. $\dfrac{(5.7 \times 10^2) \times (3.45 \times 10^5)}{3.0 \times 10^{-3}} = \dfrac{19.665 \times 10^7}{3.0 \times 10^{-3}} = 6.555 \times 10^{10}$

CRITICAL THINKING
1. complete blood count;   **2.** centimeter;   **3.** white blood count;   **4.** square meters;   **5.** red blood count;
6. milliliters;
7. $500,000 = 5 \times 10^5$ U

8. $\dfrac{6 \times 10^6}{5 \times 10^5} = 1.2 \times 10^1$ doses $= 12$ doses

CHAPTER 5

PRACTICE EXERCISE 5A
1. a. 0.625; **b.** 0.01; **c.** 0.25; **d.** 0.009; **e.** 1.75; **f.** 0.015
2. a. 65%; **b.** 12.5%; **c.** 33.3%; **d.** 0.45%;
e. 20%; **f.** 140%

PRACTICE EXERCISE 5B
1. 10%;   **2.** 25%;   **3.** 1%;   **4.** 0.4%

LEARNING ACTIVITIES
1. 0.9% NaCl; **2.** 9 g NaCl, enough to fill to 1000 ml;
3. a. 4.5 g; **b.** enough to fill to 1000 ml;
4. a. 100 ml; **b.** 400 ml; **5.** 60 g/100 ml

CHAPTER REVIEW EXERCISES
1. a. 27.2%; **b.** 0.9%; **c.** 70%; **d.** 0.01%;
  e. 132%; **f.** 250%
2. a. 0.132; **b.** 0.00045; **c.** 0.1; **d.** 1.68; **e.** 1; **f.** 0.007
3. a. 1:4 = $\frac{1}{4}$ = 0.25 = 25%; **b.** 1:8 = $\frac{1}{8}$ = 0.125 = 12.5%;
  c. 1:500 = 1/500 = 0.002 = 0.2%;
  d. 1:10000 = 1/10000 = 0.0001 = 0.01%
4. 1000 × 0.10 = 100; **5.** 250 × 0.009 = 2.25;
6. 132.8 × 0.25 = 33.2; **7.** 0.50 × 0.20 = 0.10 = 10%

CRITICAL THINKING
1. 500 cm³ × 0.09 = 45 cm³; 500 cm³ + 45 cm³ = 545 cm³
2. 36/45 = 0.80 = 80%
3. 1000 ml × 0.40 = 400 ml cresol;
  100 ml − 400 ml = 600 ml
4. 30 ounces × 0.60 = 18 ounces
5. 250 ml × $\frac{0.9\ g}{100\ ml}$ = 2.25 g
6. 250 ml × 0.50 = 125 ml Ensure;
  250 ml − 125 ml = 125 ml
7. 152.4 g × 0.05 = 7.62 g dextrose;
  152.4 g − 7.62 g = 144.78 g water
8. 2:250 = 2/250 = 0.008 = 0.8%, not isotonic (0.9%)
9. 38.6 g/0.03 = 1287 ml
10. 4000 ml × 0.02 = 80 ml; 4000 ml − 80 ml = 3920 ml

CHAPTER 6

PRACTICE EXERCISE 6A
1. $\frac{3\ ft}{1\ yd}$ or $\frac{1\ yd}{3\ ft}$ **2.** $\frac{16\ ounces}{1\ lb}$ or $\frac{1\ lb}{16\ ounces}$

3. $\frac{5,280\ ft}{1\ mi}$ or $\frac{1\ mi}{5280\ ft}$ **4.** $\frac{60\ min}{1\ hr}$ or $\frac{1\ hr}{60\ min}$

LEARNING ACTIVITIES
1. $\frac{6\ oz}{1} \times \frac{30\ cc}{1\ oz}$ = 180 cc

2. $\frac{10\ ounces}{1} \times \frac{1\ C}{8\ oz} = \frac{10\ C}{8} = 1\frac{1}{4}$ C

CHAPTER REVIEW EXERCISES
1. $\frac{3\ lb}{1} \times \frac{16\ oz}{1\ lb}$ = 48 oz

2. $\frac{5\ ft}{1} \times \frac{12\ in}{1\ ft}$ = 60 in

3. $\frac{2\ days}{1} \times \frac{24\ hrs}{1\ day}$ = 48 hrs

4. $\frac{240\ sec}{1} \times \frac{1\ min}{60\ sec}$ = 4 min

5. $\frac{130\ wks}{1} \times \frac{1\ yr}{52\ wks} = \frac{130}{52}$ yr = 2$\frac{1}{2}$ yr

6. $\frac{2.5\ hr}{1} \times \frac{60\ min}{1\ hr}$ = 150 min

7. $\frac{5\ yd}{1} \times \frac{3\ ft}{1\ yd}$ = 15 ft

8. $\frac{80\ in}{1} \times \frac{1\ ft}{12\ in} = \frac{80}{12}$ ft = 6 $\frac{2}{3}$ ft

9. $\frac{3.5\ min}{1} \times \frac{60\ sec}{1\ min}$ = 210 sec

10. $\frac{270\ min}{1} \times \frac{1\ hr}{60\ min}$ = 4.5 hr = 4$\frac{1}{2}$ hr

11. $\frac{256\ oz}{1} \times \frac{1\ lb}{16\ oz}$ = 16 lb

12. $\frac{10\ yd}{1} \times \frac{3\ ft}{1\ yd} \times \frac{12\ in}{1\ ft}$ = 360 in

13. $\frac{75\ ft}{1} \times \frac{1\ yd}{3\ ft}$ = 25 yd

14. $\frac{144\ hr}{1} \times \frac{1\ day}{24\ hr}$ = 6 days

15. $\frac{17\ weeks}{1} \times \frac{7\ days}{1\ week}$ = 119 days

16. $\frac{3\ hr}{1} \times \frac{60\ min}{1\ hr} \times \frac{60\ sec}{1\ min}$ = 10,800 sec

17. $\frac{60\ hr}{1} \times \frac{60\ min}{1\ hr}$ = 3600 min

18. $\frac{2\ wks}{1} \times \frac{7\ days}{1\ wk} \times \frac{24\ hr}{1\ day} \times \frac{60\ min}{1\ hr}$ = 20,160 min

19. $\frac{13104\ hrs}{1} \times \frac{1\ day}{24\ hr} \times \frac{1\ wk}{7\ day} \times \frac{1\ yr}{52\ wk} = \frac{13104}{8736}$ yr =
  1$\frac{1}{2}$ yr or 1.5 yr

20. $\frac{4\ wk}{1} \times \frac{7\ day}{1\ wk} \times \frac{24\ hr}{1\ day} \times \frac{60\ min}{1\ hr} \times \frac{60\ sec}{1\ min}$ = 2,419,200 sec

CRITICAL THINKING
1. hour; **2.** minute; **3.** every; **4.** every day;
5. every hour; **6.** total parenteral nutrition;
7. units; **8.** solution; **9.** every other day
10. a. First, check the name, room number, and nutrition
    number on the requisition with the food on the tray.
    Second, check the name and room number, and
    the identification bracelet with the information on
    the requisition slip. Third, check the nutrition
    requisition slip against the patient's identification
    bracelet.

  b. $\frac{4\ \mathfrak{Z}}{1} \times \frac{30\ cc}{1\ \mathfrak{Z}}$ = 120 cc

   $\frac{1\ glass}{1} \times \frac{8\ \mathfrak{Z}}{1\ glass} \times \frac{30\ cc}{1\ \mathfrak{Z}}$ = 240 cc

   $\frac{0.5\ glass}{1} \times \frac{8\ \mathfrak{Z}}{1\ glass} \times \frac{30\ cc}{1\ \mathfrak{Z}}$ = 120 cc

   $\frac{0.5\ C}{1} \times \frac{8\ \mathfrak{Z}}{1\ C} \times \frac{30\ cc}{1\ \mathfrak{Z}}$ = 120 cc

  c. 120 cc + 240 cc + 120 cc + 120 cc = 600 cc

CHAPTER 7

PRACTICE EXERCISE 7A
1. 16 ounces; **2.** 32 T; **3.** 320 $\mathfrak{Z}$; **4.** 4$\frac{1}{2}$ C

LEARNING ACTIVITIES
3. 1 quart soda; **4. a.** 96$\frac{1}{2}$ t; **b.** 12 C; **c.** 4.3 oz, 3.7 oz

CHAPTER REVIEW EXERCISES

1. $\dfrac{3/2\ T}{1}\times\dfrac{3\ t}{1\ T}=\dfrac{9}{2}\ t=4\frac{1}{2}\ t$

2. $\dfrac{12\ ℥}{1}\times\dfrac{1\ C}{8\ ℥}=1\frac{1}{2}\ C$

3. $\dfrac{4\ T}{1}\times\dfrac{1\ ℥}{2\ T}=2\ ℥$

4. $\dfrac{3\ qts}{1}\times\dfrac{2\ pt}{1\ qt}=6\ pt$

5. a. $\dfrac{3\ C}{1}\times\dfrac{8\ ℥}{1\ C}=24\ ℥$

   b. $\dfrac{3\ C}{1}\times\dfrac{8\ ℥}{1\ C}\times\dfrac{2\ T}{1\ ℥}=48\ T$

   c. $\dfrac{3\ C}{1}\times\dfrac{8\ ℥}{1\ C}\times\dfrac{2\ T}{1\ ℥}\times\dfrac{3\ t}{1\ T}=144\ t$

6. a. $\dfrac{144\ T}{1}\times\dfrac{3\ t}{1\ T}=432\ t$

   b. $\dfrac{144\ T}{1}\times\dfrac{1\ ℥}{2\ T}=72\ ℥$

   c. $\dfrac{144\ T}{1}\times\dfrac{1\ ℥}{2\ T}\times\dfrac{1\ C}{8\ ℥}=9\ C$

   d. $\dfrac{144\ T}{1}\times\dfrac{1\ ℥}{2\ T}\times\dfrac{1\ C}{8\ ℥}\times\dfrac{1\ pt}{2\ C}\times\dfrac{1\ qt}{2\ pt}=2\frac{1}{4}\ qt$

7. a. $\dfrac{3/2\ gal}{1}\times\dfrac{4\ qt}{1\ gal}=6\ qt$

   b. $\dfrac{3/2\ gal}{1}\times\dfrac{4\ qt}{1\ gal}\times\dfrac{2\ pt}{1\ qt}=12\ pt$

   c. $\dfrac{3/2\ gal}{1}\times\dfrac{4\ qt}{1\ gal}\times\dfrac{2\ pt}{1\ qt}\times\dfrac{2\ C}{1\ pt}=24\ C$

   d. $\dfrac{3/2\ gal}{1}\times\dfrac{4\ qt}{1\ gal}\times\dfrac{2\ pt}{1\ qt}\times\dfrac{2\ C}{1\ pt}\times\dfrac{8\ ℥}{1\ C}\times\dfrac{2\ T}{1\ ℥}\times\dfrac{3\ t}{1\ T}=1152\ t$

8. a. $\dfrac{1{,}200\ t}{1}\times\dfrac{1\ T}{3\ t}=400\ T$

   b. $\dfrac{1{,}200\ t}{1}\times\dfrac{1\ T}{3\ t}\times\dfrac{1\ ℥}{2\ T}\times\dfrac{1\ C}{8\ ℥}=25\ C$

   c. $\dfrac{1{,}200\ t}{1}\times\dfrac{1\ T}{3\ t}\times\dfrac{1\ ℥}{2\ T}\times\dfrac{1\ C}{8\ ℥}\times\dfrac{1\ pt}{2\ C}\times\dfrac{1\ qt}{2\ pt}=6\frac{1}{4}\ qt$

   d. $\dfrac{1{,}200\ t}{1}\times\dfrac{1\ T}{3\ t}\times\dfrac{1\ ℥}{2\ T}\times\dfrac{1\ C}{8\ ℥}\times\dfrac{1\ pt}{2\ C}=12\frac{1}{2}\ pt$

CRITICAL THINKING

1. $\dfrac{5\ mg}{1}\times\dfrac{1\ ℥}{30\ mg}\times\dfrac{2\ T}{1\ ℥}\times\dfrac{3\ t}{1\ T}=1\ t$

2. $\dfrac{8\ ounces}{1}\times\dfrac{2\ T}{1\ oz}\times\dfrac{3\ t}{1\ T}=48\ t$

3. $\dfrac{25\ mg}{1}\times\dfrac{1\ oz}{50\ mg}\times\dfrac{2\ T}{1\ oz}=1\ T$

4. $\dfrac{1\ gal}{1}\times\dfrac{4\ qts}{1\ gal}\times\dfrac{2\ pts}{1\ qt}\times\dfrac{2\ C}{1\ pt}\times\dfrac{8\ oz}{1\ C}\times\dfrac{1\ soak}{32\ oz}=4\ soaks$

5. $\dfrac{1\ gal}{1}\times\dfrac{4\ qts}{1\ gal}\times\dfrac{2\ pts}{1\ qt}\times\dfrac{2\ C}{1\ pt}\times\dfrac{8\ oz}{1\ C}\times\dfrac{1\ day}{8\ oz}=16\ days$

CHAPTER 8

PRACTICE EXERCISE 8A
1. a. xxiv; b. xxvii; c. iss; d. XLVIII; e. CLXXX; f. MCMXCVI
2. a. 39; b. 3; c. 78; d. 98; e. 2½; f. 1492

LEARNING ACTIVITIES
1. 1 minim; 2. 1 grain; 3. 1 fluid dram, 1 dram, They are parallel equivalents.
4. 8 drams, f ʒ i; 5. $\dfrac{1\ f℥}{1}\times\dfrac{8\ f ʒ}{1\ f℥}\times\dfrac{60\ gr}{1\ f ʒ}=480\ gr$
6. gr CDLXXX

CHAPTER REVIEW EXERCISES
1. a. ii; b. xxiv; c. xviii; d. xxix; e. XLV; f. iss; g. CXLIX; h. CCXL; i. ixss; j. CDXCIX
2. a. 4; b. 9; c. ½; d. 48; e. 2½; f. 91; g. 111; h. 344; i. 299; j. 1994

3. a. $\dfrac{12\ ʒ}{1}\times\dfrac{1\ ℥}{8\ ʒ}=1.5\ ℥$ or ℥ iss

   b. $\dfrac{12\ ʒ}{1}\times\dfrac{60\ m}{1\ ʒ}=720\ m$

   c. $\dfrac{12\ ʒ}{1}\times\dfrac{60\ gr}{1\ ʒ}=720\ gr$

4. a. $\dfrac{240\ gr}{1}\times\dfrac{1\ ʒ}{60\ gr}=4\ ʒ=ʒ\ iv$

   b. $\dfrac{240\ gr}{1}\times\dfrac{1\ ʒ}{60\ gr}\times\dfrac{1\ ℥}{8\ ʒ}=\frac{1}{2}\ ℥=℥\ ss$

5. a. $\dfrac{\frac{1}{2}\ ℥}{1}\times\dfrac{8\ ʒ}{1\ ℥}=4\ ʒ=ʒ\ iv$

   b. $\dfrac{\frac{1}{2}\ ℥}{1}\times\dfrac{8\ ʒ}{1\ ℥}\times\dfrac{60\ gr}{1\ ʒ}=240\ gr=gr\ CCXL$

6. a. $\dfrac{3\ ℥}{1}\times\dfrac{8\ ʒ}{1\ ℥}\times\dfrac{60\ gr}{1\ ʒ}=1440\ gr=gr\ MCDXL$

   b. $\dfrac{3\ ℥}{1}\times\dfrac{8\ ʒ}{1\ ℥}=24\ ʒ=ʒ\ XXIV$

   c. $\dfrac{3\ ℥}{1}\times\dfrac{8\ ʒ}{1\ ℥}\times\dfrac{60\ m}{1\ ʒ}\times\dfrac{1\ gtt}{1\ m}=1440\ gtt=gtt\ MCDXL$

7. $\dfrac{180\ gr}{1}\times\dfrac{1\ ʒ}{60\ gr}=3\ ʒ=ʒ\ iii$

8. $\dfrac{24\ ʒ}{1}\times\dfrac{1\ ℥}{8\ ʒ}=3\ ℥$ or ℥ iii

9. $\dfrac{90\ m}{1}\times\dfrac{1\ f ʒ}{60\ m}=1\frac{1}{2}\ f ʒ=f ʒ\ iss$

10. $\dfrac{10\ f℥}{1}\times\dfrac{1\ f℥}{8\ ℥}=1.25\ f℥$

CRITICAL THINKING

1. $\dfrac{\frac{1}{2}\ ℥}{1}\times\dfrac{60\ m}{1\ ℥}=30\ m=m\ XXX$

2. $\dfrac{\frac{1}{2}\ gr}{1}\times\dfrac{1\ tab}{\frac{1}{4}\ gr}=\dfrac{1/2}{1/4}\ tab=2\ tabs$

3. Minims

4. a. $\dfrac{10 \text{ gr}}{1} \times \dfrac{1 \text{ tab}}{5 \text{ gr}} = 2 \text{ tab}$

b. $\dfrac{1 \text{ dose}}{2 \text{ tabs}} \times \dfrac{50 \text{ tabs}}{1 \text{ bottle}} = 25 \text{ doses/bottle}$

CHAPTER 9

PRACTICE EXERCISE 9A
1. larger;   **2.** smaller;   **3.** smaller, 100 times, 100 cm = 1 m;   **4.** 1,000 mg = 1 g;
5. 1,000,000 mcg = 1 g

PRACTICE EXERCISE 9B
1. 100 cm;   **2.** 1 L;   **3.** 1,000 g;   **4.** 1 mg;
5. 1,000 mg;   **6.** 10 dl

PRACTICE EXERCISE 9C
1. 900 mg, (L-S);   **2.** 3 mg, (L-S);   **3.** 0.2 g, (S-L);
4. 1.5 g (S-L)

LEARNING ACTIVITIES
1. a. centimeters; **b.** millimeters; **c.** 100 cm;
d. 1000 mm; **e.** 10 mm = 1 cm
2. Answers will vary;   **3.** Answers will vary;
4. 50 cc (1 ℥ = 30 cc);   **5.** Answers will vary;   **6.** 20 g

CHAPTER REVIEW EXERCISES

1. $\dfrac{343 \text{ cm}}{1} \times \dfrac{1 \text{ m}}{100 \text{ cm}} = 3.43 \text{ m}$

2. $\dfrac{1.3 \text{ kg}}{1} \times \dfrac{1,000 \text{ g}}{1 \text{ kg}} = 1,300 \text{ g}$

3. $\dfrac{250 \text{ ml}}{1} \times \dfrac{1 \text{ cc}}{1 \text{ ml}} = 250 \text{ cc}$

4. $\dfrac{1250 \text{ ml}}{1} \times \dfrac{1 \text{ L}}{1,000 \text{ ml}} = 1.250 \text{ L}$

5. $\dfrac{2.4 \text{ m}}{1} \times \dfrac{1000 \text{ mm}}{1 \text{ m}} = 2400 \text{ mm}$

6. $\dfrac{75 \text{ mg}}{1} \times \dfrac{1 \text{ g}}{1,000 \text{ mg}} = 0.075 \text{ g}$

7. $\dfrac{2.7 \text{ L}}{1} \times \dfrac{1,000 \text{ ml}}{1 \text{ L}} = 2700 \text{ ml}$

8. $\dfrac{5,000 \text{ mcg}}{1} \times \dfrac{1 \text{ mg}}{1,000 \text{ mcg}} = 5 \text{ mg}$

9. $\dfrac{1.35 \text{ m}}{1} \times \dfrac{1,000 \text{ mm}}{1 \text{ m}} = 1,350 \text{ mm}$

10. $\dfrac{1.5 \text{ g}}{1} \times \dfrac{1,000 \text{ mg}}{1 \text{ g}} = 1,500 \text{ g}$

11. $\dfrac{500 \text{ m}}{1} \times \dfrac{1 \text{ km}}{1,000 \text{ m}} = 0.5 \text{ km}$

12. $\dfrac{5 \text{ L}}{1} \times \dfrac{1,000 \text{ ml}}{1 \text{ L}} \times \dfrac{1 \text{ cc}}{1 \text{ ml}} = 5,000 \text{ cc}$

13. $\dfrac{20 \text{ g}}{1} \times \dfrac{1,000 \text{ mg}}{1 \text{ g}} \times \dfrac{1,000 \text{ mcg}}{1 \text{ mg}} = 20,000,000 \text{ mcg}$

CRITICAL THINKING

1. $\dfrac{0.25 \text{ g}}{1} \times \dfrac{1 \text{ tab}}{0.5 \text{ g}} = 0.5 \text{ tab}$ **2.** mg;

3. $\dfrac{0.5 \text{ g}}{1} \times \dfrac{1,000 \text{ mg}}{1 \text{ g}} \times \dfrac{1 \text{ tab}}{500 \text{ mg}} = 1 \text{ tab}$;   **4.** 1 g;

5. 250 mg/5 ml   **6.** approximately 125 ml

7. $\dfrac{9 \text{ g}}{11} \times \dfrac{1 \text{ ml}}{1 \text{ g}} \times \dfrac{11}{1,000 \text{ ml}} = 0.009 = 0.9\%$ (normal saline)

CHAPTER 10

PRACTICE EXERCISE 10A
1. 1½ C;   **2.** 40 ℥ ;   **3.** 4 t;   **4.** 3 t;   **5.** 1 pt;   **6.** 2 qt;
7. ½ C;   **8.** 6 T;   **9.** 18 t;   **10.** 4 T

PRACTICE EXERCISE 10B
1. 2 ml;   **2.** 8 ml;   **3.** 240 ml;   **4.** 600 mg;   **5.** 2 g;
6. 30 mg;   **7.** 4 g;   **8.** 32 cc;   **9.** 30 cc;   **10.** 0.8 cc

PRACTICE EXERCISE 10C
1. 10 cc;   **2.** 240 cc;   **3.** 2 L;   **4.** 2,000 ml;   **5.** 2.5 ml;
6. 120 ml;   **7.** 120 ml;   **8.** 15 ml;   **9.** 0.5 L;   **10.** 2 L

PRACTICE EXERCISE 10D
1. 220 lb;   **2.** 45.5 kg;   **3.** 100 kg is larger because 1 kilogram is larger than 1 pound;   **4.** 65 kg;   **5.** 88.6 kg

PRACTICE EXERCISE 10E
1. 88 kg;   **2.** 87.9 kg;   **3.** 0.01 ml;   **4.** 0.07 ml;
5. 22 gtt;   **6.** 67 gtt

PRACTICE EXERCISE 10F
1. 16;   **2.** 6 C;   **3.** 2 ml, 2 cc;   **4.** 3 t;   **5.** 1 ℥ ;   **6.** 2 cc;
7. 60,000 mg;   **8.** 96 ℥ ;   **9.** A kilogram is larger.

CHAPTER REVIEW EXERCISES

1. $\dfrac{3 \text{ C}}{1} \times \dfrac{8 \text{ ℥}}{1 \text{ C}} \times \dfrac{8 \text{ f℥}}{1 \text{ ℥}} = 192 \text{ f℥}$

2. $\dfrac{5 \text{ gr}}{1} \times \dfrac{60 \text{ mg}}{1 \text{ gr}} = 300 \text{ mg}$

3. $\dfrac{40 \text{ ℥}}{1} \times \dfrac{30 \text{ ml}}{1 \text{ ℥}} = 1,200 \text{ ml}$

4. $\dfrac{4 \text{ ℥}}{1} \times \dfrac{1 \text{ t}}{1 \text{ ℥}} = 4 \text{ t}$

5. $\dfrac{44 \text{ ml}}{1} \times \dfrac{1 \text{ ℥}}{4 \text{ ml}} = 11 \text{ ℥}$

6. $\dfrac{75 \text{ kg}}{1} \times \dfrac{2.2 \text{ lb}}{1 \text{ kg}} = 165 \text{ lb}$

7. $\dfrac{3 \text{ ℥}}{1} \times \dfrac{1 \text{ t}}{1 \text{ ℥}} \times \dfrac{1 \text{ T}}{3 \text{ t}} = 1 \text{ T}$

8. $\dfrac{1/300 \text{ gr}}{1} \times \dfrac{60 \text{ mg}}{1 \text{ gr}} = 0.2 \text{ mg}$;

$\dfrac{0.2 \text{ mg}}{1} \times \dfrac{1 \text{ ml}}{0.5 \text{ g}} = 0.4 \text{ ml}$

9. $\dfrac{205 \text{ lb}}{1} \times \dfrac{1 \text{ kg}}{2.2 \text{ lb}} = 93.2 \text{ kg}$, No.

10. $\frac{1\ T}{1} \times \frac{1\ ʒ}{2\ T} \times \frac{30\ ml}{1\ ʒ} \times \frac{1\ cc}{1\ ml} = 15\ cc$

$\frac{1\ T}{1} \times \frac{3\ t}{1\ T} \times \frac{1\ ʒ}{1\ t} = 3\ ʒ$

11. $\frac{180\ gr}{1} \times \frac{1\ g}{15\ gr} = 12\ g$

12. $\frac{165\ lb}{1} \times \frac{1\ kg}{2.2\ lb} \times \frac{2.5\ mg}{1\ kg} = 187.5\ mg$

CRITICAL THINKING

1. The 10 ml is more correct. The ʒ = 1 t is roughly an equivalent. The mistake made by the lab partner is in not going from household directly to metric. It is a bad idea to make a conversion and use all three systems (it is also unnecessary) as it leads to increased inaccuracy.

2. $\frac{1\ t}{1} \times \frac{1\ ʒ}{1\ t} \times \frac{60\ ♏}{1\ ʒ} = 60\ ♏$

3. $\frac{1\ t}{1} \times \frac{5\ ml}{1\ t} \times \frac{12.5\ mg}{5\ ml} = 12.5\ mg$

4. $\frac{154\ lb}{1} \times \frac{1\ kg}{2.2\ lb} \times \frac{50\ mg}{1\ kg} \times \frac{1\ g}{1,000\ mg} = 3.5\ g$

5. $\frac{7\ mg}{1} \times \frac{1\ ʒ}{42\ mg} \times \frac{2\ T}{1\ ʒ} \times \frac{3\ t}{1\ T} = 1\ t$

6. $\frac{6\ mg}{1} \times \frac{1\ ʒ}{30\ mg} = 0.2\ ʒ$

7. $\frac{250\ mg}{1} \times \frac{5\ ml}{125\ mg} \times \frac{1\ t}{5\ ml} = 2\ t$

8. $\frac{160\ mg}{1} \times \frac{15\ ml}{80\ mg} \times \frac{1\ t}{5\ ml} \times \frac{1\ T}{3\ t} = 2\ T$

9. 1 tsp = 5 cc
1 tbsp = 15 ml
1 oz = 30 cc
1 cup = 240 cc

$\frac{4\ ʒ}{1} \times \frac{30\ cc}{1\ ʒ} = 120\ cc$

$\frac{1\ glass}{1} \times \frac{8\ ʒ}{1\ glass} \times \frac{30\ cc}{1\ ʒ} = 240\ cc$

$\frac{2\ T}{1} \times \frac{15\ cc}{1\ T} = 30\ cc$

$\frac{0.5\ C}{1} \times \frac{240\ cc}{1\ C} = 120\ cc$

$120\ cc + 240\ cc + 30\ cc + 120\ cc = 510\ cc$

CHAPTER 11

PRACTICE EXERCISE 11A
1. 50 mg/tablet; **2.** 20 mg/5 ml; **3.** gr X/3 ml;
4. 100,000 U/ml; **5.** 250 mg/ml; **6.** 500 mg/capsule;
7. 100 U/ml; **8.** 2 mEq/ml

LEARNING ACTIVITIES 11
9. 125 mcg or 0.125 mg; **11.** 500 mcg;
12. Lanoxin 125 mcg
13. 1 g/10 ml because 20 ml of solution po will be easier to administer and easier for patient to drink rather than 80 ml of 125 mg/5 ml.

14. For patient convenience, administer two 5 mg tablets.
15. Administer 2 ml of 50 mg/ml as it will be more comfortable for the patient.

CHAPTER REVIEW EXERCISES
1. 40 mg of propranolol hydrochloride orally twice a day.
2. 50 mg of Demerol given intramuscularly every 4 hours as needed for pain.
3. Two 325 mg tablets of acetaminophen given orally immediately.
4. 2 drops of pilocarpine in both eyes every 3 hours.
5. 0.25 mg of Digoxin elixir given orally each day.
6. 30 mEq of K-Lor given orally twice a day.
7. 6,000 U of heparin administered subcutaneously every 4 hours.
8. 15 U of insulin given subcutaneously each day at 7:30 A.M.
9. 10 gr of aspirin given orally every 4 hours as needed for temperature over 101°.
10. 10 mg of prednisone given orally every other day.

CRITICAL THINKING
1.

Mass	Volume/quantity
a. 10 mg	5 ml
b. 200 mg	tablet
c. 1,000 U	1 ml
d. 1,000,000 U	1 ml
e. 5 g	100 ml

2.

Name	Dosage	Route	Frequency
a. Codeine	60 mg	orally	every 3 hours as needed
b. Benadryl	30 mg	orally	3 times a day
c. Iron sulfate	300 mg	orally	4 times a day
d. Atropine	1/100 gr	IM	immediately
e. Vancomycin	1 gram	IV minibag	every 12 hours

3.

Mass	How supplied	Generic	Trade Name
a. 150 million units	oral suspension	Nystatin powder	Nilstat
b. 60 mg	tablets	Pseudoephedrine Hydrochloride	Sudafed
c. 30 mg	capsules	Extended Phenytoin Sodium capsules	Dilantin
d. 100 USP	50 ml	Cyclosporine	Sandimmune
e. 100000 U	oral suspension	Nystatin Oral Suspension	Mycostatin

4. Pour contents into glass and add at least 4 ounces cold water or juice. Stir until dissolved.
5. Administer one 0.5 mg tablet for patient convenience.
6. $\frac{0.25\ gr}{1} \times \frac{60\ mg}{1\ gr} = 15\ mg$; Administer 1.0 ml of 15 mg/ml SC.
7. Question if the medication you have found is the same as the one ordered. Consult references, pharmacist, or resource nurse.

CHAPTER 12

PRACTICE EXERCISE 12A
1. John; **2.** Patient is blind; **3.** Allergic to penicillin and ASA (aspirin); **4.** March 4 at 9 A.M.; **5.** yes;
6. Elixophyllin 0.4 g PO b.i.d.
   Acetaminophen 650 mg PO q 4h
7. Acetaminophen 650 mg PO

LEARNING ACTIVITIES
1. May offer a choice of: Meperidine HCL 25 mg IM
   Hydroxyzine 25 mg IM
   Acetaminophen 650 mg po
   Meperidine 75 mg po
   Naproxen 500 mg
2. That was a one-time order—no prescription for that. Call physician for a new order.
3. May have choice of: Acetaminophen 650 mg po
   Meperidine 75 mg po
   Naproxen 500 mg po

CHAPTER REVIEW EXERCISES
1. Answers will vary depending on institution.
2. KCL   3/4 @ 1800
   Metronidazole   3/4 @ 0900
   Procan SR   3/4 @ 0800
   Levothyroxine Na   3/4 @ 0900
   Vitamin A   3/4 @ 0900
   Vitamin C   3/4 @ 0900
   Ofloxacin   3/4 @ 1800

CRITICAL THINKING
1. Investigate, seek clarification, contact the nurse previously assigned to patient. Administration of previous dose must be clarified before proceeding.
2. Because every medication must be given in accordance with the five rights of medication administration.
3. When removing the medication package from the drawer, prior to pouring the medication, and after preparing the medication.
4. The physician's original sheet.

CHAPTER 13

PRACTICE EXERCISE 13A
1. 2 tablets;   **2.** 1.3 ml;   **3.** 2 tablets

LEARNING EXERCISES
1. 1 ounce
2. $\dfrac{15 \text{ mg}}{1} \times \dfrac{5 \text{ ml}}{12.5 \text{ mg}} = 6$ ml; No, use a syringe and squeeze into a cup.
3. a. None; **b.** $\dfrac{5 \text{ mg}}{1} \times \dfrac{1 \text{ tab}}{10 \text{ mg}} = \frac{1}{2}$ tablet
   c. 0900

CHAPTER REVIEW EXERCISES
1. $\dfrac{0.5 \text{ g}}{1} \times \dfrac{1,000 \text{ mg}}{1 \text{ g}} \times \dfrac{1 \text{ cap}}{500 \text{ mg}} = 1$ cap
2. $\dfrac{4 \text{ mg}}{1} \times \dfrac{1 \text{ tab}}{2 \text{ mg}} = 2$ tab

3. $\dfrac{0.25 \text{ mg}}{1} \times \dfrac{1 \text{ tab}}{0.125 \text{ mg}} = 2$ tab
4. $\dfrac{800 \text{ mg}}{1} \times \dfrac{1 \text{ tab}}{400 \text{ mg}} = 2$ tab
5. $\dfrac{1,000,000 \text{ U}}{1} \times \dfrac{1 \text{ ml}}{100,000 \text{ U}} = 10$ ml
6. $\dfrac{200 \text{ mg}}{1} \times \dfrac{1 \text{ cap}}{100 \text{ mg}} = 2$ cap
7. $\dfrac{0.4 \text{ g}}{1} \times \dfrac{1,000 \text{ mg}}{1 \text{ g}} \times \dfrac{1 \text{ cap}}{200 \text{ mg}} = 2$ cap
8. $\dfrac{10 \text{ mg}}{1} \times \dfrac{5 \text{ ml}}{15 \text{ mg}} = 3.3$ ml
9. $\dfrac{0.25 \text{ g}}{1} \times \dfrac{1000 \text{ mg}}{1 \text{ g}} \times \dfrac{1 \text{ tab}}{250 \text{ mg}} = 1$ tab
10. 1000 mg tablets
11. $\dfrac{25 \text{ mg}}{1} \times \dfrac{5 \text{ ml}}{10 \text{ mg}} = 12.5$ ml
12. $\dfrac{0.125 \text{ mg}}{1} \times \dfrac{1 \text{ tab}}{0.25 \text{ mg}} = \frac{1}{2}$ tab
13. $\dfrac{200 \text{ mg}}{1} \times \dfrac{1 \text{ tab}}{100 \text{ mg}} = 2$ tab
14. $\dfrac{15 \text{ mg}}{1} \times \dfrac{10 \text{ ml}}{20 \text{ mg}} = 7.5$ ml
15. $\dfrac{0.1 \text{ mg}}{1} \times \dfrac{1,000 \text{ mcg}}{1 \text{ mg}} \times \dfrac{1 \text{ tab}}{100 \text{ mcg}} = 1$ tab

CRITICAL THINKING
1. Question the amount. Go back and check the order and the strength you have been supplied. Ask a colleague to check your calculation. Two tablets to two and one-half tablets are the usual amount of oral medication administered.
2. Verify that the patient matches with the name. Verify identity and secure a name band to wrist.
3. Go back and check the order and the strength of the tablets you have been supplied.
4. Question the order. Check the order and the form of medication you have been supplied. If you are to give one half, then contact the pharmacy for further clarification of the form supplied.
5. Draw up into a 5 cc syringe and squirt into a cup.

CHAPTER 14

PRACTICE EXERCISES 14A
1. 0.3 cc;   **2.** 1 ml;   **3.** 1 ml;   **4.** 1 ml;   **5.** 0.6 ml

LEARNING ACTIVITIES
6. 0.9 ml, 12 ♏ , 20 U
7. a. 2 g; **b.** sterile water, 99 ml; **c.** 1 g/50 ml;
   d. 100 ml; **e.** 49 ml

CHAPTER REVIEW EXERCISES
1. $\dfrac{1/5 \text{ gr}}{1} \times \dfrac{60 \text{ mg}}{1 \text{ gr}} \times \dfrac{1 \text{ ml}}{10 \text{ mg}} = 1.2$ ml
2. $\dfrac{50 \text{ mg}}{1} \times \dfrac{1 \text{ ml}}{25 \text{ mg}} = 2$ ml

3. $\dfrac{300 \text{ mg}}{1} \times \dfrac{2 \text{ ml}}{300 \text{ mg}} = 2 \text{ ml}$

4. a. Intramuscular

   b. $\dfrac{250 \text{ mg}}{1} \times \dfrac{1 \text{ ml}}{250 \text{ mg}} = 1 \text{ ml}$

5. a. Intramuscular; **b.** $\dfrac{1,200,000 \text{ U}}{1} \times \dfrac{2 \text{ ml}}{600,000 \text{ U}} = 4 \text{ ml}$;

   c. once; **d.** 600,00 U/2 ml in a tubex; given as 2 ml per injection site in 2 sites since amount exceeds 0.5–2.5 ml

CRITICAL THINKING

1. A 1 ml insulin syringe will be used.

2. A 2.0 ml injection will be given intramuscularly, although given the patient's age and weight, the needle can be a smaller size because there will be less fatty tissue. A large muscle mass (such as gluteus) will be used as an injection site.

3. Deltoid

4. $\dfrac{5,000 \text{ U}}{1} \times \dfrac{1 \text{ ml}}{10,000 \text{ U}} = 0.5 \text{ ml}$;

Check most recent lab report regarding coagulation time.

CHAPTER 15

PRACTICE EXERCISE 15A

1. a. 1½ tablets; **b.** 150 mg; **2.** 3,750 mcg; **3.** 9 mg;
4. 5,818 units ≈ 5800 units (round to the nearest 100);
5. 6,800 units; **6.** 164 mg; **7.** 1200 mg; **8.** 205 mcg

PRACTICE EXERCISES 15B

1. a. 1.42 m²; **b.** approximately equal (191.7 mg);
2. a. 1.91 m²; **b.** 95.5 mg ≈ 90 mg; **3.** 5.1 g ≈ 5.7 g;
4. 722.5 mg ≈ 725 mg; **5.** 42.5 mg ≈ 40 mg; **6.** 170 mg;
340 mg ≈ 350 mg; **7. a.** yes; **b.** 260 mg ≈ 250 mg

PRACTICE EXERCISE 15C

1. 2.7 ml; **2. a.** 65 kg; **b.** 5,200 U;
3. a. 55 kg; **b.** 1,100 mg; **4.** 6,800 U

PRACTICE EXERCISE 15D

1. a. 1.81 m²; b. 452.5 mg; **c.** 1,357.5 mg/day;
2. a. 7 ml; **b.** yes; **3.** yes

LEARNING ACTIVITIES

1. 18 ml; **2. a.** 15 mg/kg; **b.** 187.5 mg; **c.** 0.5 ml;
3. a. 264 mg/day; **b.** 1.4 ml

CHAPTER REVIEW EXERCISES

1. $\dfrac{180 \text{ lb}}{1} \times \dfrac{1 \text{ kg}}{2.2 \text{ lbs}} \times \dfrac{0.01 \text{ mg}}{1 \text{ kg}} = 81.8 \text{ mg}$

2. $\dfrac{110 \text{ lb}}{1} \times \dfrac{1 \text{ kg}}{2.2 \text{ lbs}} \times \dfrac{2.5 \text{ mg}}{1 \text{ kg}} = 125 \text{ mg}$

3. $\dfrac{132 \text{ lb}}{1} \times \dfrac{1 \text{ kg}}{2.2 \text{ lb}} \times \dfrac{0.15 \text{ mg}}{1 \text{ kg}} = 9 \text{ mg}$

4. a. $\dfrac{155 \text{ lb}}{1} \times \dfrac{1 \text{ kg}}{2.2 \text{ lbs}} \times \dfrac{2.5 \text{ mg}}{1 \text{ kg}} \times \dfrac{1 \text{ tab}}{50 \text{ mg}} = 3\dfrac{1}{2} \text{ tab}$

   b. $\dfrac{1.7 \text{ m}^2}{1 \text{ dose}} \times \dfrac{90 \text{ mg}}{1 \text{ m}^2} = 153 \text{ mg/dose}$

   c. $\dfrac{153 \text{ mg}}{1 \text{ dose}} \times \dfrac{1 \text{ tab}}{50 \text{ mg}} = 3 \text{ tab}$

CRITICAL THINKING

1. 60 kg and 200 cm → 1.81 m²

$\dfrac{1.81 \text{ m}^2}{1} \times \dfrac{250 \text{ mg}}{1 \text{ m}^2} = 452.5 \text{ mg}$

2. Minimum dose: $\dfrac{130 \text{ lb}}{1} \times \dfrac{1 \text{ kg}}{2.2 \text{ lbs}} \times \dfrac{0.05 \text{ mg}}{1 \text{ kg}} = 2.95 \text{ mg}$

Maximum dose: $\dfrac{130 \text{ lb}}{1} \times \dfrac{1 \text{ kg}}{2.2 \text{ lb}} \times \dfrac{0.2 \text{ mg}}{1 \text{ kg}} = 11.8 \text{ mg}$

Yes, it is in the safe range.

3. a. 50 kg + 2.5 kg · 12 = 80 kg

   b. $\dfrac{80 \text{ kg}}{1} \times \dfrac{2 \text{ mg}}{1 \text{ kg}} = 160 \text{ mg}$

   c. $\dfrac{80 \text{ kg}}{1} \times \dfrac{1 \text{ mg}}{1 \text{ kg}} = 80 \text{ mg}$

   d. $\dfrac{80 \text{ mg}}{\text{dose}} \times \dfrac{3 \text{ doses}}{1 \text{ day}} = \dfrac{240 \text{ mg}}{\text{day}} = 240 \text{ mg/day}$

4. Ordered: $\dfrac{0.5 \text{ mcg}}{1 \text{ dose}} \times \dfrac{12 \text{ doses}}{1 \text{ day}} = 6 \text{ mcg/day}$

Lower-range value:

$\dfrac{220 \text{ lb}}{1 \text{ day}} \times \dfrac{1 \text{ kg}}{2.2 \text{ lbs}} \times \dfrac{0.04 \text{ mcg}}{1 \text{ kg}} = 4 \text{ mcg/day}$

Upper-range value:

$\dfrac{220 \text{ lb}}{1} \times \dfrac{1 \text{ kg}}{2.2 \text{ lb}} \times \dfrac{0.5 \text{ mcg}}{1 \text{ kg}} = 5 \text{ mcg/day}$

The order is not within the recommended range.

5. a. $\dfrac{100 \text{ mg}}{1 \text{ dose}} \times \dfrac{3 \text{ doses}}{1 \text{ day}} = 300 \text{ mg/day}$

   b. Lower-range value:

$\dfrac{185 \text{ lb}}{1 \text{ day}} \times \dfrac{1 \text{ kg}}{2.2 \text{ lb}} \times \dfrac{3 \text{ mg}}{1 \text{ kg}} = 252.3 \text{ mg/day}$

Upper-range value:

$\dfrac{185 \text{ lb}}{1} \times \dfrac{1 \text{ kg}}{2.2 \text{ lb}} \times \dfrac{5 \text{ mg}}{1 \text{ kg}} = 420.5 \text{ mg day}$

This order is within range.

   c. $\dfrac{300 \text{ mg}}{1 \text{ day}} \times \dfrac{1 \text{ ml}}{40 \text{ mg}} \times \dfrac{1 \text{ day}}{3 \text{ doses}} = 2.5 \text{ ml/dose}$

6. a. $\dfrac{140 \text{ mg}}{1} \times \dfrac{1 \text{ ml}}{20 \text{ mg}} = 7 \text{ ml}$

   b. Ordered: 140 mg/day
Lower-range value:

$\dfrac{1.5 \text{ m}^2}{1 \text{ day}} \times \dfrac{50 \text{ mg}}{1 \text{ m}^2} = 75 \text{ mg/day}$

Upper-range value:

$\dfrac{1.5 \text{ m}^2}{1 \text{ day}} \times \dfrac{100 \text{ mg}}{1 \text{ m}^2} = 150 \text{ mg/day}$

The order is within range.

CHAPTER 16

PRACTICE EXERCISE 16A
1. a. 3,750 mcg; 3.75 mg; **2. a.** 1½ tablets; **b.** 150 mg;
3. a. 100 mg/kg/day; **b.** 500 mg/dose; **c.** 1.25 ml

LEARNING ACTIVITIES
1. 1.08 m^2; **2. a.** 0.68 m^2; **b.** 102 mg; **c.** 306 mg/day

CHAPTER REVIEW EXERCISES
1. a. $\frac{80 \text{ mg}}{1 \text{ tab}} \times \frac{2 \text{ tab}}{6 \text{ hrs}} \times \frac{24 \text{ hrs}}{1 \text{ day}} \times \frac{1 \text{ g}}{1,000 \text{ mg}} = 0.64$ g/day; yes

b. $\frac{40 \text{ lb}}{1 \text{ dose}} \times \frac{1 \text{ kg}}{2.2 \text{ lb}} \times \frac{10 \text{ mg}}{1 \text{ kg}} = 182$ mg/dose

Keep dose the same.

2. a. $\frac{30 \text{ lb}}{1 \text{ day}} \times \frac{1 \text{ kg}}{2.2 \text{ lb}} \times \frac{4 \text{ mg}}{1 \text{ kg}} = 55$ mg/day

b. $\frac{30 \text{ lb}}{1 \text{ day}} \times \frac{1 \text{ kg}}{2.2 \text{ lb}} \times \frac{4 \text{ mg}}{1 \text{ kg}} \times \frac{1 \text{ ml}}{65 \text{ mg}} = 0.8$ mL/day

3. $\frac{70 \text{ lb}}{1} \times \frac{1 \text{ kg}}{2.2 \text{ lb}} \times \frac{0.06 \text{ mg}}{1 \text{ kg}} \times \frac{1 \text{ ml}}{1 \text{ mg}} = 1.9$ ml

4. a. $\frac{72 \text{ lb}}{1} \times \frac{1 \text{ kg}}{2.2 \text{ lb}} \times \frac{6 \text{ mg}}{1 \text{ kg}} = 196.4$ mg; one 200 mg capsule

b. $\frac{72 \text{ lb}}{1} \times \frac{1 \text{ kg}}{2.2 \text{ lb}} \times \frac{3 \text{ mg}}{1 \text{ kg}} = 98.2$ mg; one 100 mg capsule

5. a. $\frac{25 \text{ lb}}{1 \text{ day}} \times \frac{1 \text{ kg}}{2.2 \text{ lb}} \times \frac{100 \text{ mg}}{1 \text{ kg}} = 1136$ mg/day

b. $\frac{25 \text{ lb}}{1 \text{ day}} \times \frac{1 \text{ kg}}{2.2 \text{ lb}} \times \frac{100 \text{ mg}}{1 \text{ kg}} \times \frac{1 \text{ g}}{1,000 \text{ mg}} \times \frac{25 \text{ mL}}{1 \text{ g}} \times \frac{1 \text{ day}}{4 \text{ doses}} =$ 7 ml/dose

6. a. $\frac{20 \text{ kg}}{1 \text{ day}} \times \frac{10 \text{ mg}}{1 \text{ kg}} = 200$ mg/day

b. $\frac{20 \text{ kg}}{1 \text{ day}} \times \frac{10 \text{ mg}}{1 \text{ kg}} \times \frac{1 \text{ day}}{4 \text{ doses}} = 50$ mg/dose

7. a. $\frac{60 \text{ lb}}{1 \text{ dose}} \times \frac{1 \text{ kg}}{2.2 \text{ lb}} \times \frac{5 \text{ mg}}{1 \text{ kg}} = 136$ mg/dose

b. Maximum daily dosage:

$\frac{60 \text{ lb}}{1 \text{ day}} \times \frac{1 \text{ kg}}{2.2 \text{ lb}} \times \frac{40 \text{ mg}}{1 \text{ kg}} = 1{,}091$ mg/day

$\frac{136 \text{ mg}}{1 \text{ dose}} \times \frac{3 \text{ doses}}{1} = 408$ mg; yes

8. a. $\frac{1{,}100 \text{ g}}{1 \text{ day}} \times \frac{1 \text{ kg}}{1{,}000 \text{ g}} \times \frac{50 \text{ mg}}{1 \text{ kg}} = 55$ mg/day

b. $\frac{1{,}100 \text{ g}}{1 \text{ day}} \times \frac{1 \text{ kg}}{1{,}000 \text{ g}} \times \frac{50 \text{ mg}}{1 \text{ kg}} \times \frac{1 \text{ day}}{4 \text{ doses}} = 14$ mg/dose

CRITICAL THINKING
1. Ordered: 2 mg

Lower-range value: $\frac{60 \text{ lb}}{1} \times \frac{1 \text{ kg}}{2.2 \text{ lb}} \times \frac{0.05 \text{ mg}}{1 \text{ kg}} = 1.36$ mg

Upper-range value: 4 mg

This dose is closer to the minimum dosage.

2. Ordered: 2 mg

Lower-range value: $\frac{36 \text{ lb}}{1} \times \frac{1 \text{ kg}}{2.2 \text{ lb}} \times \frac{0.05 \text{ mg}}{1 \text{ kg}} = 0.82$ mg

Upper-range value: $\frac{36 \text{ lb}}{1} \times \frac{1 \text{ kg}}{2.2 \text{ lb}} \times \frac{0.2 \text{ mg}}{1 \text{ kg}} = 3.27$ mg

The order is within range.

3. a. $\frac{36 \text{ lb}}{1} \times \frac{1 \text{ kg}}{2.2 \text{ lb}} \times \frac{0.1 \text{ mg}}{1 \text{ kg}} = 1.6$ mg

b. 0.4 ml of 4 mg/ml

4. a. $\frac{57.5 \text{ lb}}{1 \text{ day}} \times \frac{1 \text{ kg}}{2.2 \text{ lb}} \times \frac{5 \text{ mg}}{1 \text{ kg}} = 131$ mg/day

b. $\frac{57.5 \text{ lb}}{1 \text{ day}} \times \frac{1 \text{ kg}}{2.2 \text{ lb}} \times \frac{5 \text{ mg}}{1 \text{ kg}} \times \frac{1 \text{ mL}}{5 \text{ mg}} \times \frac{1 \text{ day}}{4 \text{ doses}} = 6.6$ ml/dose

CHAPTER 17

PRACTICE EXERCISE 17A
1. 31 gtt/min; **2.** 16 gtt/min; **3.** 17 gtt/min;
4. 30 gtt/min, 25 gtt/min; **5.** 25 gtt/min; **6.** 20 gtt/min;
7. 60 gtt/min; **8.** 21 gtt/min; **9.** 50 gtt/min, 31 gtt/min;
10. 27 gtt/min

PRACTICE EXERCISES 17B
1. 42 cc/hr; **2.** 125 cc/hr; **3.** 63 cc/hr; **4.** 50 cc/hr;
5. 143 cc/hr; **6.** 200 cc/hr **7.** 83 cc/hr; **8.** 100 cc/hr;
9. 100 cc/hr; **10.** 300 cc/hr

CHAPTER REVIEW EXERCISES
1. a. 1,000 cc; **b.** Dextrose 5% NS with 20 mEq KCL;
c. 8 hr; **d.** 15 gtt/cc infusion set;

e. $\frac{1{,}000 \text{ cc}}{8 \text{ hr}} = 125$ cc/hr

$\frac{1000 \text{ cc}}{8 \text{ hr}} \times \frac{15 \text{ gtt}}{1 \text{ cc}} \times \frac{1 \text{ hr}}{60 \text{ min}} = 31$ gtt/min

2. a. 1000 cc; **b.** Dextrose 5% NS; **c.** 13.3 hr;
d. 10 gtt/cc infusion set; **e.** 75 cc/hr;

$\frac{75 \text{ cc}}{1 \text{ hr}} \times \frac{10 \text{ gtt}}{1 \text{ cc}} \times \frac{1 \text{ hr}}{60 \text{ min}} = 13$ gtt/min

3. a. 1000 cc; **b.** Dextrose 5% ½NS; **c.** 12.5 hrs;
d. 10 gtt/cc infusion set; **e.** 80 cc/hr;

$\frac{80 \text{ cc}}{1 \text{ hr}} \times \frac{10 \text{ gtt}}{1 \text{ cc}} \times \frac{1 \text{ hr}}{60 \text{ min}} = 13$ gtt/min

4. a. 1,000 cc; **b.** Dextrose 5% NS with 40 mEq KCL;
c. 10 hr; **d.** microdrip infusion set; **e.** 100 cc/hr;

$\frac{100 \text{ cc}}{1 \text{ hr}} \times \frac{60 \text{ gtt}}{1 \text{ cc}} \times \frac{1 \text{ hr}}{60 \text{ min}} = 100$ gtt/min

5. a. 1000 cc; **b.** Dextrose 5% ½NS with 40 mEq KCL;
c. 13.3 hr; **d.** infusion pump; **e.** 75 cc/hr

6. a. 50 cc; **b.** Dextrose 5% water with 60 mEq KCL;
c. 5 hrs; **d.** infusion pump;

e. $\frac{50 \text{ cc}}{5 \text{ hr}} = 10$ cc/hr

7. a. 700 cc; **b.** ¾ strength Ensure; **c.** 6.4 hr;
d. feeding pump; **e.** 110 cc/hr

8. a. 50 cc; **b.** 300 mg Tagamet in NS; **c.** 20 min;

d. infusion pump; **e.** $\frac{50 \text{ cc}}{20 \text{ min}} \times \frac{60 \text{ min}}{1 \text{ hr}} = 150$ cc/hr

9. a. 500 cc; **b.** ½ strength osmolyte; **c.** 14.3 hr;
d. feeding pump; **e.** 35 cc/hr

10. a. 1000 cc TPN, 500 cc Lipids; **b.** TPN and lipids;
c. TPN is 10.6 hr, lipids is 16.1 hrs; **d.** central line
infusion; **e.** TPN is 94 cc/hr and lipids is 31 cc/hr

11. 2100 hr; 1700 hr;

$$\frac{1,000 \text{ cc}}{8 \text{ hr}} \times \frac{10 \text{ gtt}}{1 \text{ cc}} \times \frac{1 \text{ hr}}{60 \text{ min}} = 21 \text{ gtt/min}$$

12. 1200 hr; 0700 hr.

CRITICAL THINKING

1. Recalculate the drip rate and adjust the roller clamp accordingly.

2. You need to know the patient's name and room number, the complete order of the infusion, the hourly rate, and the volume to be infused at the beginning of the shift.

3. $\dfrac{100 \text{ cc}}{1 \text{ hr}} \times 2 \text{ hr} = 200 \text{ cc}$; on time

4. $\dfrac{100 \text{ cc}}{1 \text{ hr}} \times \dfrac{20 \text{ gtt}}{1 \text{ ml}} \times \dfrac{1 \text{ hr}}{60 \text{ min}} = 33 \text{ gtt/min}$

$\dfrac{100 \text{ ml}}{30 \text{ min}} \times \dfrac{20 \text{ gtt}}{1 \text{ ml}} = 67 \text{ gtt/min}$; 0830

5. $\dfrac{100 \text{ cc}}{10 \text{ hr}} = 100 \text{ cc/hr}$;

$\dfrac{250 \text{ cc}}{250 \text{ mg}} \times \dfrac{20 \text{ mg}}{30 \text{ min}} \times \dfrac{60 \text{ min}}{1 \text{ hr}} = 40 \text{ cc/hr}$

$\dfrac{250 \text{ cc}}{1} \times \dfrac{1 \text{ hr}}{40 \text{ cc}} = 6.25 \text{ hr}$

CHAPTER 18

PRACTICE EXERCISE 18A

1. 30 cc/hr; **2.** 60 cc/hr; **3.** 100 cc/hr; **4.** 35 cc/hr;
5. 3 cc/hr; **6.** 30 cc/hr, 75 cc/hr; **7.** 15 ml/hr; **8.** 3 ml/hr;
9. 90 ml/hr

CHAPTER REVIEW EXERCISES

1. a. 140 mg/hr; **b.** 500 cc/hr; **2.** $\dfrac{500 \text{ cc}}{24 \text{ hr}} = 21 \text{ cc/hr}$;

3. 500 cc/hr **4.** $\dfrac{250 \text{ cc}}{30 \text{ min}} \times \dfrac{60 \text{ min}}{1 \text{ hr}} = 500 \text{ c/hr}$;

5. 500 cc/hr; **6.** 250 cc/hr

CRITICAL THINKING

1. a. 500 cc; **b.** 500 cc NS with 40 mg Amphotericin;
  c. 38.5 hr

  d. $\dfrac{134 \text{ lb}}{1 \text{ day}} \times \dfrac{1 \text{ kg}}{2.2 \text{ lb}} \times \dfrac{0.5 \text{ mg}}{1 \text{ kg}} \times \dfrac{1 \text{ day}}{24 \text{ hr}} \times \dfrac{500 \text{ cc}}{50 \text{ mg}} = 13 \text{ cc/hr}$

2. a. 500 cc; **b.** 500 cc NS with heparin drip of 1200 U

  c. 16.7 hr; **d.** $\dfrac{1200 \text{ U}}{1 \text{ hr}} \times \dfrac{500 \text{ cc}}{20,000 \text{ U}} = 30 \text{ cc/hr}$

3. a. 500 ml; **b.** heparin solution; **c.** 22.2 hr;

  d. $\dfrac{500 \text{ ml}}{20,000 \text{ U}} \times \dfrac{900 \text{ U}}{1 \text{ hr}} = 22.5 \text{ ml/hr}$

CHAPTER 19

PRACTICE EXERCISE 19A

1. 2; **2.** 5; **3.** 3; **4.** 7; **5.** 4; **6.** 3; **7.** 2; **8.** 6

PRACTICE EXERCISE 19B

1. 34,800 mi; **2.** 5440 g; **3.** 0.00231 kg;
4. 4,570,000 mi; **5.** 0.0123 kg; **6.** 5,000 g;
7. 0.100 L; **8.** 0.00377 g

PRACTICE EXERCISE 19C

1. 12.7 g; **2.** 1.24 kg; **3.** 80.2 g; **4.** 9.4 m²;
5. 6.2 cm²; **6.** 1×10^{15} mm²; **7.** 1,100 cm²;
8. 4.0 doses

CHAPTER 20

PRACTICE EXERCISE 20A

1. 192 f℥; **2.** 300 mg; **3.** 1200 ml; **4.** 4 t; **5.** 11¼ ℥;
6. 165 lb; **7.** 1 T; **8.** 0.2 mg, 0.4 ml; **9.** 15 cc, ℥ iii;
10. 187.5 mg/day

PRACTICE EXERCISE 20B

1. 1 capsule; **2.** 2 tablets; **3.** 2 tablets; **4.** 1 tablet;
5. 2 tablets; **6.** 1 ml; **7.** 1.2 ml; **8.** 2 ml; **9.** 2 ml

CHAPTER 21

PRACTICE EXERCISE 21A

1. 22.2°C; **2.** 105.1°F; **3.** −17.8°C; **4.** 41°F;
5. 37.8°C; **6.** 102.2°F; **7.** 305 K; **8.** 310.8 K

CHAPTER 22

PRACTICE EXERCISE 22A

1. 4; **2.** 1; **3.** −2; **4.** 7; **5.** 7; **6.** −3

PRACTICE EXERCISES 22B

1. beer—more acidic; tomato juice—more acidic; milk—more of a neutral effect; **2.** higher than normal

CHAPTER 23

PRACTICE EXERCISE 23A

Ca	40.1 amu	40.1 g
Na	23.0 amu	23.0 g
K	39.1 amu	39.1 g
S	32.1 amu	32.1 g
F	19.0 amu	19.0 g
Fe	55.8 amu	55.8 g
Zn	65.4 amu	65.4 g
I	126.9 amu	126.9 g

PRACTICE EXERCISE 23B

1. 58.5 g; **2.** 85.0 g; **3.** 6.02×10^{23} molecules

PRACTICE EXERCISE 23C

1. 2.22 moles; **2.** 44.0 g; **3.** 41.3 g; **4.** 1.91 moles;
5. 293 g; **6.** 6.9 moles; **7.** 2.11×10^{24} atoms;
8. 200.0 moles

POST-TEST

PART I

1. kilogram; **2.** 29½; **3a.** −5; **3b.** 1; **3c.** 10;
3d. −6; **3e.** 14.2201; **3f.** 4.673; **3g.** 1.1011;
3h. 22; **3i.** 1 1/12; **3j.** 17/25; **3k.** 17; **4a.** 0.021;
4b. 0.0045; **5.** 5%; **6a.** 6.392×10^{3};
6b. 6.392×10^{-4}; **7.** 7×10^{9}; **8.** 100.0°F;

9a. $\dfrac{8 \text{ ℥}}{1} \times \dfrac{30 \text{ ml}}{1 \text{ ℥}} = 240 \text{ ml}$

9b. $\dfrac{2 \text{ g}}{1} \times \dfrac{1{,}000 \text{ mg}}{1 \text{ g}} \times \dfrac{1{,}000 \text{ mcg}}{1 \text{ mg}} = 2{,}000{,}000 \text{ mcg}$

9c. $\dfrac{15 \text{ kg}}{1} \times \dfrac{2.2 \text{ lb}}{1 \text{ kg}} = 33 \text{ lb}$

9d. $\dfrac{1 \text{ C}}{1} \times \dfrac{8 \text{ ʒ}}{1 \text{ C}} \times \dfrac{2 \text{ T}}{1 \text{ ʒ}} = 16 \text{ T}$

9e. $\dfrac{1.5 \text{ gr}}{1} \times \dfrac{60 \text{ mg}}{1 \text{ gr}} = 90 \text{ mg}$

9f. $\dfrac{1 \text{ ʒ}}{1} \times \dfrac{8 \text{ ʒ}}{1 \text{ ʒ}} \times \dfrac{60 \text{ ♏}}{1 \text{ ʒ}} = 480 \text{ ♏}$

PART II

1. 12.5 ml;   **2.** 1.7 ml;   **3a.** 3.5 ml;   **3b.** 1.4 ml;
4a. 131 mg/day;   **4b.** 1.3 ml/dose;   **5a.** 85 kg;
5b. Yes. Range for this patient would be between 1,700 and 4,250 mg/day. Patient is receiving 3,000 mg/day.;
6a. 3,600 cm^2;   **6b.** 700,000 cm^3;   **6c.** 2 m;
7a. No, the on-hand contains 473 ml;   **7b.** 2 ml;   **8a.** 2.5 g;
8b. Enough to fill to 500 ml;   **9a.** 160 ml;   **9b.** 640 ml;
10a. 125 gtt/min;   **10b.** too slow (should be 375 ml in bag);   **11.** 0.8 ml;   **12a.** 398 mg;   **12b.** 100 cc/hr;
12c. 33 gtt/min;   **13a.** 56.1 g;   **13b.** 9 moles;
13c. 1.5×10^{24} moles

Index

This exciting CD-ROM is an interactive multimedia presentation that has been designed to enhance self-paced learning and provide you with a comprehensive learning package. Reduce any test anxiety you may experience by practicing at your own pace.

Features include:

- Tutorial to help you get started
- 300-word glossary
- Audio pronunciation of drug names
- Testing assessment tool with scoring capabilities
- Review questions with answers and rationales
- Practice problems with answers and rationales
- Critical thinking skills
- Color photographs
- 160 Drug labels
- Audio pronunciation of common sound-alike drug names
- Intuitive and attractive interface
- Help feature
- Toll-free technical support
- Plus Flash!™, an electronic flash card program

CD-ROM Set-up Instructions

Hardware Requirements

- 33 MHz 386 w/4MB of RAM
- Recommended 486 w/8MB of RAM
- Windows™ 3.1 or later; sound card
- VGA with 256 color display
- Double-spin CD-ROM drive
- 4MB free disc space

Installation

Before you run the installation program, check the system requirements noted above. This program will take approximately 4 megabytes of disc space.

Windows™ 3.1

To install the Applying Medication Math Skills: A Dimensional Analysis Approach CD-ROM, start Windows™. Insert the disc in the CD-ROM drive. From the Program Manager, click on "File," then "Run." Type "D:\SETUP" or "E:\SETUP" and press OK. The drive letter indicated depends on the drive designated for the computers CD-ROM drive.

Windows™ 95

Insert the disc in the CD-ROM drive. Select "Start" and "Run:" Type "D:\SETUP" or "E:\SETUP" and press OK. The drive letter indicated depends on the drive designated for the computers CD-ROM drive. Installation of video playback software is not required in Windows™ 95.

Sounds in Windows™ 3.1

If sound does not play while running the Applying Medication Math Skills: A Dimensional Analysis Approach CD-ROM within Windows™ 3.1, check to be sure that your sound card is set up according to the manufacturer's instructions.

The MCI-CD Audio Driver must be installed. From the Main Group in Windows™ Program Manager, open Control Panel and select the "Drivers" option. Scroll through the installed drivers list. If [MCI] CD Audio is not installed, you will need your original Windows™ installation discs to proceed. Select "Add" and select the [MCI] CD Audio driver from the list.

Starting *Medication Math Skills*

1. Make sure your CD-ROM drive is turned on and insert CD (label side up).
2. Locate the *Medication Math Skills* group in Program Manager.
3. Open the program by double-clicking on the *Medication Math* icon.

Technical Support

Call 1-800-477-3692 8:00 A.M. to 6:00 P.M. Eastern Standard Time *or* Fax 1-518-464-0301 24 hrs. a day